Children and
Exercise IX

International Series on Sport Sciences

Series Editors: **Richard C. Nelson and Chauncey A. Morehouse**

The principal focus of this series is on reference works derived primarily from international congress and symposium proceedings. These should be of particular interest to researchers, clinicians, students, physical educators, and coaches involved in the growing field of sport science. The Series Editors are Professors Richard C. Nelson and Chauncey A. Morehouse of The Pennsylvania State University. The series includes the eight major divisions of sport science: biomechanics, history, medicine, pedagogy, philosophy, physiology, psychology, and sociology.

Each volume in the series is published in English but is written by authors of several countries. The series, therefore, is truly international in scope and, because many of the authors normally publish their work in languages other than English, the series volumes are a resource for information that is often difficult if not impossible to obtain elsewhere. Organizers of international congresses in the sport sciences desiring detailed information concerning the use of this series for publication and distribution of official proceedings are requested to contact the Series Editors. Manuscripts prepared by several authors from various countries consisting of information of international interest will also be considered for publication.

The *International Series on Sport Sciences* serves not only as a valuable source of authoritative, up-to-date information but also helps to foster better understanding among sport scientists on an international level. It provides an effective medium through which researchers, teachers, and coaches may develop better communications with individuals in countries throughout the world who have similar professional interests.

Volume 1: **BIOMECHANICS IV** (Fourth International Seminar on Biomechanics) *Nelson and Morehouse* (Out of print)

Volume 2: **SWIMMING II** (Second International Seminar on Biomechanics of Swimming) *Lewillie and Clarys*

Volume 3: **CHILD IN SPORT AND PHYSICAL ACTIVITY** (First International Symposium on the Participation of Children in Sport) *Albinson and Andrew*

Volume 4: **SPORT PEDAGOGY: Content and Methodology** (First International Symposium on Sport Pedagogy) *Haag*

Volume 5: **SKIING SAFETY II** (Second International Conference on Ski Trauma and Skiing Safety) *Figueras*

Volume 6: **SWIMMING MEDICINE IV** (Fourth International Congress on Swimming Medicine) *Eriksson and Furburg*

Volume 7: **NUTRITION, PHYSICAL FITNESS, AND HEALTH** *Pařízková and Rogozkin*

Volume 8: **SWIMMING III** (Third International Symposium of Biomechanics in Swimming) *Terauds and Bedingfield*

Volume 9: **KINANTHROPOMETRY II** (Second International Seminar on Kinanthropometry) *Ostyn, Beunen, and Simons*

Volume 10: **CHILDREN AND EXERCISE IX** (Ninth Symposium on Pediatric Work Physiology) *Berg and Eriksson*

Forthcoming volumes:

Volume 11: **BIOCHEMISTRY OF EXERCISE IV** (Fourth International Symposium on Biochemistry of Exercise) *Poortmans*

Volume 12: **SKIING SAFETY III** (Third International Conference on Ski Trauma and Skiing Safety) *Lamont*

SWIMMING MEDICINE V (Fifth International Congress on Swimming Medicine)

PHYSICAL TRAINING AND EXERCISE MEDICINE (Fifth Puijo Symposium—Physical Training in Health Promotion and Medical Care) *Hänninen*

International Series
on Sport Sciences, Volume 10

CHILDREN AND EXERCISE IX

Edited by:

Kristina Berg, M.D.
Children's Clinic
Centrallasarettet
Mölndal, Sweden
and
Bengt O. Eriksson, M.D.
Department of Pediatrics
East Hospital
Göteborg, Sweden

Series Editors:

Richard C. Nelson, Ph.D.
and
Chauncey A. Morehouse, Ph.D.
The Pennsylvania State University
University Park, Pennsylvania

University Park Press
Baltimore

UNIVERSITY PARK PRESS
International Publishers in Science, Medicine, and Education
233 East Redwood Street
Baltimore, Maryland 21202

Copyright © 1980 by University Park Press

Composed by University Park Press, Typesetting Division

Manufactured in the United States of America by Universal
Lithographers, Inc., and The Maple Press Company.

This volume represents the proceedings of the IXth International Congress on
Pediatric Work Physiology, held in Marstrand, Sweden, in 1978.

Library of Congress Cataloging in Publication Data

International Congress on Pediatric Work Physiology, 9th, Marstrand,
Sweden, 1978. Children and exercise IX.

(International series on sport sciences; v. 10)
"Proceedings of the IX International Congress on Pediatric Work Physiology,
Marstrand, Sweden, 1978."
1. Motor ability in children—Congresses. 2. Physical fitness for children—
Congresses. 3. Exercise for children—Congresses. 4. Exercise—Physiological
aspects—Congresses. 5. Children—Physiology—Congresses. I. Berg, Kristina.
II. Eriksson, Bengt. III. Title. IV. Series. [DNLM: 1. Exertion—In infancy and
childhood—Congresses. 2. Handicapped—Congresses. 3. Physical education
and training—Congresses. 4. Child development—Congresses.
W3 IN636F 9th 1978c / WE103 I565 1978c]
RJ133.I57 1978 612'.044 79-6359
ISBN 0-8391-1591-1

Contents

HABITUAL PHYSICAL ACTIVITY

MUSCLE DEVELOPMENT, STRUCTURE, AND FUNCTION

Contributors

Kari Antila Cardiorespiratory Research Unit, University of Turku, 20520 Turku 52, Finland *(128)*

Erling Asmussen Laboratory for the Theory of Gymnastics, August Krogh Institute, University of Copenhagen, Universitetsparken 13, DK 2100 Copenhagen ∅, Denmark *(69)*

Oded Bar-Or Ambrose Cardiorespiratory Unit, McMaster University Medical Centre, 1200 Main Street West, Hamilton, Ontario, Canada *(139)*

Z. Bartůněk Department of Physiology, Faculty of Physical Education and Sport, Charles University, Újezd 450, 118 07 Prague 1, Czechoslovakia *(175)*

S. Bartůňková Department of Physiology, Faculty of Physical Education and Sport, Charles University, Újezd 450, 118 07 Prague 1, Czechoslovakia *(175)*

C. Bastanier Klinik fur Herz- und Kreislauferkrankungen im Kindesalter, Deutschen Herzzentrum München, Lothstrasse 11, 8000 München 2, Federal Republic of Germany *(377)*

Mette Behrendt Hansen Laboratory for the Theory of Gymnastics, August Krogh Institute, University of Copenhagen, Universitetsparken 13, DK 2100 Copenhagen ∅, Denmark *(69)*

Gaston Beunen Instituut voor Lichamelijke Opleiding, Katholeike Universiteit Leuven, Tervuursevest 101, B 3030 Heverlee, Belgium *(41)*

Sture Bevegård Department of Clinical Physiology, Södersjukhuset, Stockholm, Sweden *(289, 294)*

Robert A. Binkhorst Department of Physiology, Medical Faculty, University of Nijmegen, Nijmegen, The Netherlands *(166, 333)*

Josef Buchberger Department of Exercise Physiology and Biometry, Institute of Physical Education, University of Graz, A-8010 Graz, Mozartgasse 14, Austria *(93)*

J. P. Cocquerez École Nationale Supérieure de l'Électronique et de ses Applications, Impasse des Chênes Pourpres, 95000 Cergy, France *(183)*

Ann-Sofie Colling-Saltin Department of Obstetrics and Gynecology, Helsingborg Hospital, 251 87 Helsingborg, Sweden *(193)*

A. B. Cramwinckel G.V.O.-Projekt, University of Nijmegen, Philips van Leydenlaan 25, Nijmegen, The Netherlands *(166)*

Gordon R. Cumming Department of Pediatrics, Health Sciences Children's Centre of Winnipeg, *and* The University of Winnipeg, Winnipeg, Manitoba, Canada *(79, 354)*

Numbers in parentheses refer to page(s) where contributors' paper(s) begin.

C. T. Mervyn Davies M.R.C. Environmental Physiology Unit, London School of Hygiene and Tropical Medicine, Keppel Street, London WC1E 7HT, England *(327)*

J. Devars École Nationale Supérieure de l'Électronique et de ses Applications, Impasse des Chênes Pourpres, 95000 Cergy, France *(183)*

Rafi Dotan Department of Research and Sports Medicine, Wingate Institute, Natanya, Israel *(139)*

D. T. Drinkwater Department of Kinesiology, Simon Fraser University, Burnaby, British Columbia, Canada *(3)*

Bengt O. Eriksson Department of Pediatrics, University of Göteborg, East Hospital, S-416 85 Göteborg, Sweden *(116, 239, 251, 289, 294)*

R. A. Faulkner College of Physical Education, University of Saskatchewan, Saskatoon, Saskatchewan, Canada *(3)*

Lars P. M. Fohlin Department of Paediatrics, Karolinska Institutet, St. Göran's Children's Hospital, S-112 81 Stockholm, Sweden *(317, 327)*

Hans Forssberg Department of Physiology III, Karolinska Institutet, Lidingövägen 1, S-114 33 Stockholm, Sweden *(13, 32)*

Jean-Pierre Fouillot Laboratoire de Physiologie, C.H.U. Cochin-Port Royal 24, Rue de Faubourg Saint Jacques, 75014 Paris, France *(183)*

Ulla Freychuss Department of Clinical Physiology, Karolinska Institutet, The Serafimer Hospital, Stockholm, Sweden *(116)*

Lars-Goran Friberg Department of Pediatric Surgery, University of Göteborg, East Hospital, S-416 85 Göteborg, Sweden *(239)*

Georgine Gaisl Department of Exercise Physiology and Biometry, Institute of Physical Education, University of Graz, A-8010 Graz, Mozartgasse 14, Austria *(93)*

Viggo Graff-Lonnevig Pediatric Clinic, Karolinska Institutet, Huddinge Hospital, S-141 86 Huddinge, Sweden *(289, 294)*

Amos Grodjinovski Wingate Teachers College for Physical Education and Sports, Wingate, Israel *(139)*

Lauri Halkola Cardiorespiratory Research Unit, University of Turku, 20520 Turku 52, Finland *(128)*

Einar Hansson Department of Pediatric Surgery, University of Göteborg, East Hospital, S-416 85 Göteborg, Sweden *(251)*

J. Heller Department of Physiology, Faculty of Physical Education and Sport, Charles University, Újezd 450, 118 07 Prague 1, Czechoslovakia *(175)*

Allan Hnatiuk Department of Pediatrics, Health Sciences Children's Centre of Winnipeg, *and* The University of Winnipeg, Winnipeg, Manitoba, Canada *(79)*

Marja-Liisa Hursti Cardiorespiratory Research Unit and Sports Medicine Research Unit, University of Turku, 20520 Turku 52, Finland *(128)*

Juhani Ilmarinen Institute of Occupational Health, Helsinki, Department of Physiology, Laajaniityntie 1, 01620 Vantaa 62, Finland *(149)*

Omri Inbar Department of Research and Sports Medicine, Wingate Institute, Natanya, Israel *(139)*

J. Javurek Laboratory for Physical Fitness Research, Faculty of Pediatrics, Charles University, Prague 5 Motol, Vúvalu 84, Czechoslovakia 15006 *(49)*

B. Kaltwasser Klinik fur Herz- und Kreislauferkrankungen im Kindesalter, Deutschen Herzzentrum München, Lothstrasse 1, 8000 München 2, Federal Republic of Germany *(347)*

Fred W. Kasch Exercise Physiology—
Physical Education Department,
San Diego State University, San
Diego, California 92182, USA
(369, 382)

Han C. G. Kemper University of
Amsterdam, Jan Swammerdam
Institute, 1 Eerste Constantijn
Huygensstraat 20, 1054 BW
Amsterdam, The Netherlands (55)

Simon de Knecht Department of
Pediatric Cardiology, Medical
Faculty, University of Nijmegen,
Nijmegen, The Netherlands (333)

Günter Koch Department of Clinical
Physiology, Centrallasarettet,
Karlskrona, Sweden, and Department of Physiology, Free University
of Berlin, Berlin, West Germany
(99, 109, 375)

Sven Kraepelien Department of
Allergology, Sach's Children's Hos-
pital, Södersjukhuset, Stockholm,
Sweden (294)

Miloš Kučera Laboratory for Physical
Fitness Research, Faculty of Pediatrics, Charles University, Prague
5 Motol, Vúvalu 84, Czechoslovakia 15006 (49)

Anita E. Lundberg Department of
Pediatrics, University of Göteborg,
Östra Sjukhuset, S-416 85
Göteborg, Sweden (23)

Anders Lundin Riksidrottsinstitutet,
Bosön, S-181 90 Lidingö, Sweden
(116)

Milos Mácek Laboratory for Physical
Fitness Research, Faculty of Pediatrics, Charles University, Prague
5 Motol, Vúvalu 84, Czechoslovakia 15006 (49, 64)

Gösta Mellgren Department of
Pediatric Surgery, University
of Göteborg, East Hospital,
S-416 85 Göteborg, Sweden (239)

Rolf Mocellin Klinik fur Herz- und
Kreislauferkrankungen im Kinde-
salter, Deutschen Herzzentrum
München, Lothstrasse 1, 8000
München 2, Federal Republic of
Germany (347)

Bodil Nielsen Laboratory for the
Theory of Gymnastics, August
Krogh Institute, University of
Copenhagen, Universitetsparken
13, DK 2100 Copenhagen Ø, Den-
mark (69)

Karin Nielsen Laboratory for the
Theory of Gymnastics, August
Krogh Institute, University of
Copenhagen, Universitetsparken
13, DK 2100 Copenhagen O, Den-
mark (69)

Svein Oseid Children's Asthma and
Allergy Institute, Voksentoppen,
Oslo 3, and Norwegian College of
Physical Education and Sport,
Voksentoppen, Oslo 8, Norway
(277)

Michel Ostyn Instituut voor
Lichamelijke Opleiding, Katholieke
Universiteit Leuven, Tervuursevest
101, B 3030 Heverlee, Belgium (41)

M. Pauer Department of Physiology,
Faculty of Physical Education and
Sports, Charles University, Újezd
450, 118 07 Prague 1, Czechoslovakia (175)

Leena Pihlakoski Cardiorespiratory
Research Unit and Sports Medicine
Unit, University of Turku, 20520
Turku 52, Finland (128)

Roland Renson Instituut voor
Lichamelijke Opleiding, Katholieke
Universiteit Leuven, Tervuursevest
101, B 3030 Heverlee, Belgium (41)

Michel Rieu Laboratoire de Physiologie, C.H.U. Cochin-Port Royal
24, Rue de Faubourg Saint Jacques,
75014 Paris, France (183)

L. Röcker Department of Physiology,
Free University of Berlin, Berlin,
West Germany (109)

William D. Ross Department of
Kinesiology, Simon Fraser Univer-
sity, Burnaby, British Columbia,
Canada (3)

Joseph Rutenfranz Institut für Ar-
beitsphysiologie an der Universität
Dortmund, Ardeystrasse 67, D-4600
Dortmund 1, Federal Republic of
Germany (149, 160)

Bengt Saltin Laboratory for the Theory of Gymnastics, August Krogh Institute, University of Copenhagen, Universitetsparken 13, DK 2100 Copenhagen Ø, Denmark *(294)*

Wim H. M. Saris G.V.O.-Projekt, University of Nijmegen, Philips van Leydenlaan 25, Nijmegen, The Netherlands *(166)*

Václav Seliger Department of Physiology, Faculty of Physical Education and Sports, Charles University, Újezd 450, 118 07 Prague 1, Czechoslovakia *(175)*

Jan Simons Instituut voor Lichamelijke Opleiding, Katholieke Universiteit Leuven, Tervuursevest 101, B 3030 Heverlee, Belgium *(41)*

Roland Singer Fachgebiet Sportwissenschaft der Technischen Hochschule, Darmstadt, Federal Republic of Germany *(160)*

Michael Sjöström Departments of Anatomy and Neurology, University of Umeå, S-901 87 Umeå, Sweden *(208)*

Jerzy Skrobak-Kaczynski Norwegian College of Physical Education and Sport, Kringsjaa, Sognveien 220, Oslo 8, Norway *(300)*

V. Sobolová Department of Physiology, Faculty of Physical Education and Sports, Charles University, Újezd 450, 118 07 Prague 1, Czechoslovakia *(175)*

Claes A. R. Thorén Department of Pediatrics, Karolinska Institutet, St. Göran's Children's Hospital, S-112 81 Stockholm, Sweden *(116, 263, 327)*

Ilkka Välimäki Cardiorespiratory Research Unit and Sports Medicine Research Unit, University of Turku, 20520 Turku 52, Finland *(128)*

A. M. van der Veen-Hezemans G.V.O.-Projekt, University of Nijmegen, Philips van Leydenlaan 25, Nijmegen, The Netherlands *(166)*

Dirk Van Gerven Instituut voor Lichamelijke Opleiding, Katholieke Universiteit Leuven, Tervuursevest 101, B 3030 Heverlee, Belgium *(41)*

F. van Waesberghe G.V.O.-Projekt, University of Nijmegen, Philips van Leydenlaan 25, Nijmegen, The Netherlands *(166)*

Tom Vavik Norwegian College of Physical Education and Sport, Kringsjaa, Sognsveien 220, Oslo 8, Norway *(300)*

Jan Vávra Laboratory for Physical Fitness Research, Faculty of Pediatrics, Charles University, Prague 5 Motol, Vúvalu 84, Czechoslovakia 15006 *(64)*

Robbert Verschuur University of Amsterdam, Jan Swammerdam Institute, 1 Eerste Constantijn Huygensstraat 20, 1054 BW Amsterdam, The Netherlands *(55)*

H. Wallberg Department of Physiology III, Karolinska Institutet, Lidingövägen 1, S-114 33 Stockholm, Sweden *(32)*

N. O. Whittingham Torrens College of Advanced Education, Adelaide, South Australia, Australia *(3)*

V. Zelenka Department of Physiology, Faculty of Physical Education and Sports, Charles University, Újezd 450, 118 07 Prague 1, Czechoslovakia *(175)*

Congress Organization

ORGANIZING COMMITTEE

Bengt O. Eriksson, M.D., Chairman
Department of Pediatrics
University of Göteborg
Östra Sjukhuset
S-416 85 Göteborg, Sweden

Kristina Berg, M.D.
Children's Clinic
Centrallasarettet
S-431 22 Mölndal, Sweden

Petter Karlberg, M.D.
Professor of Pediatrics
Dean of Medical Faculty
University of Göteborg
Östra Sjukhuset
S-416 85 Göteborg, Sweden

Kerstin Edvinsson, Secretary
Department of Pediatrics
University of Göteborg
Östra Sjukhuset
S-416 85 Göteborg, Sweden

EDITORIAL BOARD

C. T. M. Davies (President,
  PWP VIII)
MCR Environmental Physiology Unit
London School of Hygiene and
  Tropical Medicine
Keppel Street
London WC1E 7HT, England

Bengt O. Eriksson, M.D. (President,
  PWP IX)

Ilka Välimäki, M.D. (President,
  PWP X)
Department of Pediatrics
University of Turku
Klinamyllynkatu 10
Turku, Finland

Sponsors

AB Findus
Fisons Sweden AB
Helcomed Norden AB
IBM Sweden AB
Mediplast AB
Mölnlycke AB
AB Stille-Werner
3M Sweden AB
Instrument AB WISEX
AB VOLVO
University of Göteborg

Preface

It becomes quite obvious when studying how children behave during daily life that the human body is perfectly designed for movement. Nevertheless, our knowledge of how children "exercise" their bodies, as well as their motivation for doing so, is rather limited. It was for this reason that a group of pediatricians and physical educators began the Pediatric Work Physiology (PWP) Congresses in 1968.

When Göteborg was given the honor of hosting the IXth PWP Congress, we attempted to organize a symposium at a high scientific level. Our intent was to provide sufficient time for discussions not only during the scientific sessions, but at other times as well. It was therefore important to find a place where the participants could easily be in touch with each other for informal discussions. We think that our choice of Marstrand, a small island north of Göteborg, was an ideal one.

It would have been impossible to organize the Congress without generous sponsorship. Therefore, we would like to express our deep gratitude to all of our sponsors.

This volume contains most of the papers presented at the Congress. The quality of this publication depends on the high standard of each of the author's presentations, and we take this opportunity to thank all contributors for their excellent work. It is our hope that the book will be both useful and well received, and that it will stimulate further scientific research in the study of children and exercise.

Kristina Berg
Bengt O. Eriksson

Introduction

The history of the Pediatric Group on Work Physiology began at a more traditional congress in Berlin. At the end of that Congress, a group of young scientists, most of them pediatricians, met in a Berlin restaurant to discuss their dissatisfaction with this type of meeting. The conclusions resulting from these discussions were condensed into six basic statements:

1. Symposia with special topics related to the development of physical performance capacity in childhood and youth are needed.
2. These symposia should bring together pediatricians and physical educators experienced in the field of work physiology.
3. The number of participants should not exceed 30 to 40.
4. The time for each presentation should be limited to 10 to 15 minutes, with unlimited time for discussion following each.
5. All discussions should occur without regard to prestige or to furthering one's professional career.
6. The symposia should be organized by a group of scientists, but not by a formal society, and the organizers should annually or bienially invite a good mixture of experienced and young scientists, mostly from European countries.

After the discussions, the group asked me to prepare the first meeting for 1968 in Dortmund. For this meeting, we invited some outstanding professors in the field of work physiology, but they were all wise enough not to come. Therefore, the basic group had to act as the experienced group.

Since the Dortmund meeting, the following symposia have been held:

PWP II—Liblice, Czechoslovakia (1969); Prof. Miloš Máček, Chairman
PWP III—Stockholm, Sweden (1970); Prof. Claes A. R. Thorén, Chairman
PWP IV—Wingate, Israel (1972); Dr. Oded Bar-Or, Chairman
PWP V—de Haan, Belgium (1973); Prof. M. Hebbelinck, Chairman
PWP VI—Sec, Czechoslovakia (1974); Prof. Miloš Máček, Chairman
PWP VII—Trois-Rivières, Québec, Canada (1975); Dr. H. Lavallée and Prof. R. Shephard, Chairmen
PWP VIII—Bisham Abbey, England (1976); Dr. C. T. Merwyn Davies, Chairman

The main topics through the years consisted of:

The influence of growth and development on physical performance capacity (PCP)
Metabolism during exercise in childhood
Body composition and PCP

Daily physical activity and PCP
Problems of physical training in youth
Exercise capacity in handicapped children
Effects of habilitation

The proceedings of most of the congresses have been printed, and it is still possible to obtain copies of PWPs III, IV, V, VI, and VII by contacting the respective chairmen.

In summary, the main idea of the Pediatric Group on Work Physiology is to promote informal scientific discussion and exchange of information about the pediatric aspects of work physiology. This volume represents the most recent contribution to the growing body of knowledge stemming from the congresses that are organized by the Group in the spirit of those discussions in Berlin.

Joseph Rutenfranz
Dortmund, Federal Republic of Germany

*In memory of Václav Seliger,
one of the pioneers in the field of exercise physiology
and sports medicine.*

Children and
Exercise IX

Body Growth, Body Composition, and Motor Learning

Anthropometric Prototypes: Ages Six to Eighteen Years

**W. D. Ross, D. T. Drinkwater,
N. O. Whittingham, and R. A. Faulkner**

Pediatric work physiology is an especially demanding area since human performance and physiological events are influenced by growth and maturation factors. Expressing strength or metabolic factors in terms of body mass may be appropriate on certain occasions for adults; however, in children, the practice is seldom adequate since there are confounding factors. Growing children do not change geometrically in size, shape, and composition. Body mass is not constituted the same at each age level. Children grow larger first in the hands and feet, then in the legs and arms and trunk, then in the hips and shoulders, and lastly in chest depth. There is also a generally increasing proportional amount of muscle. This kind of differential growth is necessary in order to overcome a concomitant increase in body mass with age. In boys, proportional skinfold values tend to decrease in the limbs and increase at the midriff sites. In girls, the proportional appendicular decline and midriff increase are inextricably affected by increases associated with sexual maturation. The exact nature of these morphological changes is currently being elucidated in longitudinal analyses. In these inquiries, evolving techniques for tridimensional graphic analyses afford a new perspective on groups and individual growth characteristics as described by Leahy et al. (1978).

Ideally, when any physiological functional variable is being studied, the research paradigm should provide for control groups matched for age and sex, or perhaps, in some instances, for maturational age. Practically, however, this situation is seldom feasible.

Basic support for the Simon Fraser Kinanthropometric Research Unit was from an operational grant for kinanthropometric research from the National Research Council of Canada.

3

One of the alternatives, as suggested by Tanner (1976), is to select a sample from a particular population as being typical of the "best off" and use this sample for developing prototypes, recognizing, however, as Tanner points out, that the selected advantageous group may mature earlier and grow taller.

SUBJECTS

With these limitations in mind, three schools judged to be middle class and having average or better than average physical activity programs were selected from the Coquitlam School District, a neighboring municipality of Vancouver, British Columbia. The project designated as the Coquitlam Growth Study quickly became known by its computer anagram, COGRO. The sample used to construct the so-called COGRO prototypes consisted of 446 girls and 473 boys ranging in age from 5.57 to 18.22 years. Subjects with physical handicaps were measured but excluded from the analysis. Participation in the project was voluntary and five potential subjects chose not to be included.

The subjects were assumed to be representative of the genetically heterogeneous population of the west coast of Canada with, perhaps, a bias toward fitness reflecting a school board policy to encourage an active lifestyle. To exemplify an abstracted version of the COGRO prototypes presented in this paper, 12 outstanding young skaters, selected on the basis of their competitive records, were compared with their appropriate COGRO age-sex prototypes.

METHODS

An experienced team of six anthropometrists obtained about 95% of the data and directly supervised the remaining portion collected by undergraduate student trainees. The measurement procedures were identical to those used in the Montreal Olympic Games Anthropological Project (MOGAP), with the addition of four items: ankle girth, head girth (slightly above glabella), neck girth (superior to laryngeal prominence), and gluteal arch height (projected measure from sacro-coccygeal fusion to floor). Designated landmarks and procedures have been described by Ross et al. (1978) and Borms et al. (1977). The figure skaters were measured by a MOGAP anthropometrist and co-author, R. A. Faulkner.

In order to determine how universal the prototype data might be, obtained mean height (stature) and weight (body mass) values for yearly age increments for each sex were compared with normative data reported for Manitoba (1970), the United States (1977), Switzerland (1977), Norway (1975), Czechoslovakia (1976), and India (1971).

The assembled data from the Coquitlam study were used to construct 26 COGRO age-sex prototypes described by mean, standard deviation, range, and raw and smoothed percentile tables using a computer protocol designed by Nie et al. (1975).

RESULTS

The obtained raw data were summarized as 26 age-sex prototypes—e.g., 6 (5.50–6.49); 7 (6.50–7.49); . . . 18 (17.50–18.49). Because the actual mean age value for each prototype was roughly at the whole year incremental value, no adjustment of the raw data was made. An extensive descriptive analysis of the obtained data is summarized in a microcarded thesis by Whittingham (1979), and reported in detail in two large addendum volumes of computer printout.

Space precludes the inclusion of a full statistical summary of the data because this involved 34 variables for each of the 26 age-sex prototypes. The composition of the sample, means, and standard deviations for height and weight are shown in Table 1. The authors will furnish similar summaries for the other 32 variables on request. Complete analyses are also available by negotiation.

Comparison of the mean COGRO height and weight values with those obtained on 60,000 girls and boys from the province of Manitoba (supplied by Victor Corrol) were as illustrated in the two graphs in Figures 1a and 1b. The COGRO data, as shown in the two graphs in Figures 1c and 1d, were similar to those reported over the same age range for U.S. children in 1977 and for Czechoslovakian children of ages 12–18 in 1976, although there was a marked departure for the latter at age 11 years.

As anticipated, mean height and weight values reported for Indian children were systematically smaller than the COGRO data. Although not displayed, Norwegian data over the same age range and Swiss data for ages 6–12 years were also similar to mean COGRO values. Thus, on the basis of graphic similarity of mean height and weight values, the COGRO prototypes appear to be a reasonable substitute for "control" samples in other countries where such comprehensive data may not be readily available.

In order to demonstrate applicability of the COGRO data, 12 outstanding young figure skaters, who had distinguished themselves by being finalists in Canadian amateur figure skating sanctioned competition in a region that routinely produces Canadian champions and international competitors, were compared with their appropriate age-sex prototype.

Twenty variables previously used in a study on figure skaters by Faulkner (1976) were used in the analyses of the figure skaters and the 11-year-old girl prototypes. In testing the hypothesis that smallness is an

Table 1.   Mean and standard deviations for height and weight for 26 age-sex prototypes

Age	Sex	N	Height (cm)		Weight (kg)	
			$\bar{x}$	σ	$\bar{x}$	σ
6	G	17	116.66	5.68	21.38	3.69
	B	15	117.04	6.30	21.75	2.98
7	G	25	122.36	5.25	23.52	3.94
	B	22	122.80	5.07	23.92	2.85
8	G	15	126.71	4.99	25.12	3.81
	B	22	129.64	6.01	27.50	4.53
9	G	30	133.41	6.56	28.74	5.02
	B	27	133.35	7.37	28.80	5.15
10	G	20	141.52	8.19	35.84	9.18
	B	21	140.14	6.99	33.23	5.90
11	G	24	145.15	7.78	39.12	10.22
	B	26	143.15	6.89	37.21	7.95
12	G	35	152.89	7.84	42.79	7.95
	B	33	149.25	6.45	42.18	8.61
13	G	37	159.33	7.00	47.92	9.44
	B	35	159.20	6.94	48.00	7.46
14	G	67	162.53	6.19	52.42	9.44
	B	76	165.52	8.64	52.60	9.69
15	G	66	163.12	6.77	53.89	7.57
	B	77	170.46	8.73	58.63	11.23
16	G	53	164.61	6.64	54.87	8.03
	B	55	174.59	8.37	62.16	8.86
17	G	47	165.13	5.69	55.76	6.79
	B	43	175.63	6.23	64.86	9.85
18	G	10	165.88	7.23	59.51	6.44
	B	21	179.04	7.66	68.82	7.70

advantage, a one-tailed t test at the 5% probability level was chosen as the level of significance. As shown in Table 2, except for age, foot length, and thigh girth, the figure skaters were shown to be significantly smaller than their prototypes, with particularly large t ratios noted for all of the skinfold comparisons.

In order to determine if, in addition to being low in skinfolds and smaller than their peers in general, the skaters showed proportionality differences, a stratagem proposed by Ross and Wilson (1974) was used. This stratagem essentially adjusts the subjects geometrically to the same stature (170.18 cm) and expresses deviations of body measures from a unisex reference human or phantom in terms of Z values based on an arbitrary human population.

Table 2. Comparison of 11-year-old girl prototypes with outstanding Canadian girl figure skaters[a]

Item	Skaters ($N=12$)	Prototype ($N=24$)	t ratio
Age (yr)	10.70 (1.1)	10.96 (0.31)	0.30
Weight (kg)	31.20 (5.6)	39.12 (10.22)	3.00 (s)[b]
Height (cm)	136.70 (9.4)	145.12 (7.78)	2.70 (s)
Sitting height (cm)	71.10 (3.4)	76.22 (4.28)	3.00 (s)
Foot length (cm)	21.50 (1.5)	21.75 (1.43)	0.50
Triceps sf. (mm)	10.20 (2.5)	14.28 (4.18)	3.70 (s)
Subscapular sf. (mm)	6.00 (1.7)	10.20 (4.5)	4.10 (s)
Suprailiac sf. (mm)	4.00 (1.0)	10.00 (5.45)	4.20 (s)
Abdominal sf. (mm)	5.20 (1.7)	13.14 (6.46)	5.60 (s)
Thigh sf. (mm)	13.60 (3.4)	23.53 (8.16)	5.10 (s)
Calf sf. (mm)	9.40 (2.5)	12.90 (5.45)	2.60 (s)
Tibial height (cm)	35.60 (3.1)	37.97 (2.46)	2.20 (s)
Biiliocr. wd. (cm)	21.50 (1.6)	23.12 (2.53)	2.30 (s)
Biepi. hum. wd. (cm)	5.51 (0.35)	5.75 (0.42)	1.80 (s)
Biepi. fem. wd. (cm)	8.10 (0.54)	8.46 (0.53)	2.10 (s)
Thigh girth (cm)	44.40 (5.1)	45.89 (5.24)	0.83
Calf girth (cm)	27.90 (1.9)	29.55 (3.14)	1.90 (s)
Chest girth (cm)	66.50 (3.8)	71.45 (6.05)	4.70 (s)
Up. arm flex g. (cm)	21.30 (1.3)	23.59 (2.68)	3.40 (s)
Up. arm length (cm)	25.70 (1.8)	27.07 (1.91)	3.20 (s)
Low. arm length (cm)	19.10 (1.9)	20.62 (1.35)	2.40 (s)

[a]d.f. = 11; critical value at 5% level = 1.782 for 1-tailed test.

[b](s) denotes significance.

Because it was obvious that figure skaters had much smaller absolute and relative skinfolds, no further analysis was made on these values. The remaining values were converted to phantom Z values by the formula:

$$Z = \left[\frac{1}{S} \quad v \left(\frac{170.18}{h} \right)^d - p \right]$$

where: Z is the standard score or proportionality value; S is the phantom standard deviation for the given variable v; v is any given variable; 170.18 is the phantom stature constant in cm; h is the subject's obtained stature or height; d is a dimensional component: 1 for lengths, breadths, girths, and skinfold thicknesses; 2 for areas or strength; 3 for mass or volume of whole body or any part; and p is the phantom value for the given variable v.

The obtained Z values for the skaters and prototypes are summarized in Table 3. These were tested for significance by a two-tailed t test. All conversions of data to Z values, both the mean and standard deviations, were calculated from the raw data using the phantom formula of Ross and Wilson (1974).

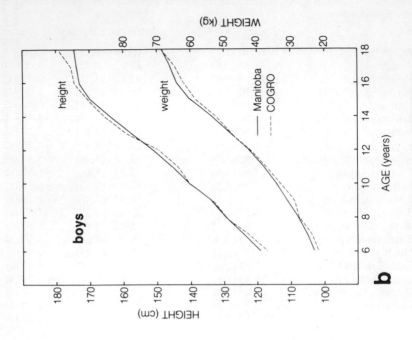

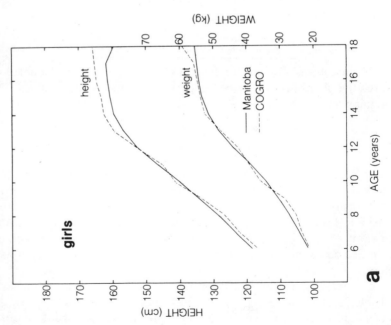

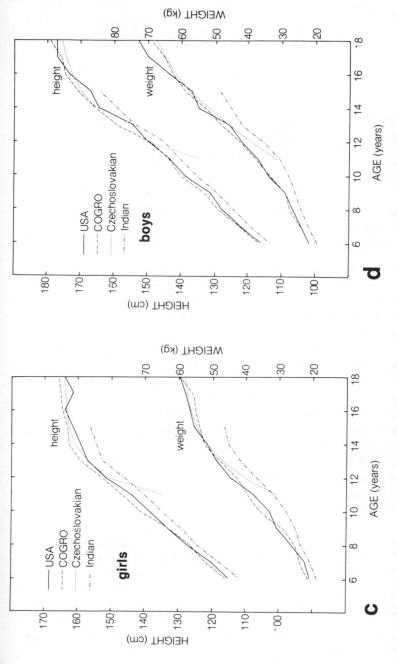

Figure 1.   a) Mean height and weight for COGRO and Manitoba girls ages 6–18 years; b) Mean height and weight for COGRO and Manitoba boys ages 6–18 years; c) Mean height and weight for Czechoslovakian, Indian, U.S., and COGRO girls ages 6–18 years; d) Mean height and weight of Czechoslovakian, Indian, U.S., and COGRO boys ages 6–18 years.

Table 3.   Standardized Z values for Canadian figure skaters and prototypes on thirteen variables

Item	Skaters	Prototype	t
Weight	−0.54 (0.64)	0.41 (0.93)	0.42
Sitting height	−0.46 (0.69)	−0.33 (0.32)	0.81
Foot length	1.04 (0.69)	0.16 (0.80)	3.28[a]
Tibial height	−1.02 (0.55)	−0.87 (0.50)	0.76
Biepi. hum. width	0.84 (1.08)	0.78 (1.24)	0.13
Biepi. fem. width	1.13 (0.67)	0.83 (0.87)	1.02
Thigh girth	−0.52 (0.67)	−0.69 (1.28)	0.33
Calf girth	−0.28 (0.88)	−0.29 (1.16)	0.02
Chest girth	−0.97 (0.71)	−0.80 (0.94)	0.52
Upper arm flex	−1.12 (0.62)	−0.74 (1.09)	0.95
Upper arm length	−0.04 (0.83)	−0.44 (0.76)	1.61
Lower arm length	−0.74 (1.18)	−0.28 (0.68)	2.23[a]
Biiliocr. width	−1.18 (0.61)	−0.99 (1.49)	0.28

[a]Significant.

The level of significance in this case was appropriate for a two-tailed test since there was no testing hypothesis as to directionality. Thus, the hypothesis was that the skaters were proportionally different to the prototypes. With 34 d.f., the critical value at the 5% level = 1.96 for a two-tailed test.

As shown in Table 3, only two Z value differences were significant for a two-tailed test at the 5% probability level—foot length and lower arm length. Thus, although in an absolute sense figure skaters were shown to differ from their age-sex peers by being significantly smaller, particularly in skinfold thicknesses, most of these differences disappeared when viewed proportionately in terms of a t ratio, as illustrated in Figure 2. The proportionally lower skinfold values may well be training effects. It is not possible from these samples to infer delayed maturity resulting from heavy training accompanied by smaller skinfolds. However, the proportionally large foot would be consistent with this phenomenon. The practical significance of the shorter forearm (lower arm) is still to be resolved.

These and other aspects of child growth remain to be explored. In this venture, the COGRO prototypes are proposed as a general reference where comprehensive local norms are not available and problems of size and proportionality appear to be otherwise inextricable.

ACKNOWLEDGMENTS

The authors gratefully acknowledge Superintendent Gordon M. Paton; Supervisor of Health and Physical Education, George Longstaff; cooperating principals and teachers of Coquitlam School District; anthropometrists R. Miller, A. Rapp,

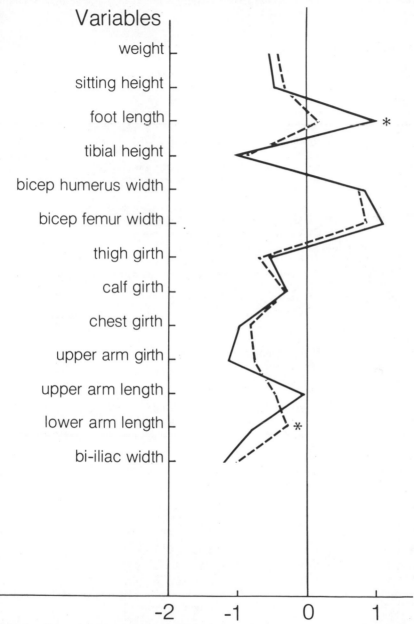

Figure 2.   Proportionality Z values for 13 variables showing a) (— — — —) deviation of pro-
totypical data for 11-year-old girls from the phantom (0); b) (————) deviation of
under-12 outstanding skaters from the phantom (0).

and R. Ward; and 36 Simon Fraser University students who contributed to the success of COGRO.

REFERENCES

Borms, J., M. Hebbelinck, J. E. L. Carter, W. D. Ross, and G. Lariviere. 1977. Standardisation of basic anthropometry in Olympic athletes—the MOGAP procedure. Paper presented at the International Symposium on Methods of Functional Anthropology, September 5-8, Prague.

Brundtland, G. H., K. Liestol, and L. Walloe. 1975. Height and weight of school children and adolescent girls and boys in Oslo, 1970. Acta Paediatr. Scand. 64: 565-573.

Corrol, V. A., and J. Dunfield. 1970. Manitoba "Fit for '70" height and weight norms. Physical Education Branch, Manitoba Department of Education, Winnipeg, Manitoba.

Faulkner, R. A. 1976. Physique characteristics of Canadian figure skaters. Microform Publication. University of Oregon, Eugene, Oregon.

Ghani, A. R., I. C. Verma, O. P. Ghai, and V. Seth. 1971. Physical growth of school children in Delphi. Indian J. Pediatr. 38:411-423.

Hamill, P. V. V. 1977. N.C.H.S. growth curves for children. D.H.E.W. Publication: (P.H.S.) 78-1650. U.S. Department of Health, Education, and Welfare, Washington, D.C.

Leahy, R. M., D. T. Drinkwater, G. W. Marshall, W. D. Ross, and A. Vajda. 1978. Computer solutions for longitudinal data: Tridimensional computer graphics in the resolution of growth curves. Paper presented at the 2nd International Seminar on Kinanthropometry, Leuven, Belgium.

Nie, N. H., C. Hull, J. C. Jenkins, A. Stenbrunner, and D. H. Bent. 1975. SPSS; Statistical Package for the Social Sciences, 2nd. Ed. McGraw-Hill Book Co., New York.

Prader, A., and H. Budliger. 1977. Body measurements, growth velocity and bone age of healthy children up to 12 years old. Helv. Paediatr. Acta (Suppl.) 37:5-45.

Ross, W. D., and N. C. Wilson. 1974. A stratagem for proportional growth assessment. Acta Paediatr. 28(Suppl. I-296):169-182.

Ross, W. D., S. R. Brown, M. Hebbelinck, and R. A. Faulkner. 1978. Kinanthropometry: Terminology and landmarks. In: R. J. Shephard and H. Lavallee (eds.), Physical Fitness Assessment Principles, Practice and Application. Charles C Thomas, Springfield, Ill.

Seliger, V., and Z. Bartunek. (eds.). 1976. Mean Values of Various Indices of Physical Fitness in the Investigation of Czechoslovak Population Aged 12-55 Years. Č.S.T.V., Praha (Č.S.S.R.).

Tanner, J. M. 1976. Population differences in body size, shape, and growth rate: A 1976 review. Arch. Dis. Child. 51:00.

Whittingham. 1979. Anthropometric prototypes for girls and boys aged 6 to 18, exemplified by structural analysis of sub-12-year-old figure skaters. Microform Publications, University of Oregon, Eugene, Ore.

Motor Learning:
A Neurophysiological Review

H. Forssberg

In order to perform a movement, an appropriate set of muscles must be activated in a proper temporal relation to one another and, simultaneously, antagonistic muscles have to be inhibited. Historically, two extreme alternatives have been used to describe the strategy of the central nervous system (CNS), one stressing central and the other peripheral factors. The latter considers a movement as being built up from smaller, discrete sequences linked together by "chain reflexes," with sensory feedback from each phase reflexively initiating each subsequent sequence. Signals from muscle receptors, tendon organs in the muscles, or receptors in skin and joints would report that the first sequence was executed and trigger the next set of muscles. In this way, several muscle groups might be linked together. By coupling the last muscle group to the first, a cyclical activity could be generated, as might be the case in walking or breathing. The idea originated mainly from an experiment by Mott and Sherrington (1895). The limb of a monkey was completely deafferented. Without muscular or cutaneous sensation, the limb was virtually paralyzed and grasp was abolished. These findings consequently led to the suggestion that afferent impulses were necessary to execute movement.

"Centralists," on the other hand, claimed that feedback induced by the movement was unnecessary for the execution of movements. They argued that the CNS already possessed sufficient information to activate the appropriate muscles. The motor output was already "programmed." When the signal arrived to induce the movement, all muscles could be activated by the program without any peripheral feedback. Some of the first supporters of the "central idea" were: Hering (1897a, 1897c) and Bickel (1897), who found that swimming and jumping movements in frogs remained after deafferentation; Brown (1911), who showed that alternating activity, as during locomotion, occurred in ankle muscles in spinal deafferented animals; Hering (1897b) and Munk (1903), who found that the monkeys used their deafferented limbs in order to grasp (Hering studied the same monkeys as Mott and Sherrington); and Lashley (1917), who studied a patient who had a gunshot injury to the spinal cord with an accidental deafferentation. Lashley found that the blindfolded patient never made a mistake in the direction and accuracy of a voluntary movement.

INNATE MOTOR PROGRAMS

From nonhuman species, there is now evidence of central motor programs executing proper movements without any peripheral feedback (Bentley and Konishi, 1978). In several elegant studies, Wilson (1961) demonstrated that a constant air stream on the head of the locust drove the deafferented wings to provide movements closely resembling the movements during ordinary flight. Detailed studies of the sense organs and EMG recordings from flight with waxed or cut wings both excluded any phasic input.

Swallowing in mammals is a very stereotyped motor act. Once it has started, it cannot be stopped or altered. About 25 different muscle groups are activated in a specific sequential order. Attempts to alter the fixed temporal sequence by denervating the different muscle groups involved have failed (Miller, 1972). The denervated muscles were silenced, but the loss of feedback induced at normal contractions did not influence the proper activation of subsequent muscle groups.

A third example of a centrally programmed motor pattern is the walking movement, as shown in Grillner's laboratory. Kittens, spinalized with a complete transection of the spinal cord at a low thoracic level one week after birth, were able to walk two days later if held with their hind limbs on a treadmill belt. Detailed studies of the movements and of the muscle activity during "spinal" locomotion showed striking similarities with intact locomotion (Grillner, 1973; Forssberg et al., 1980a, 1980b). The results suggest that the basic walking movements may be generated by the spinal cord without any supraspinal contribution. However, descending systems from the brainstem control these autonomous circuits, driving the locomotor activity slower or faster. They even initiate galloping (Shik et al., 1966). A noradrenergic descending system is probably contributing to the effects (Forssberg and Grillner, 1973; Grillner and Shik, 1973; Jordan and Steeves, 1975). By deafferentation studies and investigations where the movements were blocked by curare and the locomotor activity initiated by noradrenergic drugs (DOPA, Clonidin) a central origin of the locomotion was demonstrated (Edgerton et al., 1976; for review see Grillner, 1975).

These results give a rather detailed model of how locomotion is performed. Like the flight of the locust or swallowing in the cat, locomotion is generated by a central motor program, which is developed before birth. Neurones are genetically connected to a network able to generate the walking movements without peripheral feedback or participation of higher structures in the CNS. These walking movements are stereotyped and only generate the basic propulsive activity. The motor program or the "locomotor generator" is controlled by supraspinal centers driving it faster or slower. Finally, locomotion is adapted to the environment by different peripheral signals (visual, vestibular, and proprioceptive).

There are many reasons to believe that the human nervous system is organized in a similar way. During the first period of human life all movements that are necessary for survival seem to be generated by innate motor programs. As soon as the infant is born, it starts to breathe. "Rooting," "sucking," and "swallowing" reflexes are programmed to secure feeding. Different "postural" and "primo" reflexes exist at birth or develop during childhood and govern early motor activity. There is now evidence that human locomotion is an innate motor program (Forssberg and Wallberg, this volume). A newborn infant held over a horizontal surface may generate stereotyped walking movements. These are irregular and primitive, but there is a continuous development of the motor pattern until the child "learns" to walk without support. This implies that the child is not learning a new motor act, i.e., constructing a new motor program. Learning in this case instead means that the child "learns" to control an already established motor program and to adapt it to the external conditions. It is likely that it is the maturation and the development of different central control organs, especially the equilibrium system, that are required for free, unsupported walking.

In addition to walking, breathing, and swallowing, there are a number of motor acts present during the first year that one might suspect are generated by innate motor programs; for example, crawling, swimming (dog paddling), climbing, grasping (Bower, 1977), sitting, and standing. Certainly these programs are present in a very primitive form from the beginning, and develop to a mature pattern after practice and influence from other motor centers. Although not established, it is tempting to believe that the human is born with a library of small motor programs, for example, flexion or extension movements in each joint. These small subskills are later linked together to form new complex skills. Each innate submotor program may then be used in a number of later "learned" motor programs (see "'Learned' Motor Programs") consisting of several subprograms.

Today children with motor disabilities are often taught each motor skill in the same order as they normally develop (Gesell and Amatruda,

1947); crawling before walking, and so on. One practical consequence of innate central motor programs might be that it is unnecessary to keep this strict order. It might be possible to teach walking (equilibrium) even if the normally preceding motor skills are absent.

"LEARNED" MOTOR PROGRAMS

Even if a large part of daily motor activities are generated by innate motor programs, the distinct trait of the motor control of primates is the capacity to elaborate completely new movements, never done before. These new movements may be slow and explorative, with enough time for peripheral feedback, or fast, complex movements where several muscle groups have to be coordinated. Also, for these faster movements it should be convenient to construct central programs executing the activity without any peripheral feedback.

The innate programs are organized at lower levels in the CNS (spinal cord, brainstem), but there is reason to assume that learned movements are organized at a higher level. Recent investigations in monkeys (Evarts and Tanji, 1974) and man (Marsden et al., 1973) have demonstrated a long loop reflex on the order of 40–50 msec under voluntary control, activating pyramidal tract neurones in the motor cortex (Evarts and Tanji, 1976) that project to the motor neurones (Fetz and Finnoccio, 1975). Such long loop reflexes could still be fast enough to feed back peripheral information contributing to the next motor sequence.

However, as shown from recent experiments, there are also "learned" central motor programs. As shown by Nottebohm (1970) bird song is a very illustrative skill showing the significance of the peripheral input in motor learning. The European chaffinch exhibits some flexibility in its song development. Normally, young birds are exposed to adult song during the first 4 months of life and begin to sing themselves at 10 months of age. Birds that are not exposed at all to adult song only exhibit rudimentary sequences. If the young nestling, however, is exposed to the adult song during the first 4 months and then isolated for the remaining months, it will learn even the proper dialect of the song. This indicates that the fully developed song pattern requires previous auditory experience of the song. The young birds must therefore construct an auditive template (memory) of the song during the first months or complement an existing template that becomes manifested with experience. Six months later the template is still intact and the young bird's own song is compared with the stored adult song. When birds were deafened after 4 months of exposure to adult song, but prior to learning to sing themselves, the song was primitive and even more impaired than that of birds never exposed to adult song. On the other hand, if deafening was delayed until the song was firmly established, the song remained remarkably stable during a long

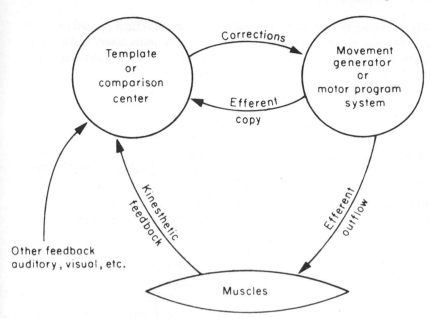

Figure 1.   A model for motor skill learning with mechanisms for error detection and correction of central motor programs (Keele and Summers, 1976).

period (Konishi, 1965). The syrinx—the vocal organ of birds—is bilaterally innervated by the hypoglossal nerve. When one side of the nerve was severed after the birds had learned a skilled song, sequences of the song dropped out, but the remaining portions of the song occurred in proper time (Nottebohm, 1970).

From these findings it is possible to construct a feasible model of the learning of the skill (Figure 1; see Bernstein, 1967, and Keele and Summers, 1976). A central motor program generates movements by efferent outflow to the muscles. The movements induce kinesthetic feedback not only from the limb, but also from the auditory, visual, and vestibular systems, depending on the task. The feedback is matched to a template and any error leads to a correction in the central motor program. Usually there is no time to correct the ongoing movement, so the program is corrected for the next time the same movement is elaborated. During the period of learning, when the central program and the template are constructed, it is important to have an intact peripheral feedback. In other words, the movements have to be trained frequently and the motor program corrected until it matches the template. At this instance the motor program seems well established, and may generate the movements without any peripheral feedback, as shown by the stability of the bird song after deafening and denervation.

In the bird song the environment is stable; the mechanics of the movement are always predictable. For many human skills, however, the environment is less predictable and one might suspect that the peripheral feedback should have a more important function. Taub and co-workers (Taub and Berman, 1968; Taub et al., 1975) demonstrated that adult deafferented monkeys were able to learn simple motor tasks. In the latter experiments, the monkeys' hands were moved to a position of visibility in front of them. As the monkeys learned the movements, they were able to see the movement of their arms and guide them to the correct position. When the monkeys had been trained, if their vision was blocked they were still able to perform the right movement without any direct feedback, although the movements were less precise. The possibility of intact afferents in dorsal or ventral roots was excluded because the nerves were stimulated with no evoked cortical responses. Taub et al. (1973) have also reported that infant monkeys both deafferented and visually blocked shortly after birth learn to walk, grasp, and climb. But, as discussed previously, these motor skills are inherited and they "learn" to control innate motor programs. Thus, it seems that primates have to use peripheral feedback to construct and learn new motor skills but that they may execute the learned movement without peripheral feedback. However, it is important to emphasize that the elegance of the normal movements is lost and that the movements are ataxic, dysmetric, and clumsy (Bossom, 1974).

EFFERENCE COPY

The notion of an efference copy originates from von Helmholst (see von Holst, 1954), who argued that the visual system had to have information about the motor commands sent to the eye muscles in order to know whether the changed image on the retina was the result of a moving eye in a stable environment or a resting eye in a moving environment. The concept of the efference copy has recently gained powerful electrophysiological support. Scratching is a spinal reflex (or innate motor program) (Sherrington, 1906) and consists of rhythmical flexion-extension movements of the hindlimb evoked by stimulation of the pinna. During scratching, ascending pathways to the cerebellum (the spinoreticular cerebellar pathway and the ventral spinocerebellar tract) convey rhythmic activity in phase with the scratching. This activity originates from the central spinal mechanism generating the efferent signals and not from the peripheral receptors, and might thus constitute an efference copy (Arshavsky et al., 1978a, b).

One possible function of the efference copy is in error detection (Figure 1). It (how the movement is planned) is thought to be compared with the peripheral feedback (how the movement is executed). Any mismatch indicates an error that may be corrected during the movement if it is slow enough, or in the motor program for the next time the movement is executed. A second important role for an efference copy might be in the coordination of several sequential motor skills to a smooth movement. It conveys information of planned but not yet executed movements. With this information, the centers coordinating the motor activities not only know what is going on (by peripheral feedback), but also which movements will be executed next. With the "feed-forward" the sequence following the next one may be designed and linked up to form a smooth continuous movement.

A hypothetical model may be constructed for motor control at a higher level. By conscious choice a certain motor skill is wanted. A "central processor" is commanded to execute the movement, but before execution the processor must receive information from the receptor systems creating a percept of the environment, of the body position in space, of the position of different parts of the body in relation to each other, and of movement parameters. This information, together with the information from the efference copy, is available at any given instance and, when commanded by an act of choice to execute the movement, all these data are coordinated by the processor and a proper motor program is chosen. The faster and the more accurate this process is, the more skilled movements are elaborated. In adults the central process time is as short as 150–200 msec, i.e., the simple reaction time. During this time the CNS prepares to execute the movement (Gurfinkel et al., 1971).

MOTOR DEVELOPMENT

The motor behavior of young children is relatively awkward when compared with that of adults, not only because they are unable to perform certain tasks. To perform more complex movements (for example writing, catching a ball, or eating) a number of subskills have to be smoothly linked together. Watching children, it appears that they are unable to integrate the necessary sequences of subskills in a rapid and accurate way; i.e., the perceptive mechanism and/or the central processes are too slow and inaccurate. Connolly (1970) let children of different ages sort cards of different colors in appropriate trays as quickly as possible. By measuring the time of movement, it was possible to determine the time of perception and central processing. In a two-choice situation, the 6-year-old child needed 1 sec, although an adult was able to execute the central process in one-third of that time. When the load increased by adding more colors and trays, the time was more prolonged for the smaller children than for the older. The younger children also showed a slower movement time, about twice as long for a 6-year-old child, as compared with adults. As the movement sequences were programmed, there were no increases in time required to distribute cards among eight as compared with two locations.

During one type of experiment, the cards had several misleading colors (without trays) along with the informative color. The increase of peripheral inflow prolonged the central time for the younger children, although the older children and the adults were uninfluenced. These findings reflect the enormous importance the perceptive mechanism has in acquiring skilled movements. Whereas the older children could filter out the irrelevant information, the younger children had great difficulty doing so.

Connolly's (1970) experiments show that there is a strong correlation between age and speed both in the central process and in the movement time up to and above 14 years of age. This means that the parts of the nervous system involved in motor control mature and develop slowly during the whole childhood; younger children are unable to learn complex and fast movement sequences where many muscle groups have to be coordinated. This is especially important in different sports, where instructors try to teach young children complex motor skills and, as a result, an incorrect motor program may be established and stored.

ACKNOWLEDGMENT

I thank Drs. Sten Grillner and Michael Zomlefer for critically reading the manuscript.

REFERENCES

Arshavsky, Y. I., I. M. Gelfand, G. N. Orlovsky, and G. A. Pavlova. 1978a. Messages conveyed by spinocerebellar pathways during scratching in the cat. I. Activity of neurones of the later reticular nucleus. Brain Res. 151:479–492.

Arshavsky, Y. I., I. M. Gelfand, G. N. Orlovsky, and G. A. Pavlova. 1978b. Messages conveyed by spinocerebellar pathways during scratching in the cat. II. Activity of neurones of the ventral spinocerebellar tract. Brain Res. 151: 493–506.

Bentley, D., and M. Konishi. 1978. Neural control of behaviour. Annu. Rev. Neurosci. 1:35–39.

Bernstein, N. 1967. The Coordination and Regulation of Movements. Pergamon Press, Oxford.

Bickel, A. 1897. Concerning the influence of the sensory nerves and the labyrinth on the movements of animals (in German). Pflugers Arch. Ges. Physiol. 67:299–344.

Bossom, J. 1974. Movement without proprioception. Brain Res. 71:285–296.

Bower, T. G. R. 1977. A Primer of Infant Development, Chap. 2. W. H. Freeman & Company, San Francisco.

Brown, T. G. 1911. The intrinsic factors in the act of progression in the mammal. Proc. R. Soc. (Biol.) 84:308–319.

Connolly, C. 1970. Response speed, temporal sequencing and information processing in children. In: C. Connolly (ed.), Mechanisms of Motor Skill Development. Academic Press, London.

Edgerton, V. R., S. Grillner, A. Sjöström, and P. Zangger. 1976. Central generation of locomotion in vertebrates. In: R. Herman, S. Grillner, P. Stein, and D.

Stuart (eds.), Neural Control of Locomotion. Vol. 18, pp. 439–464. Plenum Publishing Corp., New York.

Evarts, E. V., and J. Tanji. 1974. Gating of motor cortex reflexes by prior instruction. Brain Res. 71:479–494.

Evarts, F. V., and J. Tanji. 1976. Reflex and intended responses in motor cortex pyramidal tract neurons of monkey. J. Neurophysiol. 39:1069–1080.

Fetz, E. E., and D. V. Finnoccio. 1975. Correlations between activity of motor cortex cells and arm muscles during operantly conditioned response patterns. Exp. Brain Res. 23:217–240.

Forssberg, H., and S. Grillner. 1973. The locomotion of the acute spinal cat injected with Clonidine i.v. Brain Res. 50:184–186.

Forssberg, H., S. Grillner, and J. Halbertsma. 1980a. The locomotion of the low spinal cat. I. Coordination within a hindlimb. Acta Physiol. Scand. In press.

Forssberg, H., S. Grillner, J. Halbertsma, and S. Rossignol. 1980b. The locomotion of the low spinal cat. II. Interlimb coordination. Acta Physiol. Scand. In press.

Gesell, A., and C. S. Amatruda. 1947. Developmental Diagnosis. Harper and Row, New York.

Grillner, S. 1973. Locomotion in the spinal cat. In: R. B. Stein, K. G. Pearson, R. S. Smith, and J. B. Redford (eds.), Control of Posture and Locomotion, pp. 515–535. Plenum Publishing Corp., New York.

Grillner, S. 1975. Locomotion in vertebrates: Central mechanisms and reflex interaction. Physiol. Rev. 55:247–304.

Grillner, S., and M. L. Shik. 1973. On the descending control of the lumbo-sacral spinal cord from the "mesencephalic locomotor region." Acta Physiol. Scand. 87:320–333.

Gurfinkel, V. S., Y. M. Kots, V. I. Krinskiy, E. I. Paltsev, A. G. Feldman, M. L. Tsetlin, and M. L. Shik. 1971. Concerning tuning before movement. In: I. M. Gelfand, V. S. Gurfinkel, S. V. Fomin, and M. L. Tsetlin (eds.), Models of the Structural-Functional Organization of Certain Biological Systems, pp. 361–372. MIT Press, Cambridge.

Hering, H. E. 1897a. Concerning interference with movements after central deafferentation (in German). Arch. Exp. Pathol. Pharmacol. 38:266–283.

Hering, H. E. 1897b. Concerning central ataxia in men and monkeys (in German). Affen. Neurologisches Centralblatt, pp. 1077–1094.

Hering, H. E. 1897c. The jumping phenomenon of frogs and its explanation through the elimination of reflexive antagonistic muscle tension (in German). Pflugers Arch. Ges. Physiol. 68:1–31.

Jordan, L. M., and J. D. Steeves. 1975. Chemical lesioning of the spinal noradrenaline pathway: Effects on locomotion in the cat. In: R. Herman, S. Grillner, P. Stein, and D. Stuart (eds.), Neural Control of Locomotion, pp. 679–774. Plenum Publishing Corp., New York.

Keele, S. W., and J. J. Summers. 1976. The structure of motor problems. In: G. E. Stelmach (ed.), Motor Control—Issues and Trends. Academic Press, Inc., New York.

Konishi, M. 1965. The role of auditory feedback in the control of vocalization in the white-crowned sparrow. Z. Tierpsychol. 22:770–783.

Lashley, K. S. 1917. The accuracy of movement in the absence of excitation from the moving organ. Am. J. Physiol. 43:169–194.

Marsden, C. D., P. A. Merton, and H. B. Morton. 1973. Latency measurements compatible with a cortical pathway for the stretch reflex in man. J. Physiol. (Lond.) 230:58p–59p.

Miller, A. J. 1972. Significance of sensory inflow to the swallowing. Brain Res. 43:147–159.

Mott, F. W., and C. S. Sherrington. 1895. Experiments upon the influence of sensory nerves upon movement and nutrition of the limbs. Preliminary communication. Proc. R. Soc. (Biol.) 57:481–488.

Munk, H. 1903. Concerning the consequences of the loss of sensation in the extremity on motility (in German). Sitzungsberichten der K. Preuss. Akad. Wissensch., pp. 1038–1077.

Nottebohm, F. 1970. Ontogeny of bird song. Science 167:950–956.

Sherrington, C. S. 1906. Observations on the scratch reflex in the spinal dog. J. Physiol. (Lond.) 34:1–50.

Shik, M. L., F. V. Severin, and G. N. Orlovsky. 1966. Control of walking and running by means of electrical stimulation of the mid-brain. Biofizika 11:659–666. (English transl., pp. 756–765).

Taub, E., and A. J. Berman. 1968. Movement and learning in the absence of sensory feedback. In: S. J. Freedman (ed.), The Neurophysiology of Spatially Oriented Behaviour, pp. 173–192. Dorsey Press, Homewood, Ill.

Taub, E., I. A. Goldberg, and P. Taub. 1975. Deafferentation in monkeys: Pointing at a target without visual feedback. Exp. Neurol. 46:178–186.

Taub, E., P. N. Perrella, and G. Barbo. 1973. Behavioral development after forelimb deafferentation on day of birth in monkeys with and without blinding. Science 181:959–960.

von Holst, E. 1954. Relations between the central nervous system and the peripheral organs. Br. J. Anim. Behav. 2:89–94.

Wilson, D. M. 1961. The central nervous control of flight in a locust. J. Exp. Biol. 38:471–490.

Normal and Delayed Walking Age: A Clinical and Muscle Morphological and Metabolic Study

A. E. Lundberg

In pediatric and developmental psychology literature there is surprisingly varied information on the age at which children start to walk independently (Table 1). To some extent, different methodological approaches explain this: some authors give median or other percentile ages, others give mean ages. Also, the definition of the term "walking independently" varies. Walking age is sometimes based on retrospectively recalled data from parents; this has been shown to be unreliable (Pyles et al., 1935; Neligan and Prudham, 1969). However, if you concentrate on prospective studies with the same definition of walking age you will also find a different median age for the start of walking in different cultural and socioeconomic populations. The early development of postural control and locomotion of children in East Africa is well known and probably explained by the active training of these activities in the East African community (Super, 1976). However, differences in walking age are also found in modern European studies made on various populations (Table 2), for which genetic factors (Hindley et al., 1966), socioeconomic factors (Neligan and Prudham, 1969), and handling and nursing factors (Pikler, 1971) have been offered as explanations. In addition—and contrary to earlier opinions—the age at which a child has acquired an ability to perform a specified motor activity does not show a normal distribution. The percentile curve has a protracted course in the older ages (Hindley et al., 1966; Neligan and Prudham, 1969; Touwen, 1975; Lundberg, 1979) (Figure 1). In population studies these "late developers" may be recruited from deviant infants. However, a similar phenomenon is found in studies in which deviant children are excluded carefully (Touwen, 1975).

Table 1.　Comparison of mean age in months for free walking as given in different standard books

Literature source	Mean age in months
Gesell and Amatruda, 1940	15.2
Brünet and Lezine, 1951	14.2
Bühler and Hetzer, 1953	16.3
Illingworth, 1960	13.0

LATE WALKING—ETIOLOGICAL AND FOLLOW-UP STUDY

Children who started to walk independently at 18 months of age or later have been followed at a special clinic at the Children's Hospital in Gothenburg. The age of 18 months for walking start represents the 98th percentile in a Swedish community (Hindley et al., 1966; Lundberg, 1979); thus, these children were "late walkers." Furthermore, to be included in the clinical material, the children had to be found to have an isolated gross motor developmental delay, as judged by the Denver Developmental Screening Test (Frankenburg and Dodds, 1967), whose etiology was unclear at 18 months of age, and to have no clinical signs of cerebral palsy, myopathy, or polyneuropathy. Sixty-five children, thirty-seven girls and twenty-eight boys, were followed. Their ages at first examination were between 9 and 26 months, and at the last examination were between 3 and 7 years.

Table 3 gives the findings at the last examination. Thirty children (about 50%) had normal general and motor development according to the Denver Developmental Screening Test. Some of them were considered to be clumsy by their parents. Approximately 25% of the group still had gross motor developmental delay, defined as an inability to perform gross motor items that 90% of the Denver standardization population had performed at the same age. Three of them had a marked gross motor developmental delay, performing at a level corresponding to three-quarters of

Table 2.　Comparison of median age in months found in different cultural and socioeconomic populations

Literature source	Median age in months	Comments
Hindley et al., 1966	13.6	Zürich
	12.4	Stockholm
Neligan and Prudham, 1969	13.8	Newcastle, social class I
	13.1	Newcastle, social class II
	12.7	Newcastle, social class III
Pikler, 1971	15.5	Budapest, self-learning

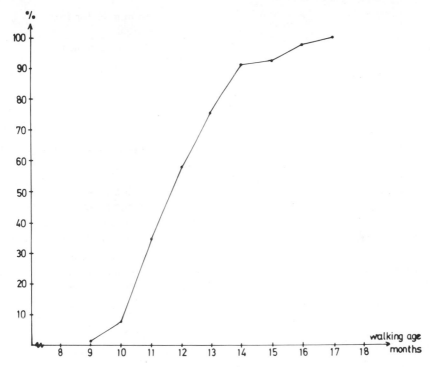

Figure 1.   Cumulative distribution of age at the start of walking in Gothenburg children (Lundberg, 1979).

their chronological age or less. However, no child in this deviant group had any other symptom or sign of upper motor lesion or neuromuscular disorder. The remainder of the group (approximately 25%) had signs of CNS disturbance. Most children were mildly mentally retarded and would need special education in the Swedish school system. The cerebral palsy group was comprised of one child with spastic hemiplegia and one with spastic diplegia. Both had minor motor handicaps. One boy had a progressive course of polyneuropathy of the hereditary type, which was identified at 24 months of age.

At follow-up, the mean and median ages in three groups were almost identical; therefore, age alone could not determine the child's performance at follow-up. Thus, the conventional pediatric examination procedure and screening failed to give a long term prognosis.

Table 4 gives some risk factors in the history of the children and the presence of these factors in the clinical groups at follow-up. Heredity for late walking was found in all groups, but heredity for shuffling (sliding on the bottom) as a way of prewalking locomotion was overrepresented in

Table 3.   Findings at last examination in 65 children with late walking syndrome

Group	Neural condition	N	Motor development	N
Group I "Normal"	No pathological signs	30	Motor and general development adequate for age	22
			Motor and general development for age but clumsy according to parents	8
Group II "Deviating"	Only gross motor development signs	19	Moderate gross motor delay	16
			Dissociated motor development without signs of CNS disorder	3
Group III "Abnormal"	Signs of CNS disorder	16	Mental retardation, mild	13
			Cerebral palsy	2
			Polyneuropathy	1
	Total	65		

the normal group and the group with only gross motor developmental delay as compared with children with normal walking age and the abnormal clinical group. Perinatal risk factors of dignity were more frequent in the abnormal group; and the occurrence of a deteriorating somatic disease between 10 and 12 months of age was overrepresented in the normal group at follow-up.

There were 15 children in the series who were identified as having similar developmental patterns and examination findings. This syndrome was called *dissociated motor development, normal variant* (Table 5). By using this term, an attempt was made to stress the isolated gross motor disturbance in the syndrome and the fairly good prognosis of it (Table 6).

Three main etiological groups of late walkers have been identified in the series (Table 7).

Table 4.   Risk factors in the histories of 65 children with gross motor delay in relation to a clinical group at follow-up[a]

	Heredity for		Perinatal	Deteriorating
Group	Shuffling	Walking	risk factors	somatic disease
I "Normal"	+	+	−	+
II "Deviant"	+	+	−	−
III "Abnormal"	−	+	+	−

[a] +, present; −, absent.

Table 5.   Gross motor developmental pattern and examination findings in the constitutional dissociated motor development syndrome

Characteristic
Late in taking sitting position Late in taking standing position
Muscle hypotonia: legs > arms Hyperflexibility of joints: legs > arms
Flabby, thin lower legs Small infantile feet
Genu recurvatum Pes planovalgus $\Big\}$ at weight

MUSCLE MORPHOLOGICAL AND METABOLIC STUDIES IN LATE WALKING SYNDROME
(Lundberg et al., 1979a, 1979b)

Needle biopsy of the lateral vastus muscle (Bergström, 1962) has been performed in 18 children with gross motor delays and late walking syndrome. The findings have been compared with the results in 25 children with normal development in whom muscle biopsies were performed under general anesthesia in connection with but before non-acute surgery, and with the results in 10 children in good health with diet-treated celiac disease [eight of them had also been examined in the untreated stage of their disease (Table 8)].

The concentrations of ATP, creatine phosphate (CP), and glycogen have been measured (Karlsson, 1971). For morphometric analysis (fiber-typing, fiber diameter measuring), histochemical stainings for measurement of ATPase and DPNH-diaphorase activities were used (Padykula and Herman, 1955; Novikoff et al., 1961).

Figure 2 gives the results of the biochemical analyses. ATP concentration was low in children with dissociated motor development (normal variant) and in children with untreated celiac disease as compared to controls, mentally retarded children, and children with treated celiac disease

Table 6.   Frequency and prognosis of the constitutional dissociated motor development syndrome

	N
Frequency in this group	15 of 65
Prognosis	
Normal motor and general development	7 of 15
Motor developmental delay	8 of 15
Symptom giving pes planovalgus	9 of 15

Table 7.   Etiological groups in 65 children with late walking age

Etiological group	N
1. Simple late walking syndrome	20
2. Symptomatic dissociated motor development syndrome	30
a) Prenatal disorders with CNS involvement	5
b) Peri- or postnatal disorders with CNS involvement	9
c) Postnatal non-neurological disorder	5
d) Mental retardation of unknown etiology	11
3. Constitutional dissociated motor development syndrome	15

($p \leq 0.01$). CP concentration followed the same pattern, and the differences were significant ($p \leq 0.05$). The glycogen concentration was also low in the disturbed groups, but only the differences between children with untreated celiac disease and children with treated celiac disease and the control group of children were significant ($p \leq 0.01$).

Mean fiber diameters of type 1 and especially type 2 fibers were smaller in children with constitutional dissociated developmental syndrome than in the other groups (Table 9). Fiber type 1 percentage was low in children with untreated celiac disease as compared both to controls and to the results in the same children at an older age during treatment of the disease (Table 10).

Finding low amounts of energy-giving substrates is nonspecific. They are affected by factors such as physical training (Karlsson et al., 1971; Eriksson et al., 1973); diseases such as rheumatoid arthritis (Nordemar et al., 1974) and Parkinson's disease (Landin et al., 1974); and conditions upsetting normal metabolism, such as starvation, acute renal failure, and abdominal surgery (Bergström et al., 1964; Hultman and Bergström, 1967, 1969). However, the combination of low amounts of energy-giving substrates and small fibers in children in good general condition indicates that constitutional dissociated motor development could be a clinical entity. The low fiber type 1 percentage before treatment in celiac disease and

Table 8.   Number of children in clinical series with gross motor delay in which muscle biochemical and morphometric analyses have been performed, and their age range at the biopsy

Group	N	Age (months)
Controls	25	2–131 (11 years)
Late walking syndromes		
General developmental delay	4	18–28
Constitutional dissociated motor		
development syndrome	6	15–24
Celiac disease		
Before treatment	8	5.5–15
During treatment	10	16–38

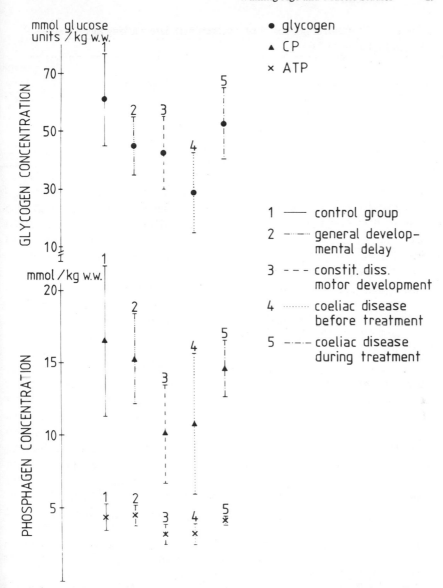

Figure 2.   Metabolic substrates in groups of children with gross motor delay and control groups.

the normalization after treatment are remarkable. Fiber composition is generally thought to be genetically determined and unaffected by age and training. Changes of fiber composition have been noted in animals after denervation, cross-innervation, and nerve stimulation (Close, 1972). An increasing type 1 percentage has been observed during growth in rats

Table 9. Comparison between mean diameter of type 1 and type 2 fibers in children with gross motor delay and controls

Clinical group	N	Mean fiber diameter[a]	
		Type 1	Type 2
General developmental delay	4	n	n
Constitutional dissociated motor development syndrome	6	↓	↓↓
Celiac disease, before treatment	10	n	↓
Celiac disease, during treatment	10	n	n

[a]n = normal, ↓ = small, ↓↓ = very small.

Table 10. Comparison between type 1 fiber percentage in children with gross motor delay and controls

Clinical series	N	Percentage	
		Mean ± SD	Sig.
General developmental delay	4	58 ± 17	N.S.
Constitutional dissociated motor development syndrome	6	52 ± 11	N.S.
Celiac disease, before treatment	10	41 ± 10	↓
Celiac disease, during treatment	10	57 ± 10	N.S.

(Kugelberg, 1976) and in humans after nerve stimulation (Munsat et al., 1976). The main factor for changing fiber composition in children with celiac disease cannot be identified in this study.

REFERENCES

Bergström, J. 1962. Muscle electrolytes in man. Scand. J. Clin. Lab. Invest. 14:Suppl. 68.

Bergström, J., H. Castenfors, E. Hultman, and T. Silander. 1964. The effect of surgery upon muscle glycogen in man. Acta Chir. Scand. 130:1.

Brünet, O., and I. Lezine. 1951. The Psychological Development of the New Infant (in French). Presses Universitaires de France, Paris.

Bühler, C., and H. Hetzer. 1953. Tests of small children from 1 to 6 years of age (in German). Johann Ambrosius Barth, München.

Close, R. I. 1972. Dynamic properties of mammalian skeletal muscles. Physiol. Rev. 52:129.

Eriksson, B., P. D. Gollnick, and B. Saltin. 1973. Muscle metabolism and enzyme activities after training in boys 11–13 years old. Acta Physiol. Scand. 87:485–497.

Frankenburg, W. K., and J. B. Dodds. 1967. The Denver Development Screening Test. J. Pediat. 71:181.

Gesell, A., and C. Amatruda. 1940. Developmental Diagnosis. Paul Hoeber, London.

Hindley, C. B., A. M. Filluzat, C. Klackenberg, D. Nicolet-Meister, and E. Sand. 1966. Differences in age of walking in five European longitudinal samples. Hum. Biol. 38:364.

Hultman, E. 1973. Energy metabolism in human muscle. J. Physiol. 231:56.

Hultman, E., and J. Bergström. 1967. Muscle glycogen synthesis in relation to diet studied in normal subjects. Acta Med. Scand. 182:109.

Hultman, E., and J. Bergström. 1969. Glycogen content in patients with renal failure. Acta Med. Scand. 186:177.

Illingworth, R. S. 1960. The Development of the Infant and Young Child. E. and S. Livingstone Ltd., Edinburgh.

Karlsson, J. 1971. Lactate and phosphagen concentrations in working muscle of man. Acta Physiol. Scand. (Suppl.):358.

Karlsson, J., B. Diamant, and B. Saltin. 1971. Muscle metabolites during submaximal and maximal exercise in man. Scand. J. Clin. Lab. Invest. 26:385.

Kugelberg, E. 1976. Adaptive transformation of rat soleus motor units during growth. J. Neurol. Sci. 27:269.

Landin, S., L. Hagenfeldt, B. Saltin, and J. J. Wahren. 1974. Muscle metabolism during exercise in patients with Parkinson's disease. Clin. Sci. Mol. Med. 47:493.

Lundberg, A. 1979. Gross and fine motor performance in healthy Swedish children aged fifteen and eighteen months. Neuropaediatrie 10:35.

Lundberg, A., B. O. Eriksson, and G. Jansson. 1979a. Muscle abnormalities in coeliac disease: Studies on gross motor development and muscle fibre composition, size and metabolic substrates. Eur. J. Pediatr. 130:93.

Lundberg, A., B. O. Eriksson, and G. Mellgren. 1979b. Metabolic substrates, muscle fibre composition and fibre size in late walking and normal children. Eur. J. Pediatr. 130:79.

Munsat, T. L., D. McNeal, and R. Waters. 1976. Effects of nerve stimulation on human muscle. Arch. Neurol. 33:608.

Neligan, G., and D. Prudham. 1969. Norms for four standard developmental milestones by sex, social class and place in family. Dev. Med. Child Neurol. 11:413.

Nordemar, R., O. Lövgren, P. Fürst, R. C. Harris, and E. Hultman. 1974. Muscle ATP content in rheumatoid arthritis—a biopsy study. Scand. J. Clin. Lab. Invest. 34:185–191.

Novikoff, A. B., W. Shin, and J. Ducker. 1961. Mitochondrial localization of oxidation enzymes: Staining results with two tetrazolium salts. J. Biophys. Biochem. Cytol. 9:47–61.

Padykula, H. A., and E. Herman. 1955. The specificity of the histochemical method of adenosine triphosphatase. J. Histochem. Cytochem. 3:170–195.

Pikler, E. 1971. Learning of motor skills on the basis of self-induced movements. In: J. Hellmuth (ed.), Exceptional Infant. Volume 2, p. 54. Butterworths, London.

Pyles, M. K., H. R. Stolz, and J. W. MacFarlane. 1935. The accuracy of mother's report on birth and developmental data. Child Dev. 6:165.

Super, M. C. 1976. Environmental effects on motor development: The case of the African infant precocity. Develop. Med. Child. Neurol. 18:561.

Touwen, B. 1975. Neurological Development in Infancy. Drukkery Grasmeijer and Wijngaard, Groningen, The Netherlands.

Infant Locomotion: A Preliminary Movement and Electromyographic Study

H. Forssberg and H. Wallberg

A newborn infant may perform walking movements if held under the arms with the feet touching a flat surface (Thomas and Autgarden, 1966). This inherited capacity will improve instead of being suppressed (which usually happens 6–8 weeks after birth) if the child is systematically trained (Zelazo et al., 1972). Preliminary data on infant walking are presented in this chapter. These data have been obtained by using an automatic system for simultaneous recording of position data (with high resolution), force data, and electromyographical data.

METHODS

Children of varying ages were held under the arms above a treadmill with their bare feet touching the belt. They were held very lightly, letting the limbs carry as much of the body weight as possible. The treadmill belt was driven manually at a speed adjusted to suit the walking movements.

There were 26 children, ranging in age from 5 hr to 6 weeks, who were tested on the treadmill. EMGs were recorded from 14 children, and recordings of movements and force reactions were done in two children. Six children, from 2 to 12 months old, were also studied with more extensive recordings. Two of these children were followed from the neonatal period.

The movements of the limb were recorded by a Selspot System (Selcom Co., Partille, Sweden). Five diodes, emitting infrared light, were glued to the pelvis, hip, knee, and heel, and to the base of the lateral toe. The diodes were lit 160 times per sec and their positions were detected by a

This study was supported by Norrbacka-Eugeniastiftelsen och Clas Groschinsky's Minnesfond.

camera with an infrared-sensitive plate in the focal plane. The x and y coordinates were continuously fed into a minicomputer (Hewlett-Packard 21 MX) and stored on a disc. The limb movements were displayed on a graphic terminal as "stick diagrams," with straight lines between the points representing the position of each diode. While walking on the treadmill, the children maintained approximately the same position in front of the camera, but in the "stick diagrams" the pelvis was plotted as if it moved with a constant speed forward, as would occur during overground walking (cf. Figures 1 and 2).

Bipolar surface electrodes were used to record EMG activity of four lower limb muscles. The muscles selected for study were the tibialis anterior (TA), the lateral head of gastrocnemius (LG), the medial hamstring group (Ham), and the quadriceps muscle group (Q). All of the electrodes were put in place by the same person and an effort was made to locate the electrodes over the same area of the muscle belly in each subject. Depending on the size of the muscles and the thickness of the subcutaneous tissue, it is possible that some crosstalk from neighboring muscles was obtained in TA and Ham. The electrodes were directly coupled to an instrumentation amplifier (2×2 cm) glued to the skin adjacent to the electrodes. The EMG could subsequently be rectified and filtered (time constant: 10 msec) (Gottlieb and Agarwal, 1970).

The reaction forces in the surface supporting the body were recorded by a Kistler force plate (Type 9261A). Each child was held and walked over the floor so that one foot struck the force plate. In this manner, the forces during two or three consecutive step cycles could be recorded. All data were fed into the computer and stored on a disc. They were also recorded on an eight-channel ink recorder (Mingograph; frequency response 1250 Hz) and on an FM tape recorder (Racal-Thermionic Ltd.; frequency response 2500 Hz).

RESULTS

All infants ($N = 26$) tested during the first 6 weeks after birth could perform at least parts of a single step (a forward swing). Fourteen infants performed complete steps, i.e., two consecutive swing phases of the same limb separated by a support phase, and two of the children were able to perform several consecutive step cycles. On different occasions (time after feeding, etc.) the ability to walk varied substantially in the same child. Therefore, the children performing worse might have been capable of walking better under some other conditions.

The walking movements differed in many respects from those seen during adult locomotion. During the swing phase, the limb was moved forward by a forceful flexion in the hip without corresponding effects in other joints. The foot was thereby lifted to an extreme degree toward the

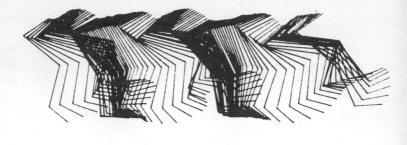

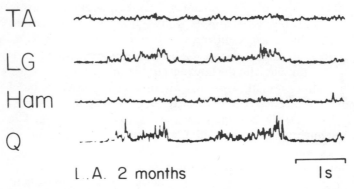

Figure 1.   Movement analysis and EMG recordings of a 2-month-old boy. A "stick diagram" is reconstructed from the coordinates of the diodes (see "Methods") during locomotion on a treadmill. Three successive positions of the diodes were averaged for each limb representation (final frequency 53 Hz). The pelvis is represented with a constant speed forward (to the right). At the bottom, the rectified and filtered EMG activity is presented (synchronized to the position of the pelvis).

end of the swing (Figure 1). As a consequence of the extreme elevation, the foot was rapidly lowered in a backward direction, producing a short-lasting contact force in the forward direction at the impact of the foot with the ground (Figure 2B). The foot was usually placed with the toes making the first contact (Figure 2B). In the beginning of the support phase the limb had a braking force (backward thrust), which was usually not followed by a forward thrust, as in adult walking. This reflects the fact that the body was moved forward by an external force (i.e., the person supporting the child). The infants carried approximately 40% of their body weight on each limb (see Figures 2A and B; body weight 5010 g). The person supporting the infant consequently carried the remaining weight, with the amount depending on whether one or two limbs supported the body. The variability is reflected in the large vertical oscillation of the body (Figure 1), with an elevation during double support and a lowering during the swing phase of either limb.

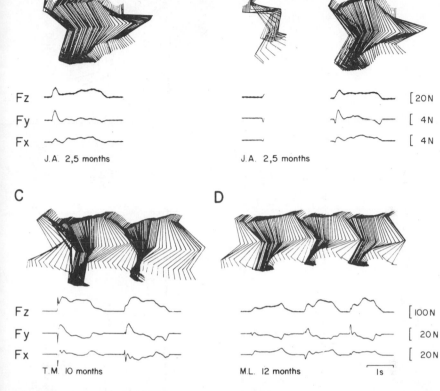

Figure 2.   Movements and force reactions of the right limb at varying ages. In each part of the figure the movements are represented as "stick diagrams" at the top (see "Methods"; 53 Hz) and the simultaneously recorded reaction forces are at the bottom (see "Methods"). Fz is the vertical force. Fy is the longitudinal-horizontal force with the backward direction of the reaction force directed upward. Fx is the transversal-horizontal force. A shows a support phase and the beginning of the following swing in a child 2.5 months old. B shows another support phase from the same child. The first sequence shows the placement of the foot. C and D are several consecutive step cycles of a 10-month- and a 12-month-old child, respectively. Note force and time calibrations.

The extensor muscles of both knee (Q) and ankle (LG) were activated in the first extension phase (E_1), (i.e., the period from when the limb starts to extend until the foot contacts the ground) and remained active during the entire support phase, with an increased activity in the beginning and in the end (Figure 3). Usually, LG was maximally activated in the beginning of the support, with a burst of activity at foot contact and with only a small increase in the activity at the end; whereas in Q the second burst of activity was comparatively larger than the first (Figure 1). The flexor muscle of the ankle (TA), as well as the hamstring muscles (Ham), usually maintained a small tonic activity during the support phase, with biphasic

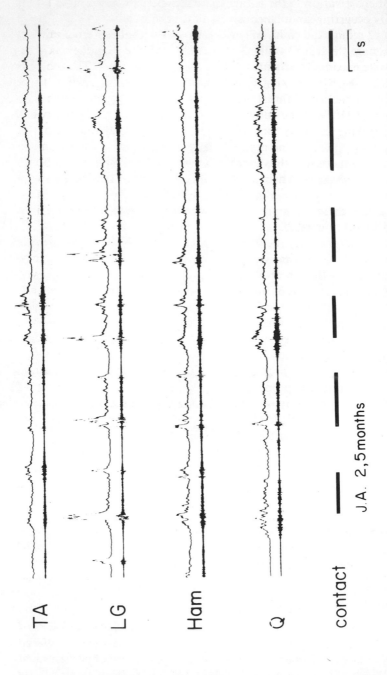

Figure 3.   EMG activity from a 10-week-old child. The activity in the four studied muscles (see "Methods") is presented in raw and in rectified and filtered forms. At the bottom are indicated the periods of foot contact calculated from the movement of the diodes at the toe and heel.

bursts in the beginning and at the end (Figure 3). Thus, there was a high degree of coactivation in the antagonistic muscles, with two main bursts of activity occurring simultaneously in all four muscles.

In a 12-month-old child, still unable to walk without external support but with more "mature" walking movements (Figure 2D), the ankle extensors were maximally activated during the end of support. The foot was placed with the heel striking first without any forward reaction force preceding the backward thrust. The forces indicated that the single limb carried about 110% of the body weight and exhibited a forceful forward thrust propelling the body forward (Figure 2D). As a consequence of the strong support, there was no need for any external agent to carry or move the body, and there was thus much less vertical oscillation of the body. The children only needed help to maintain equilibrium. During the swing phase the limb was no longer lifted so high, but instead was quickly lifted to a maximum early in the swing and then smoothly lowered as the limb moved forward (Figure 2D).

During early infancy (below 6 months) the walking movements were highly irregular. After some steps the child might suddenly stop with one limb in prolonged flexion or with both limbs on the belt, often followed by a concomitant flexion of both limbs. All children had inadequate adduction, often resulting in the forward-swinging limb becoming entangled with the other limb. However, it is important to note that, even during this early period, sequences of more "mature" movements would appear; for example, a proper placement of the limb on the ground with no forward peak preceding the normal backward thrust (Figure 2A), or a forward thrust (Figure 2B) propelling the body forward. In the children in whom the walking capacity was not suppressed, there seemed to be a continuous stabilization and development of the walking movements. Sequences of the more mature pattern appeared more frequently with increasing age. In Figure 2C the recordings from a 10-month-old boy are presented. In the first swing phase, the foot was elevated until the end of the swing and then lowered, with a backward impact on the ground (first support phase). During the second support phase, there was no negative peak preceding the backward thrust and the forward thrust was strong. During the swing the foot was slowly lowered after an initial elevation. Hence, in the same sequence there were steps resembling the early infant locomotion together with more mature steps.

DISCUSSION

The recordings from infant locomotion have shown a typical form of walking. It may be characterized by an extreme forward swing, induced mainly by a flexion of the hip followed by a rapid placement of the front part of the foot with an accompanying ankle extensor activity (partly resembling a Prussian march) and a support phase where the limb can neither fully support the body nor propel it forward.

What kind of neural activity do these immature walking movements reflect? Kittens whose spinal cords have been transected (a lesion at T_{12}) 1 week after birth can perform well coordinated locomotor movements with the hindlimbs some days after the operation (Grillner, 1973; Forssberg et al., 1980a, 1980b). Monkeys deafferentated and blinded on the day of birth can still develop the ability to use the forelimbs for ambulation (Taub et al., 1973). It is now generally accepted that throughout the animal kingdom—from swimming fish to walking monkeys—the stereotyped ambulatory activity is generated by innate central motor programs (see Grillner, 1975). The neural network generating the basic activity seems to be organized in the spinal cord and may be responsible for the pattern of muscle activity without any supraspinal contribution. These spinal networks are, however, turned on and switched off from higher centers. It is therefore likely that the immature walking movements during infancy reflect the activity in a spinal "locomotor generator" that acts autonomously with only minor influence from higher centers. Its early appearance only some minutes after birth (see Thomas and Autgarden, 1966) indicates that the walking capacity is inherited and present without earlier practice. The fact that the extensor muscles were active prior to foot contact shows that the extensor activity is not reflexively induced by the contact, an assumption often made. It favors a central origin of the activity.

Normally, the walking capacity disappears 6–8 weeks after birth and a walking pattern closely resembling that of adulthood develops when the child "learns" to walk freely. A second question might therefore be: Does infant locomotion utilize the same neuronal apparatus as the later "learned" walk or is it an independent phenomenon?

During infant locomotion all four muscles recorded showed a biphasic activation, with bursts of activity during the shifts between the swing and the support phases and vice versa. Usually the activity was irregular and a high degree of coactivation occurred. The net force output from the muscles was not sufficient to support or to move the infant forward. Although the pattern was not fully differentiated, the muscles were active during the same periods as during adult locomotion (i.e., when the body was accelerated and decelerated). Considering the high degree of coactivation (see "Methods") during infancy it might seem puzzling that the limb moved at all. However, quantitative differences in the degree of activation remain between antagonistic muscles and there is, of course, no direct relationship between muscle activity (EMG), force (length-tension and force-velocity diagrams), and movement (see Bernstein, 1967), which depends on the position of the limb. A given pattern of muscular activation at the end of the support will inevitably produce a different movement than a similar activation would at the end of the swing.

As noted earlier (Zelazo et al., 1972) and confirmed in this study, the walking capacity was not suppressed in all children. Some continuously developed the more mature pattern seen prior to the time when children walk freely. The finding of a more mature pattern in the same walking sequence as an immature pattern (Figure 2C) indicates that the same basic activity is present, but that it is transformed gradually as the child grows. Concurrent with the maturation of the higher centers, these children begin to control and influence the "locomotor generator," which acts almost autonomously in the earlier stage. The suppression of the walking capacity normally seen might be an effect of the neural rearrangement required. It is interesting that the ankle extensor was activated prior to foot contact with a digitigrade support. After maturation there is a suppression of the early ankle extensor activity concurrent with a proper initial heel contact. To our knowledge the human walk is the only one in which the heel first makes contact with the ground (even though the bear is known to have a plantigrade foot contact). A plantigrade walk is more effective in lengthening the step during bipedal locomotion. Thus, in its initial form human locomotion might be programmed for a digitigrade pattern, as it was for most of our mammalian ancestors and only with maturation does the walk pattern evolve. It can be noted that some children, when walking freely, also use a digitigrade walk even when they can place the heel during standing (habitual toe walkers).

ACKNOWLEDGMENT

Thanks are given to Drs. Sten Grillner and Avis Cohen for critically reading this manuscript.

REFERENCES

Bernstein, N. 1967. The Coordination and Regulation of Movements. Pergamon Press, Oxford.

Forssberg, H., S. Grillner, and J. Halbertsma. 1980a. The locomotion of the low spinal cat. I. Coordination within a hindlimb. Acta Physiol. Scand. In press.

Forssberg, H., S. Grillner, J. Halbertsma, and S. Rossignol. 1980b. The locomotion of the low spinal cat. II. Interlimb coordination. Acta Physiol. Scand. In press.

Gottlieb, G. L., and G. C. Agarwal. 1970. Filtering of electromyographic signals. Am. J. Phys. Med. 49:142–146.

Grillner, S. 1973. Locomotion in the cat. In: R. B. Stein, K. G. Pearson, R. S. Smith, and J. B. Redford (eds.), Control of Posture and Locomotion, pp. 515–535. Plenum Publishing Corp., New York.

Grillner, S. 1975. Locomotion in vertebrates: Central mechanisms and reflex interaction. Physiol. Rev. 55:247–304.

Taub, E., P. N. Perrella, and G. Barbo. 1973. Behavioral development after fore-limb deafferentation on day of birth in monkeys with and without blinding. Science 181:959–960.

Thomas, A., and S. Autgarden. 1966. Locomotion from pre- to postnatal life. Clin. Prev. Med. 24.

Zelazo, P. R., N. A. Zelazo, and S. Kolb. 1972. Walking in newborn. Science 176:314–315.

Learning Effects in Repeated Measurements Designs

G. Beunen, J. Simons, M. Ostyn,
R. Renson, and D. Van Gerven

Tanner (1951) indicated the precise nature of the merits of longitudinal, mixed longitudinal, and cross-sectional growth studies and set forth the statistical treatment of each type of data. More recently, Schaie (1965) concluded that the discrepancies and contradictions in the conclusions derived from longitudinal and cross-sectional studies are consequences of the violation of assumptions implicit in these research designs. He proposed a model for research on behavioral changes over time. This developmental model assumes that a response is a function of the age of the organism, the cohort to which the organism belongs, and the time at which the measurement occurs. These components are by no means independent and their confounding dictates the methods available for their separate and joint analyses. In cross-sectional designs developmental differences are confounded with cohort differences, and in longitudinal designs developmental differences are confounded with time-of-measurement differences.

In the Nijmegen growth study (Prahl-Andersen and Kowalski, 1973; van 't Hof, et al., 1977) a mixed longitudinal design was chosen for the study of developmental changes to circumvent the difficulties inherent in each of these approaches. The same design was also chosen for the Project Growth and Health in Teenagers (Kemper and van 't Hof, 1977).

Because in the Leuven growth study two separate studies were conducted simultaneously, the design of this study resembles that proposed by van 't Hof et al. (1977). Consequently some of the components of the

The Leuven Boys Growth Study was supported by grants received from the Ministries of Dutch and French Culture, Administrations of Physical Education, Sports and Open Air Activities, and from the Ministry of Public Health and Family, all of the Belgian Government.

model proposed by Schaie (1965) can be isolated. In the present study we investigated the presence of test or learning effects in the repeated measurements of anthropometric measures and motor abilities.

METHODS

The data were from a mixed longitudinal study of the physical fitness of Belgian school boys (Leuven Boys Growth Study). This growth study consisted of a 6-year investigation of a representative sample of Belgian school boys, ages $12\pm$ to $20\pm$ years. The testing program started in 1969 and ended in 1974. A total of 21,174 examinations were conducted. In addition to anthropometric measurements, skeletal maturity, somatotype, motor ability, sports participation, and sociocultural determinants were studied. A description of the measuring procedures is given by Simons et al. (1978).

The present study is concerned with results for 1055 17-year-old boys from the same cohort (1955–56) who were measured and tested at the same time (January to March, 1973). The sample of 17-year-old boys was subdivided into five groups according to the number of test sessions in which they participated. There were 13% who were tested once, 20% twice, 13.5% three times, 16.5% four times, and 37% five times. To test the hypothesis that the number of tests participated in influences the results of 17 anthropometric measures and nine motor abilities, the differences between these five groups were tested for their significance by means of analysis of variance and covariance techniques using the computer programs ONE WAY and ANOVA (hierarchical approach) described by Nie et al. (1975).

Comments on Methods

Before describing in detail the results obtained in this study, it seems necessary to clarify the design of the Leuven Boys Growth Study. In this study a pure longitudinal study was conducted simultaneously with a cross-sectional one. This resulted in a mixed longitudinal study with four cohorts (the number of subjects in the other cohorts was very small) and six measurement times at yearly intervals. This design differed somewhat from the one proposed by van 't Hof et al. (1977) because at each time of measurement (see Figure 1) several subsamples were tested in each cohort. The number of subsamples equaled the number of years that the study was continued.

In 1973, the fifth year of the study, for example, four cohorts were tested, including boys ages 16 through 19 years. But in each of the age groups a number of boys were tested for the first time, some for the second, and others for the third, fourth, or fifth time. In 1974, six such subsamples were present since this was the sixth year of the study.

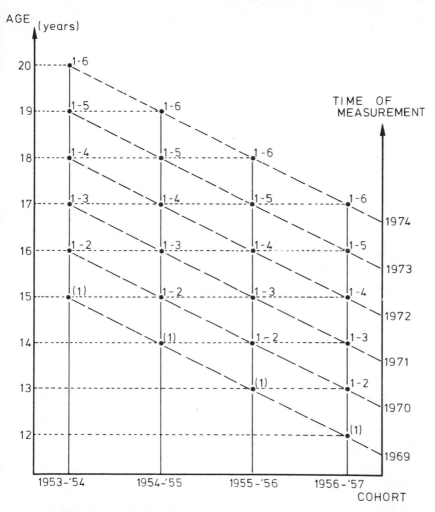

Figure 1. The design of the Leuven Boys Growth Study with four cohorts and six repeated measurements (adapted from the model proposed by van 't Hof et al., 1977). Key: 1 = all boys tested for the first time; 1-2, 1-3, 1-4, 1-5, 1-6 = some boys tested for the first time, others for the second, third, fourth, fifth, or sixth time.

This design enabled us to study the testing or learning effects due to test participation. In the present investigation, for example, the 17-year-old boys from the 1955–56 year who were tested in 1973 were studied. As can be seen in Figure 1, this sample consisted of five subsamples according to the number of times the boys had already participated in the study. From Figure 1 it can also be noted that this sample of 17-year-old boys was only a part (about 40%) of the total sample of 17-year-old boys tested in the Leuven Boys Growth Study.

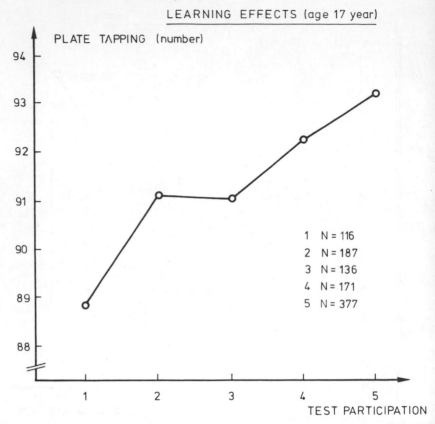

Figure 2.   Learning effects in plate tapping (speed of limb movement) for 17-year-old boys.

RESULTS

The differences between the five test participation groups were analyzed using a one-way analysis of variance with test participation as the independent variable and the different motor abilities and anthropometric measures as the dependent variables. Significant differences were found for four of the eight motor ability tests, for the pulse frequency after exercise and also for four anthropometric variables. But it was also found that the five groups differed somewhat in chronological age, skeletal age, and sociocultural background. In previous studies (Beunen et al., 1978; Renson et al., 1978) the relationships between these variables and motor abilities and anthropometric measurements were demonstrated. Therefore, a two-way analysis of covariance was carried out with profession of the father and test participation as the independent variables and skeletal and chronological age as the covariates. From this analysis it appeared that testing or learning effects disturbed neither the anthropometric results

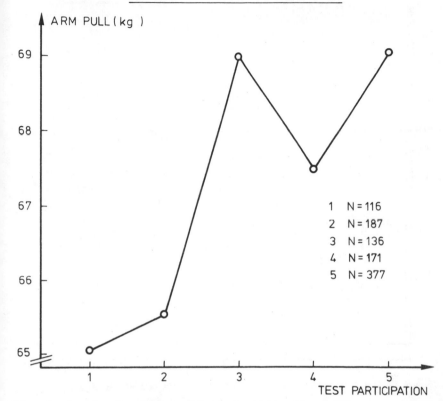

LEARNING EFFECTS (age 17 year)

Figure 3.   Learning effects in arm pull (static strength) for 17-year-old boys.

(except for bicondylar humerus) nor four of the eight motor test results. However, significant differences were found for the four remaining motor tests and for the pulse frequency after exercise. For speed of limb movement (plate tapping) a nearly linear increase was found as a function of the number of tests participated in (Figure 2). For static strength (arm pull) and trunk strength (leg lifts) the results show a marked increase from the first to the third test participation; thereafter they remained at the same level (Figures 3 and 4). The largest increase for running speed (shuttle run) occurred between the first and second test participation; afterwards only a small continual increase was noted (Figure 5).

DISCUSSION

Significant differences between five test participation groups were present in four of the eight motor tests, in pulse frequency after a 1-min step test, and in bicondylar humerus width. However, the significant difference for pulse frequency after a 1-min step test disappeared when, instead of socio-

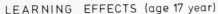

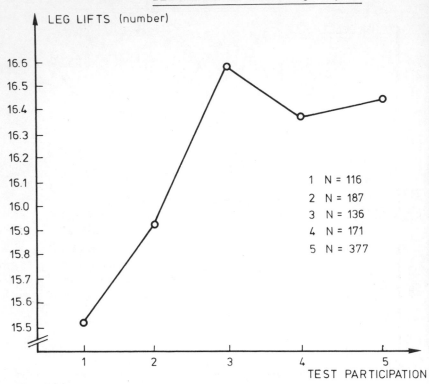

Figure 4.   Learning effects in leg lifts (trunk strength) for 17-year-old boys.

professional status, the school type was introduced as the first independent variable. The significant differences found for the four motor abilities and bicondylar humerus width were also present in this analysis. Consequently, it seemed justified to accept a learning effect for these four motor abilities and a testing effect for bicondylar humerus width. We were not surprised to find such effects for motor abilities where the subject had to learn how to perform the task. As can be seen from Figures 2 through 5, the largest increase also occurred between the first and the third test participations. Why, however, a testing effect was found in the bicondylar humerus diameter remains unanswered.

These findings add additional problems to the analysis of individual growth patterns of motor abilities. Although for some abilities, a significant learning effect is to be expected, it is not known to what extent such a learning effect interferes with the growth component on an individual basis.

In conclusion, it can be stated that the developmental model proposed by Schaie (1965), and further developed and adapted by van 't Hof et al. (1977), leads to the separation of certain effects that cannot be iso-

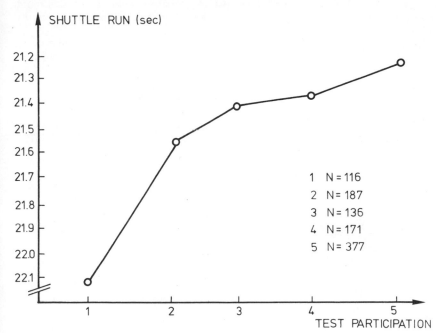

Figure 5.   Learning effects in shuttle run (running speed) for 17-year-old boys.

lated in pure longitudinal or cross-sectional designs. Furthermore, this study indicates that at least one of the components of this developmental model—namely, the testing or learning component—has a significant effect on some motor abilities.

REFERENCES

Beunen, G., M. Ostyn, J. Simons, D. Van Gerven, P. Swalus, and G. De Beul. 1978. A correlational analysis of skeletal maturity, anthropometric measures and motor fitness of boys 12 through 16. In: F. L. Landry and W. A. R. Orban (eds.), Biomechanics of Sports and Kinanthropometry. International Congress of Physical Activity Sciences, Vol. 6, pp. 343–349. Symposia Specialists, Miami.

Kemper, H. C. G., and M. A. van 't Hof. 1977. Project Growth and Health in Teenagers (in Dutch). Tijdschr. Sociale Geneeskunde 55:445–451.

Nie, N. H., C. H. Hull, J. G. Jenkins, K. Steinbrenner, D. H. Bent. 1975. SPSS. Statistical Package for the Social Sciences, 2nd Ed. McGraw-Hill Book Co., New York.

Prahl-Andersen, B., and C. J. Kowalski. 1973. A mixed longitudinal, interdisciplinary study of the growth and development of Dutch children. Growth 37:281–295.

Renson, R., G. Beunen, L. de Witte, M. Ostyn, J. Simons, and D. Van Gerven. 1980. The social spectrum of the physical fitness of 12 to 19 year old boys. In: M.

Ostyn, G. Beunen, and J. Simons (eds.), Kinanthropometry II. International Series on Sport Sciences, Vol. 9, pp. 104–118. University Park Press, Baltimore.

Schaie, K. W. 1965. A general model for the study of developmental problems. Psychol. Bull. 64:92–107.

Simons, J., G. Beunen, R. Renson, and D. Van Gerven. 1978. The Leuven boys growth study. Profile charts and growth curves. Report. Studiecentrum van de Fysieke Ontwikkeling bij Jongeren. Instituut voor Lichamelijke Opleiding. Katholieke Universiteit Leuven, Leuven, Belgium.

Tanner, J. M. 1951. Some notes on the reporting of growth data. Hum. Biol. 23: 93–159.

van 't Hof, M. A., M. J. Roede, and C. J. Kowalski. 1977. A mixed longitudinal data analysis model. Hum. Biol. 49:165–179.

A Method for Estimation of the Changes in Bipedal Locomotion

M. Kučera, M. Máček, and J. Javurck

Bipedal locomotion is a cyclic movement; each cycle involves a series of actions and intermediate positions between two identical positions in which the body rests on the same foot. Thus bipedal locomotion is a part of gross motor development, and its quality expresses the maturity of the developing organism. Movement in early childhood is characterized by quick bursts of consecutive movements. The highest level of locomotion is running, or mastery of the nonsupport phase of the step. The start of walking is currently used in pediatric practice as an important sign of the child's development. However, there are very few studies concerned with the history of the evolution of walking.

The data in the literature indicate differences in the times of starting to run, ranging from 12 months to 5 years of age in healthy children. The reason for this is the great difficulty in proving the exact start of the non-support phase of locomotion. There are different methods for the exact recording of the step and the run; for technical and psychological reasons it has been difficult to use these methods with small children. The child fears every outside intervention, and his standard level of motor development is retarded by this influence. Because of this the method used in this study, described by Groh (1972) and Bauman (1972) for use with adults, was modified for recording by the use of a hidden camera.

The purpose of this study was to determine the start of children's locomotion involving the nonsupport phase. An attempt was made to follow the evolution of motor development in early childhood and correlate it with body development and chronological age.

METHODS

A total of 188 healthy children were included in this study. All children were selected by random sampling, with 50% from the city of Prague and

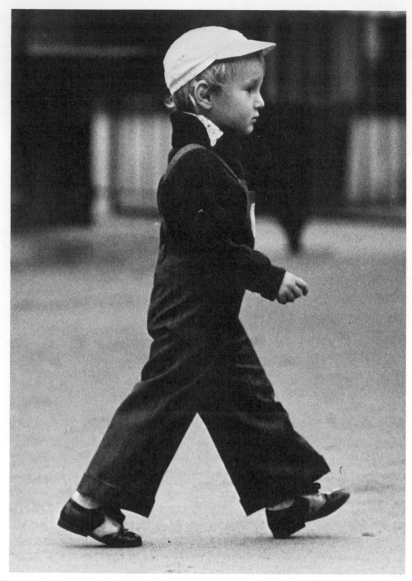

Figure 1.   Photograph of a child, 34 months old, without the nonsupport phase of loco-motion.

50% from the country. The average values for weight and height corre-sponded well with the average of the Czechoslovakian population.

Photographing the spontaneous movements of children was done with a hidden camera, 8 mm Supra Quartz (speed 36 fps), and photo-graphic apparatus Cannon QL 17 with a Leica motor (speed 20 fps). Both

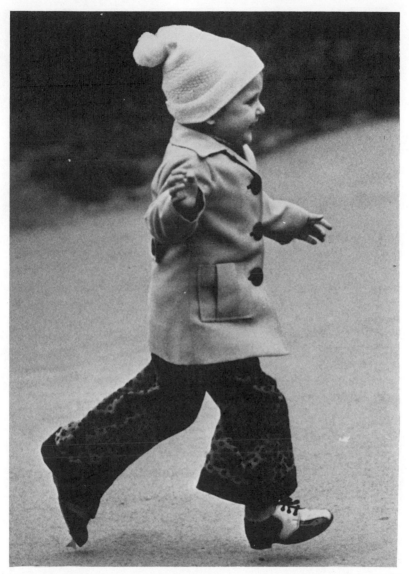

Figure 2.   Photograph of a child, 36 months of age, with the nonsupport phase of locomotion.

cameras were placed 10 m perpendicular to the line of motion; the existence of the nonsupport phase was thus determined in our sample. In
Figure 1 (taken with the Leica motor camera), of a 34-month-old child, no
nonsupport phase was found; but in Figure 2 a nonsupport phase was recorded for a girl 36 months old.

Table 1.   The characteristics of the group
at the onset of the nonsupport phase of
locomotion

	$\bar{x}$	SD
Age (months)	32.88	2.16
Body height (cm)	92.55	6.58
Body weight (kg)	13.45	1.61

RESULTS AND CONCLUSION

A type of locomotor activity—running, or the nonsupport phase of steps—was studied in a series of normal healthy children. The age of onset of the nonsupport phase varied from 2 to 5 years. Photographing of spontaneous movements was performed by the hidden camera method. The nonsupport phase of the motion pattern was used as the criterion. Most children mastered the run at the age of 32.88 months, at which age they had a body height of 92.55 cm and a body weight of 13.45 kg (Table 1).

The time of the onset running can be used as an indicator of maturity not only of the locomotion system, but also for the degree of general development of the organism. The determination of the qualitative jumps in bipedal locomotion time can be used as a method for studying the child's development. This latter is related to body weight, body height, and age. We can recommend this determination as the screening method of early diagnosis of motor development in toddlers and preschool children.

REFERENCES

Bauman, W. 1972. Methods of biomechanical research (in German). Z. Orthop. 110:831–833.
Groh, H. 1972. Biomechanics of exercise (in German). Z. Orthop. 110:823–830.
Kučera, M. 1978. Qualitative changes of bipedal locomotion in children (in German). Med. Sport 18:244–247.

Physical
Working Capacity

Measurement of Aerobic Power in Teenagers

H. C. G. Kemper and R. Verschuur

Since 1976 a multiple longitudinal study called "Growth and Health of Teenagers" has been carried out in two secondary schools in the Amsterdam area (Kemper and van't Hof, 1978). The purpose is to describe the course of physical and mental development of children during their teens. The multiple longitudinal design implies four repeated measurements (1976, 1977, 1978, and 1979) on two age groups (birth years 1963 and 1964) in one school, and four independent measurements on the same age groups in a second school. Maximal oxygen uptake is measured in order to evaluate the health status of these growing Dutch youngsters, with respect to their endurance fitness, and to compare it with similar data from other countries.

In this article cross-sectional data on the measurement of maximal oxygen uptake of 13- and 14-year-olds in the first year of the study are reported.

SUBJECTS AND METHODS

The subjects in the first year of this longitudinal study were all the pupils of the first and second forms of two secondary schools in the Amsterdam area. There were 120 boys and 123 girls 13 years of age and 64 boys and 78 girls 14 years of age who were measured in this first year. All the testing took place during regular school hours in a mobile laboratory placed near the school. The pupils were asked not to eat for 90 minutes prior to the test.

This study is part of a research project "Growth and Health of Teenagers," supported by grants from the Praeventiefonds (Prevention Fund) and S.V.O. (Foundation for Educational Research) in The Hague (Project Number 0255).

The anthropometric variables measured (Table 1) included: standing height; body weight; lean body mass, calculated from skinfold thicknesses at four sites (biceps, triceps subscapular, and suprailiac); and weight, according to Durnin and Rahaman (1967). Leg volume was determined according to the method of Jones and Pearson (1970), using circumferences of the left leg at seven heights, and multiplied by two to include the right leg. Leg volume was corrected for fat content (LV lean) using four skinfold thicknesses, two at the calf and two at the thigh (Jones and Pearson, 1970).

Prior to the exercise tests, heart rate and systolic and diastolic blood pressures were measured with the subject sitting on a chair. No attempt was made to obtain basal conditions. Maximal oxygen uptake of each subject was determined during running on a treadmill (Quinton model 18-54) after the method of Bar-Or and Zwiren (1975). The procedure was the following (Figure 1):

1. A submaximal test, consisting of three 2-min runs at a constant speed ($8 \text{ km} \cdot \text{h}^{-1}$) with increasing slope (0%, 2.5%, and 5%) to allow the pupils to get used to the treadmill and the mouthpiece and to warm up.
2. A maximal test in which the slope was increased every 2 min by 2.5% or 5%, depending on the heart rate of the subject. The test was continued until complete exhaustion was reached. Each boy or girl was urged, with verbal encouragement, to exercise to his or her maximum.

In general, the criterion for the attainment of $\dot{V}_{O_2 \text{ max}}$ was that the $\dot{V}_{O_2}$ showed no further rise with increased work load ($< 10\%$). The secondary criteria, added to evaluate the quality of the test values, were based on heart rate ($> 95\%$ of maximum), respiratory gas exchange ratio (> 1.0), and minute volume ventilation (liters, BTPS) per kg of body weight (> 1.6) (Åstrand, 1952).

Oxygen uptake was analyzed throughout the test by the open circuit technique. Expired air was collected in a 10-liter high speed, low resistance, dry gasometer (Parkinson Cowan CD4) via a two-way low resistance breathing valve with a dead air space of 35 ml. Samples of mixed expired air were continuously withdrawn from the gasometer, dried by tampons (Amira-extra), and analyzed for F_EO_2 by a paramagnetic oxygen analyzer (Servomex) and F_ECO_2 by an infrared carbon dioxide analyzer (Mijnhardt).

A gasometer and gas analyzers and a number of electronic calculators were built into a removable 19-inch apparatus, called an ergoanalyzer (Mijnhardt B.V.). The ergoanalyzer continuously and automatically analyzed the expired air collected and printed the calculated oxygen uptake, corrected for standard temperature and barometric pressure, on a minute-to-minute basis (Kemper et al., 1976).

Table 1. Means and standard deviations of anthropometric measurements of 13- and 14-year-old boys and girls

		Age (years)	Height (cm)		Weight (kg)		LBM (kg)		LV (l)		LV (lean) (l)	
	N		$\bar{X}$	SD	$\bar{X}$	SD	$\bar{X}$	SD	$\bar{X}$	SD	$\bar{X}$	SD
Boys	120	13	158.5	±7.3	43.1	±6.1	36.2	±4.5	9.9	±1.7	8.1	±1.3
	64	14	165.6	±7.4	48.5	±6.9	41.1	±5.4	11.1	±1.7	9.2	±1.4
Girls	123	13	160.4	±7.3	46.5	±8.4	35.1	±4.8	11.5	±2.3	8.9	±1.5
	78	14	164.9	±6.3	51.5	±8.1	38.4	±4.4	12.7	±2.4	9.7	±1.6

LBM, lean body mass; LV, leg volume; LV (lean), lean leg volume.

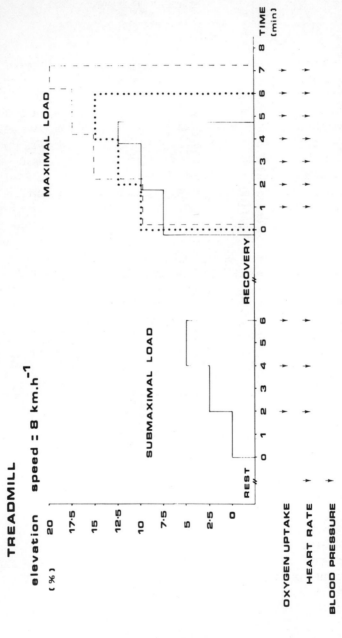

Figure 1.   Protocol of submaximal and maximal exercise test on the treadmill. The arrows indicate time of measurements of oxygen uptake, heart rate, and arterial blood pressure.

Heart rates were monitored telemetrically throughout the exercise, using chest electrodes in conjunction with an ECG pen recorder (Siemens Telecust 36).

RESULTS

The mean and standard deviation of the $\dot{V}O_{2\,max}$ values are presented in Table 2. $\dot{V}O_{2\,max}$ is given in absolute values (liters$\cdot$min^{-1}) as well as in relation to body weight, lean body mass, leg volume, and lean leg volume.

The results of the statistical testing (Student's t test) of the differences between the mean values of the two age groups and of the two sexes of the same age are summarized in Table 3. Comparison of the age groups revealed that in boys only the absolute value of the $\dot{V}O_{2\,max}$ was significantly different; it was higher in the 14- than in the 13-year-olds. In girls all mean values, except in relation to lean leg volume, were significantly different. The 14-year-old girls had a higher absolute $\dot{V}O_{2\,max}$ but lower relative values than the 13-year-olds. Comparison of the mean values of boys and girls of the same age showed significantly higher $\dot{V}O_{2\,max}$ values in boys, in absolute as well as in all the relative values.

For each criterion the percentage of pupils that achieved maximum work load is given in Table 4. The major criterion—a leveling-off in oxygen uptake—was observed in 77% of the boys and in 84% of the girls. When an absolute increase of less than 150 ml in the last 2 min of the load (Åstrand, 1952) or an increase less than 2.1 ml$\cdot$kg$^{-1}\cdot$min^{-1} (Taylor et al., 1955) were used as criteria, 44% of the pupils reach a plateau in oxygen uptake. This value is in accordance with the results of Cunningham et al. (1977) in boys of the same age.

DISCUSSION

It has been stated that $\dot{V}O_{2\,max}$ rises with age from 6 to 15 years and that, at any age, girls have a lower $\dot{V}O_{2\,max}$ than boys (Godfrey, 1974). However, the reason for measuring aerobic power is to evaluate a person's functional aerobic power; therefore, statements about absolute $\dot{V}O_{2\,max}$ values are of little importance, because they give no information about the functional aerobic power.

Aerobic power, therefore, should be expressed in relative values. In these teenagers, the 14-year-olds had higher absolute values than the 13-year-olds; but in relation to body dimensions the differences in boys disappear, and in girls the older ones have even lower values (see Tables 2 and 3). The higher absolute values of the 14-year-olds were apparently due to growth in body dimensions.

Various attempts have been made to narrow the scatter of $\dot{V}O_{2\,max}$ results with age and sex. Davies et al. (1972) investigated this relation with

Table 2. Means and standard deviations of $\dot{V}O_{2\,max}$ values for 13- and 14-year-old boys and girls[a]

	N	Age (years)	l·min⁻¹ STPD		ml·min⁻¹·kg⁻¹ b.w.		ml·min⁻¹·kg⁻¹ LBM		ml·min⁻¹·l⁻¹ LV		ml·min⁻¹·l⁻¹ LV (lean)	
			$\bar{X}$	SD	$\bar{X}$	SD	$\bar{X}$	SD	$\bar{X}$	SD	$\bar{X}$	SD
Boys	120	13	2.54	±0.32	59.3	±5.4	70.5	±5.9	260	±30	318	±32
	64	14	2.82	±0.36	58.8	±6.8	69.3	±6.9	259	±34	311	±35
Girls	123	13	2.39	±0.30	52.2	±6.5	68.5	±6.5	213	±30	271	±31
	78	14	2.54	±0.32	50.0	±5.6	66.4	±6.1	204	±27	265	±29

[a]Data are given in absolute values and per kg of body weight (b.w.), per kg of lean body mass (LBM), per liter of leg volume (LV), and per liter of lean leg volume (LV (lean)).

Table 3.   Significant differences between age groups and sex groups on Student's
t test

$\dot{V}O_{2\,max}$ (STPD)	Age 13 vs 14		Boys vs Girls	
	Boys	Girls	Age 13	Age 14
l•min^{-1}	$p < 0.01$	$p < 0.01$	$p < 0.01$	$p < 0.01$
ml•min^{-1}•kg^{-1} b.w.		$p < 0.01$	$p < 0.01$	$p < 0.05$
ml•min^{-1}•kg^{-1} LBM		$p < 0.05$	$p < 0.05$	$p < 0.01$
ml•min^{-1}•l^{-1} LV		$p < 0.05$	$p < 0.01$	$p < 0.01$
ml•min^{-1}•l^{-1} LV (lean)			$p < 0.01$	$p < 0.01$

b.w. = body weight, LBM = lean body mass, LV = leg volume, LV (lean) = lean leg volume.

three parameters of body composition: weight, lean body mass, and lean leg volume. From their results, it can be seen that weight and lean body mass reduce the variation in age range, but significant sex differences remain. However, when they related $\dot{V}O_{2\,max}$ to lean leg volume, the variation throughout the age range became much less and the difference between the sexes was no longer apparent.

In these 13- and 14-year-old populations, comparison of the sexes showed significantly higher $\dot{V}O_{2\,max}$ values in boys, both in absolute and relative values; this was also the case when $\dot{V}O_{2\,max}$ was related to lean leg volume (See Table 3). This lack of agreement may be caused by the difference in exercise tests. The $\dot{V}O_{2\,max}$ value is probably related to the muscle mass involved in the exercise test. Davies et al. (1972) tested with a bicycle ergometer, where the children exercised almost exclusively with their legs, whereas in this study children were running on a treadmill using more, and partly different, muscles than in bicycling.

From the three secondary criteria that were used to support the attainment of maximal work level, heart rate ($> 95\%$ of f_h max) and respiratory exchange ratio ($R > 1.0$) show that the percentage of pupils who met these criteria ranged from 77% to 90%. Ventilation volume per unit of body weight (> 1.6 liters•kg^{-1}), however, demonstrated the lowest percentages, especially in the girls, with 44% (see Table 4). This low percent-

Table 4.   Percentage of boys and girls who met the four $\dot{V}O_{2\,max}$ criteria[a]

$\dot{V}O_{2\,max}$ criteria	Boys (%)	Girls (%)
$\Delta \dot{V}O_2$ ($< 10\%$)	77	84
$f_{h\,max}$ ($> 95\%$)	81	79
R (> 1.0)	85	90
$\dot{V}_E$•kg^{-1} (> 1.6)	72	44

[a]$\Delta \dot{V}O_2$ = increase in oxygen uptake with increasing load, $f_{h\,max}$ = maximal heart rate, R = respiratory exchange ratio, $\dot{V}_E$•kg^{-1} = expiratory minute ventilation per kg of body weight.

Table 5. Comparison of maximal aerobic power in 13- and 14-year-old girls with values from other studies

			$\dot{V}O_{2\,max}$ $(ml\cdot kg^{-1}\cdot min^{-1})$	
Country	Reference	Load	13 years	14 years
Sweden	Åstrand (1952)	Bicycle	53[a]	52[a]
Japan	Ikai et al. (1970)	Treadmill	43	38
Norway	Hermansen (1973)	Treadmill	52	50
Č.S.S.R.	Seliger et al. (1976)	Bicycle	43[a]	42[a]
The Netherlands	Kemper et al. (1976)	Treadmill	52	50

[a]In cases of bicycle loads, mean values have been increased by 10%.

age was probably due to the higher body weight of the girls with respect to their height, compared with the boys.

In Tables 5 and 6 a comparison is made of maximal aerobic power measured as $\dot{V}O_{2\,max}$ related to body weight with our data and those of 13- and 14-year-old boys and girls from other countries. The difficulty in comparing the results with other studies are numerous, because of differences in methods. Since treadmill running provides about a 10% higher $\dot{V}O_{2\,max}$ in the same subjects than bicycling, in case of $\dot{V}O_2$ values measured on a bicycle we raised the mean values by 10% (W.H.O., 1968). In both boys and girls, our mean $\dot{V}O_{2\,max}$ values were quite high, compared with other studies. The only available data in the Netherlands were from boys in 1968 (Bink and Wafelbakker, 1968) and they were lower.

Lack of daily physical activity is supposed to be one of the causes of a bad state of health and lack of fitness in many adults in modern industrialized countries. Comparison of these $\dot{V}O_{2\,max}$ data with teenagers from the early studies of Robinson (1938) and Åstrand (1952) do suggest that, at least in Norway (Hermansen, 1973) and the Netherlands, the fall in endurance fitness is not yet clear at this age. This may be due to the fact that most of the pupils use their bicycles for transportation to and from school.

Table 6. Comparison of maximal aerobic power in 13- and 14-year-old boys with values from other studies

			$\dot{V}O_{2\,max}$ $(ml\cdot kg^{-1}\cdot min^{-1})$	
Country	Reference	Load	13 years	14 years
U.S.A.	Robinson (1938)	Treadmill	48	42
Sweden	Åstrand (1952)	Bicycle	62[a]	64[a]
The Netherlands	Bink et al. (1968)	Bicycle	56[a]	56[a]
Canada	Mirwald et al. (1969)	Treadmill	59	59
Japan	Ikai et al. (1970)	Treadmill	52	51
Norway	Hermansen (1973)	Treadmill	63	63
Č.S.S.R.	Seliger et al. (1976)	Bicycle	54[a]	54[a]
The Netherlands	Kemper et al. (1976)	Treadmill	59	59

[a]In cases of bicycle loads, mean values have been increased by 10%.

REFERENCES

Åstrand, P -O. 1952. Experimental Studies of Physical Working Capacity in Relation to Sex and Age. Munksgaard, Copenhagen.

Bar-Or, O., and L. D. Zwiren. 1975. Maximal oxygen consumption test during arm exercise—reliability and validity. J. Appl. Physiol. 38:424–426.

Bink, B., and F. Wafelbakker. 1968. Physical working capacity at maximum levels of work of boys 12–18 years of age. Internal Report N.I.P.G. (T.N.O.).

Cunningham, D. A., et al. 1977. Reliability and reproducibility of maximal oxygen uptake measurement in children. Med. Sci. Sports 9(2):104–108.

Davies, C. T. M., C. Barnes, and S. Godfrey. 1972. Body composition and maximal exercise performance in children. Hum. Biol. 44:195–214.

Durnin, J. V. G. A., and M. M. Rahaman. 1967. The assessment of the amount of fat in the human body from measurements of skinfold thickness. Br. J. Nutr. 21:681–689.

Godfrey, S. 1974. Exercise Testing in Children: Applications in Health and Disease. W. B. Saunders, London.

Hermansen, L. 1973. Oxygen transport during exercise in human subjects. Acta Physiol. Scand. Suppl. 399.

Ikai, M., and K. Kitagawa. 1970. Maximum oxygen uptake of Japanese related to sex and age. Res. J. Phys. Educ. 14:137–142.

Jones, P. R. M., and J. Pearson. 1970. Anthropometric determination of leg fat and muscle plus bone volumes in young male and female adults. J. Physiol. 204:63P–64P.

Kemper, H. C. G., R. A. Binkhorst, R. Verschuur, and A. C. A. Vissers. 1976. Reliability of the Ergo-analyzer. J. Cardiovasc. Pulmon. Technol. 4:27–30.

Kemper, H. C. G., and M. A. van't Hof. 1978. Design of a multiple longitudinal study of growth and health in teenagers. Eur. J. Pediatr. 129:147–155.

Mirwald, R. L., D. A. Bailey, and C. Weese. 1977. Problems in the assessment of maximal aerobic power in a longitudinal growth study. In: R. Bauss and K. Roth (eds.), Motor Development, Problems and Results in Longitudinal Studies (in German), pp. 65–76. Darmstadt.

Robinson, S. 1938. Experimental studies of physical fitness in relation to age. Arbeitsphysiologie 10:252–323.

Seliger, V., and Z. Bartunek (eds.). 1976. Mean Values of Various Indices of Physical Fitness in the Investigation of Czechoslovak Population Aged 12–55 Years. SČTV, Praha.

Taylor, H. L., E. Buskirk, and A. Henschel. 1955. Maximal oxygen intake as an objective measure of cardiorespiratory performances. J. Appl. Physiol. 8: 73–80.

World Health Organization. 1968. Exercise Tests in Relation to Cardiovascular Function. W.H.O. Tech. Rep. Ser. No. 388. Geneva.

Oxygen Uptake and Heart Rate with Transition from Rest to Maximal Exercise in Prepubertal Boys

M. Máček and J. Vávra

Transient oxygen uptake at the onset of exercise has been studied by several authors with different results. Margaria et al. (1965) and Di Prampero et al. (1970) have shown that the curve is exponential with the time for half value occurring at 30 sec regardless of the work load. Others, such as Whipp and Wassermann (1972) and Hagberg et al. (1978), found that the transient $\dot{V}O_2$ response may vary with the maximum oxygen uptake of the individual; in those with higher maximum oxygen uptake the time to half value is shorter, at the same submaximal work load. The intensity of the work load may also influence the time to half value; with higher loads this index may be achieved after a longer time interval.

The purpose of this study was to examine the effect of maximal load on the initial kinetics of oxygen uptake in prepubertal boys and to examine the relationship between the kinetics of this oxygen response and the initial oxygen deficit.

METHODS

There were 21 healthy boys, ages 10–11 years, who served as subjects for this study (Table 1). All the boys were volunteers who participated in extracurricular games and sports for approximately 6 hr weekly. All the tests were performed on a bicycle ergometer in a sitting position using the Douglas bag technique. The volume of expired air was measured on a Tissot spirometer and oxygen and carbon dioxide concentrations were measured using a Beckman oxygen analyzer and infrared CO_2 analyzer HB, respectively. Heart rate was determined from ECG records. The experimental arrangement consisted of the estimation of the maximal oxygen uptake on a bicycle ergometer by the conventional Douglas bag method. After 1 week, the maximal work load used in the first exami-

Table 1.   Characteristics of the group of
subjects ($N = 21$)

	$\bar{x}$	SD
Age (years)	10.5	0.6
Weight (kg)	31.3	8.4
Height (cm)	137.9	11.4
$\dot{V}_{O_2 \, max}$ (ml•min•kg^{-1})	52.8	7.8

nation was applied repeatedly without any warm-up until the point of exhaustion was reached. During this time the expired air was collected separately in Douglas bags in 30-sec intervals during the first 2 min of exercise; after that 1-min samples were gathered until the cessation of maximal exercise. The heart rate was recorded every 30 sec.

CALCULATIONS

For estimation of the oxygen deficit and the magnitude of the aerobic and anaerobic energy metabolism, the ideal oxygen demands for full coverage of energy demands by aerobic processes were calculated. For this purpose, the following formula was used:

$$\text{Ideal } \dot{V}_{O_2} = \text{resting } \dot{V}_{O_2} + W \cdot 12.7$$

where $12.7 =$ the correction factor among the physical units, caloric equivalent for oxygen, and mechanical efficiency for muscular work and $W =$ the work load in watts. The mechanical efficiency of the muscular work was assumed to be 23%. The oxygen deficit was obtained by subtracting the actual oxygen uptake, minus the resting oxygen consumption, from the ideal oxygen consumption. The changes in aerobic and anaerobic contribution to the energy demands at subsequent time intervals of 30 sec were calculated in a similar manner.

RESULTS

In the first half-minute of exercise, the percentage of oxygen uptake was $56.4 \pm 7\%$ of $\dot{V}_{O_2 \, max}$; in the second half-minute $85.4 \pm 10\%$ was reached; in the third half-minute this value was $98 \pm 10\%$; and it was $99 \pm 5\%$ in the fourth half-minute. In the third or in the fourth half-minute, the $\dot{V}_{O_2 \, max}$ was reached (Figure 1). The half time of the maximal oxygen uptake was not measured directly, but from graphic and planimetric analysis this value was lower than in adults, being less than 20 sec. Figure 2 displays the negative correlation of the oxygen deficit and the percentage of oxygen uptake in the first half-minute of exercise ($p < 0.01$). The steeper increase of the oxygen consumption in the first 30 sec of exercise results in a lower oxygen deficit.

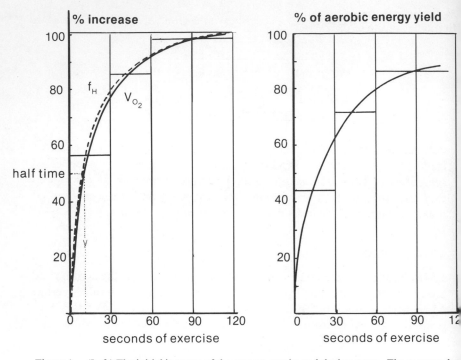

Figure 1. (Left) The initial increase of the oxygen uptake and the heart rate. The measured values of $\dot{V}O_2$ in following half-minutes are depicted by horizontal lines. The curve of oxygen uptake was obtained by graphical construction. (Right) The percentage of aerobic energy participation on the total energy demands of the work in the respective half-minutes.

During the first 30 sec the ratio of aerobic to anaerobic energy yield was 44:56, in the second half-minute the aerobic part was predominant with the ratio of 73:27, and in the second minute of exercise, the ratio increased to 86:14.

The heart rate increase was very steep from the pre-exercise value of 77 ± 9 b.p.m. to 158 ± 13 b.p.m. at the 30th second of exercise up to the maximal value of 182 ± 7 b.p.m. at the end of the second minute.

DISCUSSION

The finding that the time to 50% of maximum oxygen uptake is reached earlier in boys than in adults is partly in agreement with a recent report of Hagberg et al. (1978). These authors found a shorter time to 50% $\dot{V}O_{2\,max}$ and more rapid adaptation in a highly trained group of young adults than in untrained subjects. As reported recently by Máček et al. (1976), the adaptation of prepubertal boys to prolonged submaximal exercise is better than that of either highly trained adults or untrained subjects. Obtained values of the time for 50% response in boys were lower at the maxi-

% Vo₂ max in the
first half minute of exercise

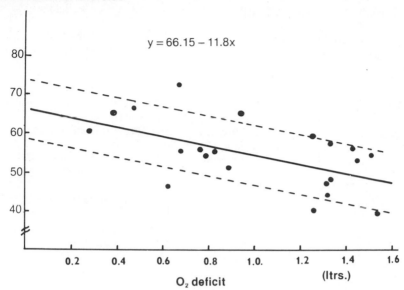

Figure 2.   The relationship between the increase of oxygen uptake in the first 30 sec and oxygen deficit during maximal exercise in boys.

mal load than those found in trained persons at submaximal and lower loads.

The hypothesis that the oxygen deficit is negatively correlated to the kinetics of the transient $\dot{V}o_2$ uptake response at the onset of exercise seems to be tenable. It is possible that the method used in this study led to these results, especially the calculation of the oxygen deficit. Work efficiency of 23% is generally accepted for submaximal exercise in the steady-state condition and it is assumed to be unchanged at maximal work load as well.

In adults, anaerobic metabolism is more important until the end of the second minute of exercise (Åstrand and Rodahl, 1970) when the ratio of aerobic to anaerobic energy yield is 50:50, but in children this ratio is already reached after 30 sec. of exercise. The earlier and faster increase of aerobic metabolism at high work intensities would help to explain the lower accumulation of lactic acid in boys. Eriksson (1972) reported that the lower values of lactic acid in children are probably caused by a rate-limiting enzyme for glycolysis. The lower amount of glycolytic enzyme, together with faster adaptation of oxygen uptake, may both contribute to the lower lactic acid value commonly found in children; or, it can be postulated that the ability for rapid mobilization of aerobic metabolism in the initial phase of exercise in children makes the high capacity of glycolysis unnecessary.

REFERENCES

Åstrand, P.-O., and K. Rodahl. 1970. Textbook of Work Physiology. McGraw-Hill Book Co., New York.

Di Prampero, P. E., C. T. M. Davies, P. Cerretelli, and R. Margaria. 1970. An analysis of O_2 debt contracted in submaximal exercise. J. Appl. Physiol. 29: 547–551.

Eriksson, B. O. 1972. Physical training, oxygen supply and muscle metabolism in 11–13 year old boys. Acta Physiol. Scand. Suppl. 384.

Hagberg, J. M., F. J. Nagee, and J. L. Carlson. 1978. Transient O_2 uptake response at the onset of exercise. J. Appl. Physiol. 44:90–92.

Máček, M., J. Vávra, and J. Novosadová. 1976. Prolonged exercise in prepubertal boys. Eur. J. Appl. Physiol. 35:291–298.

Margaria, R., F. Mangili, F. Cuttica, and P. Cerretelli. 1965. The kinetics of the oxygen consumption at the onset of muscular exercise in man. Ergonomics 8:49–54.

Whipp, B. J., and K. Wassermann. 1972. Oxygen uptake kinetics for various intensities of constant-load work. J. Appl. Physiol. 33:351–356.

Training of "Functional Muscular Strength" in Girls 7–19 Years Old

B. Nielsen, K. Nielsen, M. Behrendt Hansen, and E. Asmussen

Force can be developed using the muscles of the body in various ways; e.g., "isometric" or "dynamic" contractions. But muscle force can also be applied in more complex motor functions, such as running and jumping, where the task requires skill and coordination as well as strength. We have defined *functional muscular strength* as the maximum muscular force that can be exerted in a definite task.

The aim of the present study was to measure and compare three manifestations of leg muscle strength in relation to body weight in girls: *isometric strength* in knee extension, and *functional muscular strength* as expressed by the height of a vertical jump, or by the acceleration in a sprint. Furthermore, the effects of different training regimens on muscular strength were studied, and the possible transfer of training among the different types of training were evaluated.

METHODS

There were 381 girls, ages 7–19 years, who were studied. A total of 249 took part in the training experiments. The girls came from two suburban schools north of Copenhagen. Their anatomical data and scoring in three strength tests were recorded twice, the first time just before the fall vacation (mid-October) and the second time immediately after a 5-week training period. The control subjects were tested twice with an interval of 6 weeks between tests.

Measurements

Body height and weight of the girls dressed in their sports suits were measured to the nearest cm or half-kg.

Table 1. Girl subjects divided into height and training groups ($N = 381$)

Training	Height groups and heights (cm)						Total number
	<134	135–144	145–154	155–164	165–174	>175	
Isometrics	8	7	8	13	14	0	50
Jumpers	10	5	10	28	27	8	88
Runners	11	8	7	21	25	3	75
Controls	0	5	11	16	4	0	36
1st Test only	7	6	8	44	54	13	132
Total	36	31	44	122	124	24	381

Isometric strength of hip-knee extension was measured in a sitting position. The subject sat on the floor and placed her feet on a vertical foot plate 25 cm above the floor. A girdle with chains on both sides that were connected to the foot plate supported the back of the girl. The lengths of the chains were adjusted until the measured angle between thigh and leg was 125°. Each chain was attached to a Collin dynamometer. The girls were instructed to press maximally against the foot plate by extension of the legs. Five trials, on each of two different days, were allowed. The highest reading was taken as the maximal functional isometric strength, and is referred to in this article as F_i.

The vertical lift of the center of gravity was measured in a vertical jump ("jump and reach"). A wind-up movement by flexing the knees was allowed. The best of five trials was used in estimating the lift of the center of gravity in the vertical jump.

Acceleration in sprint running was measured by means of three adjustable photocell systems placed at hip height. Accelerations were calculated using the time recordings from the three photocell systems placed at 0, 2, and 4 meters from the starting line. The subjects made a standing start after a countdown and ran 10 m as fast as possible.

Training

The girls were divided into six groups according to height (Table 1). Each height group was divided into:

1. "Isometrics" who trained with isometric knee extensions.
2. "Jumpers" who trained using vertical jumps.
3. "Runners" who trained by sprinting.

The girls trained for 5 weeks, three times per week. All training took place during the physical education periods at school, or immediately after school hours. The training sessions were initiated with a 6–8 min general warm-up program followed by 12 min of the specific training program.

It is difficult to quantitatively compare the training programs. However, all girls performed maximally during the 12-min training sessions. In each session, the "isometrics" subjects performed 24 maximal voluntary contractions with both legs together, the "jumpers" exerted their maximal functional strength by jumping 80 times, and the "runners" took about 100 steps in 10 starts, employing maximal force with each leg.

Calculations

The height, b, of a vertical jump depends on the velocity, v, of the body achieved at the take off:

$$b = \frac{v^2}{2g} \tag{1}$$

where g is the acceleration due to gravity. To obtain this velocity the muscles must exert force on the body and transfer kinetic energy to the body mass, m. The work of the muscles is the product of the average force, f, exerted over the distance, d, through which the center of gravity is lifted, usually from a semisquatting position to a toe-standing position:

$$f \cdot d = \frac{1}{2}mv^2$$

By rearranging and inserting into Equation 1 we get:

$$b = \frac{f \cdot d}{m \cdot g} \tag{2}$$

The distance, d, over which the extensors were active was measured in the subjects and found to be one-seventh of the body height. The height of the jump, (b in Equation 2) as defined in these experiments was greater than the measured score, due to the knee bending before the jump. This extra lift of the center of gravity was estimated to be one-eighth of the body height. Thus, the functional strength in vertical jumps (F_j) can be calculated from Equation 2 as:

$$F_j = \frac{mass \cdot g \cdot (score + 1/8\ height)}{1/7\ height} \tag{3}$$

From the acceleration in the sprint, the functional strength in sprints (F_s) was calculated from the general definition of force as:

$$F_s = body\ mass \cdot measured\ acceleration \tag{4}$$

The data were treated statistically, using standard nonparametric methods.

RESULTS

Figure 1a-d presents the median values of weight (body mass), isometric strength, lift in the vertical jump, and acceleration for all subjects before the training, plotted against body height. The plots are double logarith-

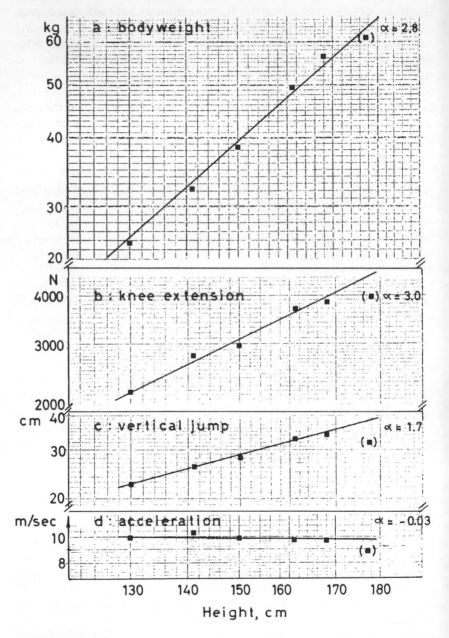

Figure 1.   Relationship between a) body weight, b) knee extension, c) vertical jump, and d) acceleration - and body height based on measurements of 381 girls. The 132 girls who did not take part in the training experiments are included. The values are medians for each height-group. The slope, α, for the best eye-fitted line is shown.

mic plots. Relationships to height, h, of the form $y = k \cdot h^\alpha$ will thus appear as straight lines in the form: $\log y = \alpha \log h + \log k'$.

The weight increases with the height as a linear function on the double log plot. The slope is 2.8; that is, the weight increases with height to the 2.8th power. The slope for isometric knee extension versus height is 3.0. The lift of the center of gravity in the vertical jump also increases with body height, $\alpha = 1.7$; i.e., as a function of $h^{1.7}$. Acceleration in the sprint, a_1 (from 0–2 m), is independent of height with $\alpha = 0.0$. The slopes calculated from all the data are shown in the graphs. (Height group 6 [> 175 cm] was not included in the calculations of the regression lines.)

The improvement in performance—within the 95% confidence limits—produced by the different types of training in the three tests are presented for all the subjects in Figure 2A. Figure 2B shows separately the training effects on the youngest and smallest (< 155 cm) of the girls. It appears that the training effect is largest in the tests for which the subjects have been specifically trained, but all types of training improved performance, except in acceleration. The same is the case with the smallest or youngest girls taken alone. The control group—for unknown reasons—performed better in acceleration (statistically significant) in the second test, but not in the knee extension and the jump tests.

Functional muscular strength (Equations 3 and 4) also increased with height. In each height group, it was also greater in an older subgroup than in a younger subgroup (Figure 3).

After training there was a parallel upward change of the curves. Generally, the results from one age group moved to the place where the next age group was before the training.

Figure 4 shows the functional strength as a percentage of isometric strength from both the first and second testings. After training, F_s and F_j constituted a smaller percentage of F_i than before training.

DISCUSSION

In this study, a dimensional analysis was applied to the results; i.e., the assumption was made that muscle strength is proportional to the transverse area of the muscles, and hence to body height squared (h^2), and that body mass and weight correspondingly are proportional to h^3. From these assumptions predictive formulas were evolved for some physical performances and for functional strength in jumping and running (see Asmussen and Heebøll-Nielsen, 1955, 1956). The predicted exponents (α, in the general formula, $y = k \cdot h^\alpha$) and the actual calculated values in this and earlier investigations are presented in Table 2.

The weight/height relationship needs no further explanation, and apparently has changed very little since 1956. On the other hand, it seems worth noting that the absolute height of the girls in relation to *age* has in-

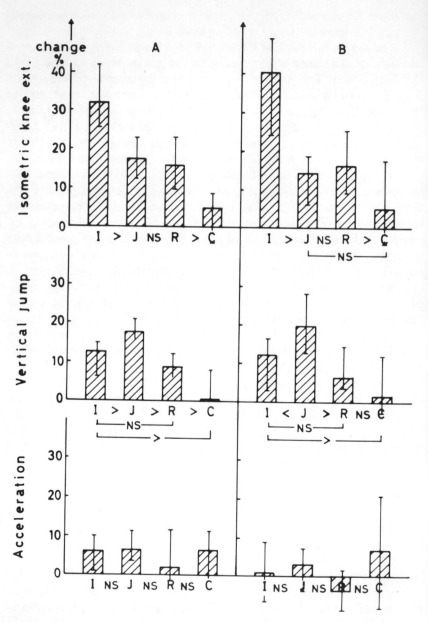

Figure 2.   Percentage change in performance in the three tests after training for the differ-ent training groups: I = isometrics, J = jumpers, R = runners, and C = controls. Median values for the groups are shown. Vertical lines are 95% confidence levels. A > B denotes a significantly greater change in A than in B; NS means a nonsignificant difference (Mann-Whitney U test, 5% significance level). Panel A includes all subjects; B includes only the smaller (< 155 cm) and younger girls.

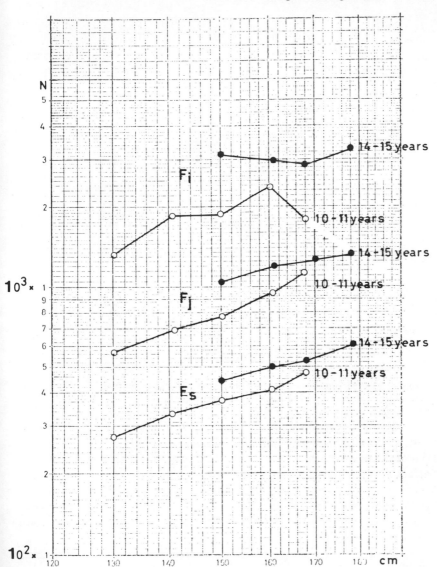

Figure 3. Isometric functional strength, F_i, and functional muscle strength in jump, F_j, and sprint, F_s, in relation to height. Two age groups, 10–11 years and 14–15 years, are shown.

creased by nearly 5 cm since 1956 [the "secular growth increase" that according to Tanner (1962) has been going on for more than a hundred years; see also Døssing (1952) and Andersen et al. (1974)]. It is apparent, however, that whereas the weight/height relationship comes quite close to the predicted values, the physical performance versus height increases at a

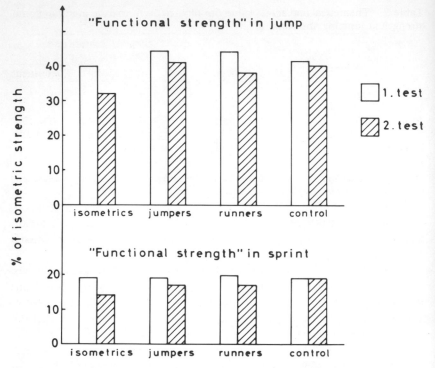

Figure 4.   Functional strength in the jump (top) and in the sprint (bottom), expressed as a percentage of isometric strength before and after training.

considerably steeper rate than expected from the dimensional analysis. This means that changes other than simple quantitative (dimensional) ones take place during growth, presumably qualitative changes due to the effect of age per se. Such changes may signify a general maturation of the central nervous system or an acquired improvement in motor skill. In both cases, one might expect them to be especially pronounced in performances demanding a high degree of motor skill, as is also indicated in Table 2.

The results of the three training programs on the performances studied in this investigation were presented in Figure 2. It can be noted that all three programs had a positive effect on isometric leg extension and on the height of a vertical jump, but there was no significant effect on acceleration in a sprint. The percentage increases in performances tended to be slightly higher if the girls below 13.5 years of age were treated separately (Figure 2B). Of greater interest is the finding that the improvement was considerably more pronounced in the test tasks that were identical with the training programs, again with the exception of the sprint training. These findings demonstrate quite clearly that strength training to a certain degree can be transferred from a training program of isometric contractions to vertical jumping and vice versa, for example. However,

Table 2. Theoretical and actual values for physical performances and functional strength in jumping and running

		Slope of relationship $\log y = \alpha \log h + k$	
	1978	1955–56	Theoretical
Height / Weight	2.80	2.88	3
Isometric F_i / Height	3.00	2.70	2
Jump / Height	1.70	1.59	0 $(1.2)^a$
Acceleration / Height	− 0.03	1.86 (boys)	− 1 $(0.2)^a$
F_j / Height	3.50	3.30 (boys)	2
F_s / Height	2.80	4.50 (boys)	2

^{a}Values in parentheses are calculated from the measured isometric strength / height and weight / height relationships in the present study.

even in these simple tests a certain skill is demanded that can only be developed if the training program is identical with the test. In other words, there is a clear specificity of muscle strength training.

Calculating the functional strength in jumping and sprinting and expressing the values as percentages of isometric strength gives the picture seen in Figure 4. It can be noted that the functional strength developed in jumping and sprint starts is only about 40% and 20%, respectively, of the maximal isometric strength. The main reason for this can probably be found in the force / velocity relationship of contracting muscles. Both in the vertical jump and in the fast stepping of a sprint start, the actual contraction times are so short (200–300 msec) that full isometric strength cannot be developed. The extra low relative value (20%) of F_s is probably due to the fact that force in running is produced by one leg at a time, whereas F_i and F_j are measured in a two-leg exertion. Figure 4 further shows that the percentage of F_i exerted as functional strength decreased as a result of the training. In the case of F_s, where no improvement in acceleration was seen (Figure 2), the reason must be that F_i has increased. The same explanation may also be given for the relative decrease in F_j, but here it can be seen that this relative decrease is much less for the group that trained in jumping.

In conclusion, it may be stated that the increase in girls' muscle strength with age is partly the result of a dimensional growth in height and weight, but it is also because of an age factor, which presumably improves neuromuscular function. Furthermore, strength training by different methods is transferable to a certain degree, but even simple tests, such as isometric strength testing, demand so much skill that a specific training effect is noticeable.

ACKNOWLEDGMENTS

We are greatly indebted to the staffs and the pupils of Holte Gymnasium and Hillerødsholm Skole, to the Medical Research Council, who financed the statistical treatment of the data, to Bjørn Andersen, M.D., who gave advice on the statistics, and to EDB programmer Jørgen Holm, who treated the data in the computer.

REFERENCES

Andersen, E., H. Andersen, B. Hutchings, M. Nyholm, B. Peitersen, J. Rosen, E. Thamdrup, and R. Wichman. 1974. Heights and weights in Danish school children in 1971–72 (in Danish). Ugeskr. Loger. 136:2796–2802.

Asmussen, E., and K. Heebøll-Nielsen. 1955. A dimensional analysis of physical performance and growth in boys. J. Appl. Physiol. 7:593–603.

Asmussen, E., and K. Heebøll-Nielsen. 1956. Physical performance and growth in children. Influence of sex, age and intelligence. J. Appl. Physiol. 8:371–380.

Døssing, J. 1952. Determination of Individual Normal Weights of School Children. Munksgaard, Copenhagen.

Tanner, M. J. 1962. Growth at Adolescence. Blackwell Scientific Publications Ltd., Oxford.

Establishment of Normal Values for Exercise Capacity in a Hospital Clinic

G. R. Cumming and A. Hnatiuk

**ESTABLISHMENT OF NORMAL VALUES FOR
EXERCISE CAPACITY IN A HOSPITAL CLINIC**

Where, when, and how should subjects be selected to establish normal values for various clinical tests? Unfortunately, tests often become clinical before the normal response is fully explored. In choosing normal subjects for exercise measurements, obvious variables to be considered include age, sex, anthropometric measurements, and past exercise habits. Token, or sometimes very careful, efforts are made to randomly select groups of subjects in order to avoid obvious biases. Another variable that needs to be standardized for clinical work in the health field is the milieu of the test itself; the physician's office, the hospital ward or clinic, or various field locations. Not only is the location important, but the method of recruiting the normal subjects and patients into the test environment should also be considered. These factors are of obvious importance in psychological testing, and performance in exercise tests has an important psychological component.

In comparing the maximal exercise capacity of children with various abnormalities to that of normal children, it has been found that the way in which the normal values were established significantly affected the results. To answer the question of how frequently children with heart defects have exercise capacities below the limits of normal children, a valid normal population was required. The primary purpose of this investigation was to compare the results of two normal groups, one selected

---

This work was supported by the Children's Hospital of Winnipeg Research Foundation.

and tested in a school setting, and the other selected and tested in a hospital clinic.

THE EXERCISE TEST

Exercise capacity was arbitrarily defined as the maximal time the subject was able to walk and/or run on a treadmill programmed to set increments in speed and grade every 3 min following the Bruce protocol. This protocol has been used in children ages 4 years and up, and, although perhaps not better than many of the other programs available, it has been found to be a suitable way of having children of all ages produce a near maximal or even exhausting physical effort in the hospital clinic setting. The treadmill speed and percentage grade must be checked frequently, and the treadmill must be level, because slight reductions in grade allow considerable increases in the walking and/or running times. The end point of the test occurs when the child stops exercising and, since this is the only measurement made to assess exercise capacity, some explanation of how the child arrives at this end point is necessary. We encourage all children to work as hard as they are able, often to the point of a few tears. The encouragement is given firmly, yet kindly. An element of competition can be established by giving above average values as goals. The technician urges "Just finish one more minute," or "Just finish this stage," or "Let me count to 20 and then you can stop," and, when the time comes to stop, "How about trying just a little longer," or, when the subject is ready to quit, "Do you really have to stop? You could be a champion if you made just another half minute." Although these urgings may be wasted on today's sophisticated teenager, they work surprisingly well on 4- to 10-year-olds. Most children are quite distressed when pushed close to an exhausting effort, and some become rather upset. However, within a minute or so of stopping most are quite happy. Many will admit that they have never worked quite so hard before, and yet 10 minutes later will claim "I wasn't really tired, it wasn't that bad." The actual stopping of the treadmill usually occurs by mutual agreement between the child and the technician, or sometimes by the child taking matters into his or her own hands and jumping off, holding onto the guard rails and refusing to let go, or clutching the technician and going limp, or purposely falling onto the belt. Occasionally a child will learn to push the emergency stop button.

OBJECTIVE END POINTS

Maximal heart rate can be used as a guide, but it is not a definitive way to assess whether a near-maximal effort was made, because maximal heart rate can vary from 180 to 234 beats/min in normal children. A digital heart rate display is very useful as a means to urge children with maximum

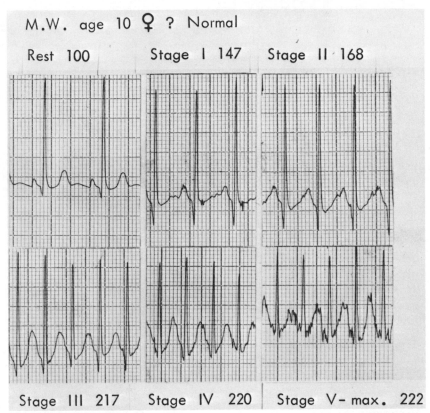

M.W. age 10 ♀ ? Normal

Rest 100   Stage I 147   Stage II 168

Stage III 217   Stage IV 220   Stage V- max. 222

Figure 1.   ECG from an exercise test in a normal girl showing capability of 6 min more exercise at higher work loads after a heart rate of over 217 was attained.

rates of less than 200 to continue exercising. One should not terminate a test at a heart rate of 180 or 200, or even 210 b.p.m. because some children can exercise at increasing loads well past any of these artificial end points, as is illustrated in Figure 1.

How the child looks at the end of the test is a very practical guide as to whether a near-maximal effort was made. The hot, sweaty, flushed child who sits exhausted in the recovery chair has obviously performed well, as have some who go beyond this and are pale with marked dyspnea, dizziness, and wobbly legs, and are literally close to exhaustion. A few will vomit, especially if they have eaten within the last 4 hours.

Another routine practice has been to draw post-exercise venous blood samples for lactate determinations. This measurement has been of limited value and probably provides no useful information beyond the experienced technician's subjective impression of whether the child has made a maximal effort or not. Figure 2 shows the lactate values of 50 consecutive tests recently performed by 6- and 7-year-olds plotted against heart rate. Some children with low heart rates had high lactates and vice

POST EXERCISE VENOUS LACTATE vs MAXIMAL
EXERCISE HEART RATE BOYS & GIRLS AGE 6&7

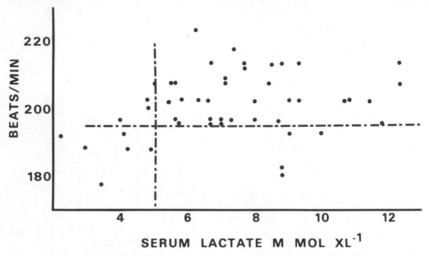

Figure 2. Serum lactate versus maximal heart rate in children with and without heart disease, ages 6 and 7 years. Four of the six subjects with both lactate < 5 mmol•liter^{-1} and heart rate < 195 b.p.m. had cyanosis.

versa. All children in this series made what was considered a maximal or near maximal effort. Four of the six subjects with both low lactates and low maximal heart rates had cyanotic heart disease and had performed a truly maximal effort. In the absence of cyanosis there was no difference between children with and without heart disease.

It is commonly stated that one should measure $\dot{V}O_2$ and look for a plateau effect in order to determine whether the person has exercised maximally or not. However, when research laboratories have reported that a plateau in $\dot{V}O_2$ occurred in less than half of all children tested on different days (Åstrand, 1962; Cumming and Friesen, 1967), and when half of those children who did show a plateau on the first test failed to show a plateau on their next test (Cunningham et al., 1977), this method for assessing whether a truly maximal effort has been made is far from satisfactory. Collection of expired air introduces another variable in that exercise time, maximal heart rate, and the effort made by some children are considerably reduced when they are forced to use a breathing apparatus.

Despite these problems of determining an exact end point, the test has been reproducible. In Figure 3, the results for two tests performed 2 to 14 days apart by 20 boys and girls are plotted. These data show a high test-retest correlation. Neither the investigator nor the subjects recalled the exact exercise times of the first tests.

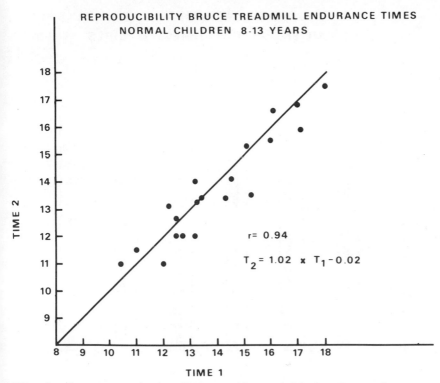

Figure 3.   Test-retest exercise times in 20 normal boys and girls, 8 to 13 years of age.

SUBJECTS

School Series

There were 209 boys and 179 girls, ages 6–13 years, who were recruited and tested in two urban schools. Parental permission was required; about 90% of the students returned the permission forms and one out of every two of those students returning the forms was tested.

Clinic Series

The results from this series have been published (Cumming et al., 1978). Subjects were obtained by testing patients seen in a hospital cardiac clinic over a period of 3 to 4 years. The patients were referred to the clinic because of suspected heart disease (usually because of a heart murmur), and after complete evaluation they received a diagnosis of a normal heart with a functional murmur.

RESULTS

Subjects were arbitrarily divided into age groups (6 to 7, 8 to 9, 10 to 12, 13 to 15, and 16 to 18 years) in order to provide a reasonable number for

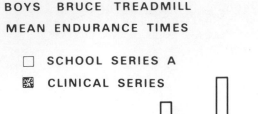

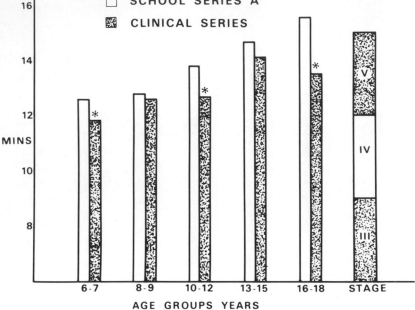

Figure 4.   Mean exercise times of boys in school series and clinic normals (* indicates statistical significance, $p < 0.05$).

each group (Table 1). Subjects ages 4 to 5 years were tested in the clinic series but not in the schools, and are not discussed in this article.

The mean exercise times for the school and clinic series are compared in Figures 4 and 5. Except for the 10- to 12-year-old girls, the mean exercise times were greater in the school series, with the difference reaching statistical significance for four of the ten age groups. The differences ranged from 1% to 16%, with a mean of 7%.

Subjects with exercise times below the 10th percentile value from the clinic series were arbitrarily considered to have a low fitness level. A comparison of these 10th percentile values in the two populations is made in Figures 6 and 7. For the boys, the school 10th percentile exercise times were 11% to 22% greater (mean 17%) than the boys in the clinic series. For the girls the 10th percentile values were 1% to 21% greater for the school series (mean 12%). With only 24 to 55 subjects in each group, only three to five subjects were below the 10th percentile; thus, the differences were possibly due to chance alone. Although it would be possible to recruit considerably more subjects in the school series, this would be logistically difficult to do in the clinic series. The consistency of the difference of

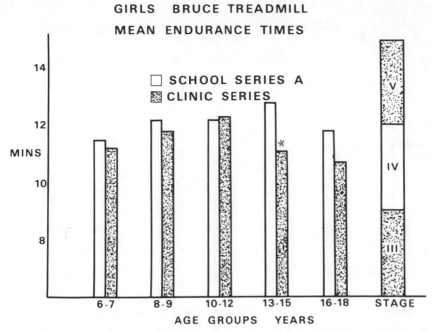

Figure 5.   Mean exercise times of girls in school series and clinic normals (* indicates statistical significance, $p < 0.05$).

the ten age and sex groups suggests that the differences are real and due to factors other than chance.

MAXIMAL HEART RATES IN
SCHOOL AND CLINIC NORMAL SUBJECTS

The maximal heart rates of the two series are compared in Table 1. The table shows that the children tested in the schools had maximal heart rates that were on the average 5 b.p.m. greater than those tested in the clinic. This difference was present in each age group and, although the difference reached statistical significance for only two groups, the direction was clear. The differences in maximal heart rate may reflect differences in motivation to work to near exhaustion. The rates were obtained using the same electrocardiograph recorder so that technical error in the measurement was unlikely. Room temperature was 2° to 3°C higher for the school tests, but this difference should not have influenced body temperature in a short test sufficiently to alter maximal heart rate.

BODY BUILD AND EXERCISE TIME

Body fat was estimated from skinfold data (Durnin and Rahaman, 1967) for the school series and lean body mass was calculated from these values.

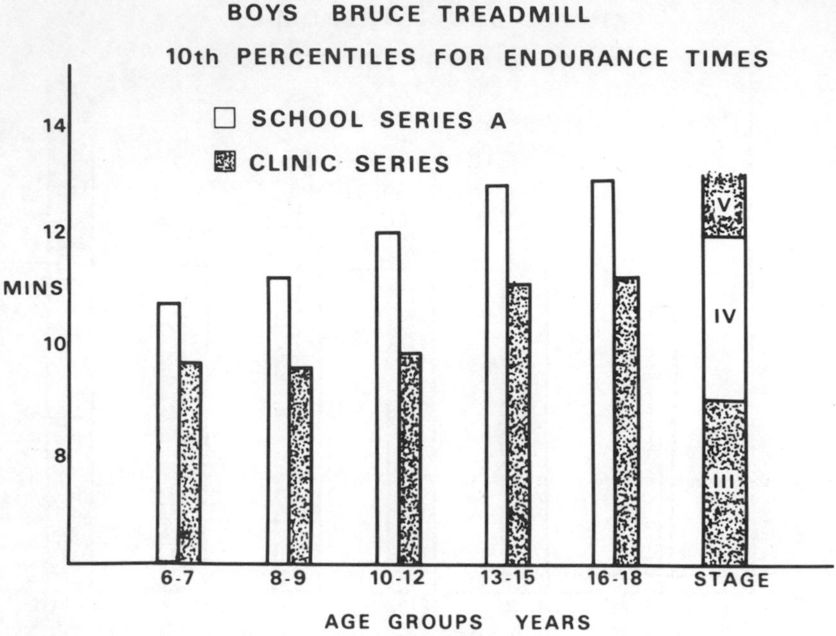

Figure 6. 10th percentile values of boys in school series A and clinic normals.

An estimate of body heaviness was obtained by calculating weight divided by height³ for both the school and the clinic series. Table 2 gives the correlation coefficients found from the linear regression of exercise time against these variables. For all age and sex groups, body fat was an important determinant of exercise time, with negative correlation coefficients ranging from -0.30 to -0.72 (mean $r = -0.54$). Significant negative correlations were also observed between exercise time and weight/height³ for all age and sex groups in school series A (mean r was -0.41). Exercise times also showed significant negative correlations with calculated lean body mass in five of the ten groups (mean correlation coefficient for these five groups was -0.29). For the clinic series, skinfolds were not measured so that correlations were obtained only for weight:height³. The mean cor-

Table 1. Maximal heart rates—school and clinic normals

Age groups	Boys				Girls			
	b.p.m.		N		b.p.m.		N	
	School	Clinic	School	Clinic	School	Clinic	School	Clinic
6–7	210 ± 8	201 ± 7	28	28	208 ± 6	202 ± 4	28	34
8–9	205 ± 9	200 ± 6	34	30	208 ± 7	206 ± 9	28	26
10–12	206 ± 8	199 ± 7	45	31	207 ± 6	204 ± 8	43	28
13–15	202 ± 7	198 ± 6	55	26	204 ± 7	196 ± 6	39	24
16–18	203 ± 9	201 ± 6	47	12	200 ± 9	193 ± 5	41	12

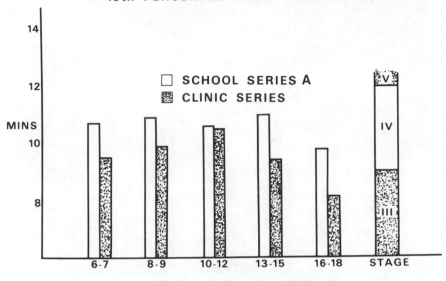

Figure 7.   10th percentile values of girls in school series A and clinic normals.

relation coefficient was −0.36, with significant negative correlation for 11 of the 12 age and sex groups. The importance of body build to exercise time for treadmill running is more dramatically illustrated by Figure 8. The older, heavily built, muscular, athletic boy had an exercise time 1.5 min less than the slim young girl beside him who engaged in no sports activities.

PHYSICAL ACTIVITY AND EXERCISE TIME

In the school subjects, physical activity was graded on a 1 to 4 scale: grade 1 indicated minimal activity other than the compulsory physical education

Table 2.   Correlation coefficients—exercise time and body fat and weight/height^3

| | School boys correlation coefficients | | School girls correlation coefficients | | Clinic-Wt/Ht^3 correlation coefficients | |
Age group	% Fat	Wt/Ht^3	% Fat	Wt/Ht^3	Boys	Girls
6–7	−0.53	−0.25	−0.67	−0.72	−0.28	−0.34
8–9	−0.60	−0.23	−0.47	−0.29	−0.05	−0.42
10–12	−0.65	−0.60	−0.67	−0.62	−0.26	−0.47
13–15	−0.45	−0.28	−0.33	−0.42	−0.43	−0.35
16–18	−0.69	−0.39	−0.30	−0.26	−0.39	−0.45

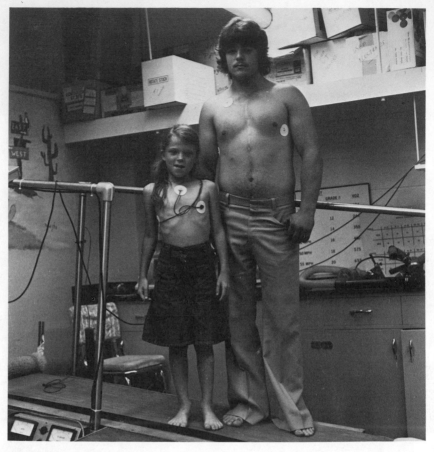

Figure 8.   Importance of the effect of body build on exercise time. An 8-year-old nonathletic girl lasted 1.5 min longer than an athletic 16-year-old boy. The girl had a ventricular septal defect, and the boy had had surgery for valvular pulmonary stenosis at age 3, but at the
time of testing had normal right ventricular pressure. The boy was actively participating in
football, weight training, and judo.

program; grade 2 indicated walking to school over 2 km, with some recreational physical activity in addition to the physical education program;
grade 3 indicated participation in competitive sports at the school level, or
a moderate personal fitness program; and grade 4 indicated frequent participation in sports, both within and outside of school, with an active running program in the sport involved, or intensive sports training, or personal fitness programs. Exercise times showed significant correlations
with this simple grading system (Table 3). The correlation was higher for
13- to 18-year-olds than for the 8- to 12-year-olds. Up to 25% of the interindividual variations in exercise times in the older group could be explained by the assigned activity rating.

PRACTICAL IMPORTANCE OF THE
DIFFERENCES BETWEEN CLINIC AND SCHOOL

Norms

Exercise times from 830 consecutive exercise tests on cardiac patients were compared to those of both the school normals and the clinic normals, and subjects with exercise time values below the 10th percentile were categorized as having a low fitness level. When the normal values in the school series were used, 49% of the tests in the cardiac children indicated a low fitness level, whereas when the clinic series of normals was used only 21% of the tests in the cardiac patients were classified as having a low fitness level. This was because the clinic normal series gave 10th percentile exercise times about 15% below the school normals. The conclusion could be that only one out of five cardiac patients has a low fitness level, or that 50% of the cardiac patients have low fitness levels, depending on which "normal" values are used. Therefore, the differences in the two normal series have definite clinical implications.

POSSIBLE REASONS FOR THE
DIFFERENCE BETWEEN CLINIC AND SCHOOL NORMALS

Possible reasons for the longer exercise times in the school series as compared to the clinic normals included a built-in bias in the selection of the subjects, a higher motivational level in the school series tests, the establishment of goals for the school test, differences in the test supervisors, and physical differences in the test procedures, such as gym clothes versus street clothes or higher room temperatures for the school tests.

It is possible that some children with low fitness levels were not tested in the school situation because the requirement for parental consent allowed some children less interested in physical activity to avoid the testing.

It is possible that the clinic group of normals included a concentration of children with low fitness levels because some of these children were taken to their physician because of inadequate performances. These refer-

Table 3. Correlation of exercise time with activity rating of schoolchildren

Age group	Correlation coefficients activity grade	
	Boys	Girls
8–12	0.28^a	0.30^a
13–18	0.50^b	0.52^b

$^a p < 0.05.$
$^b p < 0.01.$

rals led to the discovery of a heart murmur, so that cardiac disease became a possible cause for fatigue or other symptoms. It has been our experience, however, that when a parent complains that their child tires easily and has what they consider below average stamina, the child more often than not has an exercise time above the 50th percentile rather than below this point. It was possible that the clinic series may have included more heavy or obese children, and that this explained the difference in exercise times. However, the mean weight:height^3 ratio was 4% lower in the clinic normals as compared to the school series; thus, longer exercise times would have been expected for the clinic groups. At present, we think that the main difference between the two groups is the difference in attitudes of the children performing the test in a clinical setting and those performing it in the school. The child who was brought to the hospital clinic by a parent often was reluctant to come, frequently had not been warned that an exercise test would be part of the investigation, and probably had every reason to have a negative attitude toward the whole affair. For many children the treadmill was a new experience; they took this as a challenge, and most appeared to want to do well, but some did not. However, in the school, the children accepted the exercise test as a special challenge, they volunteered to do the test, they wanted to show their friends and school authorities that they were fit, and they did not wish to let the school down. The motivational climate was clearly very different, and this may have been the reason for the higher maximal heart rates in the school series.

SCHOOL SUBJECTS BROUGHT TO THE HOSPITAL LABORATORY

Because higher values were obtained in the school tests, a second series of tests with school children was arranged by having 60 children brought from the school to the hospital laboratory for testing. The mean results for these children were slightly higher than for the school series tested in the schools (with a significant difference in only one of six age groups). The exercise times of this second school series were higher than those in the clinic series of normals, with the difference being significant in four of the six groups. This second school series was probably a "super" select group of school children because only the more adventuresome (and perhaps more fit) children volunteered to leave the normal surroundings of the school and brave the uncertainties of a medical clinic. This was not considered a suitable normal population either.

One way to solve this dilemma would be to randomly select a suitable school series from the school records, and, without the children's knowledge, arrange a clinic visit with the parents for the exercise test; this way the impact of the test on the child would be similar to that of the patients making an actual clinic visit. This experiment would be difficult to arrange and has not been done.

WHICH NORMAL SUBJECTS TO USE
FOR EVALUATING CLINIC PATIENTS

The use of the clinic normals' data is preferred because these data were collected by the same technicians, under the same motivational conditions, over the same time period, and in the same physical environment; the tests were also given in a random order to the patients.

Further support for use of the clinic normals comes from a comparison of the exercise times of patients with no heart disease, or insignificant heart disease. Patients with previous acute rheumatic fever but no cardiac involvement had a normal distribution of exercise times as compared to the clinic normals. Patients with very small ventricular septal defects unlikely to cause any impairment had a normal distribution of exercise times when compared to the clinic normals. Up to 30% of the subjects in these groups had exercise times below the 10th percentile when compared to the school normals, thus providing further evidence that the school normals are too high for clinic use.

REFERENCES

Åstrand, P.-O. 1952. Experimental Studies of Physical Working Capacity in Relation to Sex and Age. Ejnar Munksgaard, Copenhagen.

Åstrand, P.-O., and I. Ryhming. 1954. A nomogram for calculation of aerobic capacity (physical fitness) from pulse rate during submaximal work. J. Appl. Physiol. 7:218–221.

Borg, G., and H. Linderholm. 1967. Perceived exertion and pulse rate during graded exercise in various age groups. Acta Med. Scand. 472:194–206.

Bruce, R. A., F. Kusumi, and D. Hosmer. 1973. Maximal oxygen intake and nomographic assessment of functional aerobic impairment in cardiovascular disease. Am. Heart J. 85:546.

Cumming, G. R., D. Everatt, and L. Hastman. 1978. Bruce treadmill test in children: Normal values in a clinic population. Am. J. Cardiol. 41:69–75.

Cumming, G. R., and W. Friesen. 1967. Bicycle ergometer measurement of maximal oxygen uptake in children. Can. J. Physiol. Pharmacol. 45:937–946.

Cumming, G. R., D. Goulding, and G. Baggley. 1969. Failure of school physical education to improve cardiorespiratory fitness. Can. Med. Assoc. J. 101:69–73.

Cunningham, D., B. M. V. Waterschoot, D. H. Paterson, M. Lefcoe, and S. P. Sangal. 1977. Reliability and reproducibility of maximal oxygen uptake measurement in children. Med. Sci. Sport 9:104–108.

Durnin, J. V. G. A., and M. M. Rahaman. 1967. The assessment of the amount of fat in the human body from measurements of skinfold thickness. Br. J. Nutr. 21:681–689.

Determination of the Aerobic and Anaerobic Thresholds of 10–11-Year-Old Boys Using Blood-Gas Analysis

G. Gaisl and J. Buchberger

In today's high-performance sports there is a trend to begin endurance training at the earliest possible age. However, sport physiological examinations point out that up to the age of 10 years it is not usually possible to train the cardiopulmonary system, and thus there is little likelihood of achieving early first-class endurance (Bar-Or and Zwiren, 1972; Wasmund and Mocellin, 1972). Not until a child is older does his growing body reach the stage where it benefits maximally from endurance training, and even then such training is too much for some children. The reason for this lies in the fact that training does not take into consideration the physiological variations in different individuals. Thus, it is justifiable to give sports instructors some physiological criteria to facilitate the maximum benefit being drawn from endurance training.

The Department of Exercise Physiology and Biometry at the University of Graz has for years been supervising a special sports secondary modern school and judging the state of training of its pupils on the basis of stress acidosis (Gaisl, 1977, 1978). In addition to this, its activity has now been expanded to include the actual control of the training.

METHODS

Subjects

Altogether, 45 pupils of the first special sports class took part in the examination, and their physical characteristics are presented in Table 1. At the time of the examination, these pupils were just finishing their third month of 8 hr of training per week.

Table 1.   The physical characteristics of subjects ($N = 45$)

	Age (years)	Height (cm)	Weight (kg)
$\bar{x}$	10.8	146.2	34.9
SD	0.4	6.0	5.2
Range	1.7	24.5	25.1

Ergometric Stress

The children were subjected to progressive stress on a mechanically braked bicycle ergometer. The number and degree of individual stages of stress, each lasting 3 min, were chosen by considering body weight, heart rate behavior, and stress acidosis. As a result, it was possible to ascertain with reasonable accuracy the aerobic-anaerobic transition and also the maximum oxygen intake.

Recording the Heart Rate

Before the test and during the last 30 sec of each stage of stress, an electrocardiogram was recorded. On the basis of the recognized relationship between heart rate and ergometric achievement, it was possible to graphically ascertain physical working capacity (PWC), according to Wahlund's method (1948), equivalent to a heart rate of 170 b.p.m.

Air Intake and Expired Air Analysis

In the last 60 sec (lower stress) and 30 sec (greater stress), respectively, of each stage of stress the expired air was collected in Douglas bags by means of a mouthpiece-valve-tube system with a very small dead space. Following this, the oxygen concentration in the air collected was determined with a polarographic Beckmann OM-11 analyzer. At the same time the volume of the air expired per time unit was measured with Elster's experimental gasometer. The drawback of ignoring carbon dioxide was largely compensated by arithmetic correction (Croonen and Binkhorst, 1974). For determining spiroergometric values, the air volumes measured under ATPS conditions were converted to BTPS conditions, and the oxygen volumes to STPD conditions.

Blood Collection and Blood-Gas Analysis

Before the test and immediately after each stage of stress, as well as 3, 6, and 10 min after the test was ended, blood was collected from the hyperemized earlobe for blood-gas analysis. With the blood-gas analyzer, Gas Check AVL, the partial pressure of carbon dioxide and pH were determined. In addition, the base excess values were ascertained on the nomogram according to the method of Thews and Harnoncourt (1972). The aerobic and anaerobic thresholds were determined in accordance with more recent works by Keul et al. (1978) and Kindermann et al. (1978).

Table 2.   Maximal oxygen intake and physical working capacity (PWC_{170})
($N = 45$)

	Maximum oxygen intake		PWC_{170}	
	(l/min)	(ml/min•kg)	(kpm/min)	(kpm/kg•min)
$\bar{x}$	1.84	53.4	496	14.3
SD	0.24	5.3	104	2.5
Range	1.22	22.1	521	12.2

RESULTS

Directly measured maximum oxygen intake, as a criterion of aerobic capacity, is given in Table 2, in addition to oxygen intake related to body weight (ml/min•kg). In the same table PWC_{170} is shown as an indirect criterion of circulation work capacity, together with PWC_{170}/kg.

Table 3 contains the achievement of the group on the bicycle ergometer in kpm/min, heart rate, and the percentage of the maximum oxygen intake on passing the aerobic and anaerobic threshold, equivalent to the increase in acid valency in the capillary blood of 2.5 mmol/liter and 4.5 mmol/liter, respectively. The aerobic-anaerobic transition extends over the range between the corresponding pairs of values.

DISCUSSION

Maximum Oxygen Intake

The mean value of 53.4 ml/kg is between the values of 41.5 ml/kg for 11-year-old boys who were poor at sports and 56.0 ml/kg for boys of the same age who were good at sports, as reported by Roth et al. (1971); and it is higher than the 49.3 ml/kg quoted by Lange-Andersen et al. (1974) for 10-year-old boys from an average cross section of the Norwegian population. It is also higher than the results of Davis et al. (1972), who found a maximum oxygen intake of 47 ml/kg in 11-year-old boys.

Physical Working Capacity (PWC_{170})

The mean value of 496 kpm/min is higher than the results reported with Canadian boys of the same age (Howell and Macnab, 1968), lower than with Finnish boys (Elo et al., 1965), and about the same as the findings of Mocellin et al. (1971) with children in West Germany.

So far little is known of the determination and interpretation of the *aerobic and anaerobic threshold* of children. Only Keul and his associates make mention of a mean heart rate of 190 at the anaerobic threshold (4 mmol/liter lactate) in children of 10 to 14 years of age (Kindermann et al., 1978). In principle, with an improvement in general endurance, the only ways to make more anaerobic energy available are by higher relative con-

Table 3.   Descriptive measures associated with aerobic and anaerobic threshold ($N=45$)

	Aerobic threshold			Anaerobic threshold		
	Work rate (kpm/min)	Heart rate (b.p.m.)	Percentage of max O_2 intake	Work rate (kpm/min)	Heart rate (b.p.m.)	Percentage of max O_2 intake
$\bar{x}$	455	161.4	64.7	614	185.5	84.2
SD	97	16.0	11.8	86	9.5	8.0
Range	375	75.0	55.3	390	51.0	33.6

sumption of the maximum oxygen intake and by increasing the heart rate. In this context, especially in children, hyperactivity of the circulatory system and the upward shift of heart rate reserve (adult athletes: 50 to 190 b.p.m.; children: 70 to 120 b.p.m.) could give the appearance of an individual who is highly trained in the field of endurance. To avoid misinterpretations, the state of training itself should be judged by other criteria.

In determining optimal training heart rate according to the aerobic or anaerobic threshold, the relative conflicting influences of "vagotomy" due to training on the one hand, and the metabolic adaptation to expanding the aerobic energy available by raising the level of circulatory stress on the other, seem to play little or no part in the resulting heart rate.

CONCLUSIONS

Determining heart rate at the so-called aerobic or anaerobic threshold (here at $\delta BE = 2.5$ or 4.5 mmol/liter) seems, with regard to empirical as well as theoretical facts, to produce useful pointers for endurance training in the case of children. Furthermore, guidance in the intensity of endurance training according to heart rate has yet another advantage, namely, that with increasing work capacity there is necessarily a leveling-off of the rise in pulse frequency in relation to the maximal oxygen intake and to achievement. With training in the same range of heart rate, the result is an automatic rise in stress intensity to match the increased work capacity.

With the pupils who took part in these tests, the results suggested a training heart rate of 175 to 195 b.p.m. for intensive endurance training, according to the individual anaerobic threshold. For longer and consequently less intensive endurance training, a training heart rate of 145 to 180 b.p.m. is recommended, depending on the aerobic threshold. The mean value is 161 b.p.m. When training, the pulse rate can only be measured after stress or during a short interruption in stress, and the sharp drop in heart rate immediately following interrupted stress must be taken into account. In adults, this drop represents 5 to 10 b.p.m. after 15 sec in the range of the anaerobic threshold, and 10 to 20 b.p.m. in the range of the aerobic threshold (Kindermann et al., 1978). The trainers of the children involved in these tests, taking into consideration the individual variability in drop in heart rates after stress, were advised to assume that the values of a training heart rate were lower by about 15 to 30 b.p.m. as a guideline.

REFERENCES

Bar-Or, O., and L. D. Zwiren. 1972. Physiological effects of increased frequency of physical education classes and of endurance conditioning on 9 to 10 year old girls and boys. Proceedings of the 4th International Symposium on Pediatric Work Physiology, pp. 183–198. Wingate Institute, Israel.

Croonen, F., and P. A. Binkhorst. 1974. Oxygen uptake calculated from expiratory volume and oxygen analysis only. Ergonomics 17:113–117.

Davis, C. T. M., C. Barnes, and S. Godfrey. 1972. Body composition and maximal exercise performance in children. Hum. Biol. 44:195–214.

Elo, O., L. Kirvonen, T. Peltonen, and J. Välimäki. 1965. Physical working capacity of normal and diabetic children. Ann. Paediatr. Fenn. 11:25–31.

Gaisl, G. 1977. The differences in the behavior of work acidosis in the laboratory and on the field in athletes of various disciplines (in German). Leibesübungen, Leibeserziehung 31:81–88.

Gaisl, G. 1978. The significance of the behavior of stress acidosis for the objectivization and supervision of the state of training and for the controlling of training procedures. Inaugural dissertation (in German). University of Graz, Graz, Austria.

Howell, M. L., and R. B. J. Macnab. 1968. The Physical Working Capacity of Canadian Children Aged 7 to 17. CAHPER, Toronto.

Keul, J., W. Kindermann, and G. Simon. 1978. The aerobic and anaerobic capacity as a basis for diagnosing achievement (in German). Leistungssport 8:22–32.

Kindermann, W., G. Simon, and J. Keul. 1978. Endurance training—determination of optimal training-heart-frequency and work capacity (in German). Leistungssport 8:34–39.

Lange-Andersen, K., V. Seliger, and J. Rutenfranz. 1974. Physical performance capacity of children in Norway. Part I. Population parameters in a rural inland community with regard to maximal aerobic power. Eur. J. Appl. Physiol. 1: 177–195.

Mocellin, R., J. Rutenfranz, and R. Singer. 1971. On the question of norm values of physical work capacity in childhood and youth (in German). Z. Kinderheilkd. 110:140–165.

Roth, W., H. Götze, and D. Urban. 1971. Results of spirometric examinations on pupils with a poor performance in sports instruction (in German). Med. Sport 11:229–232.

Thews, G., and K. Harnoncourt. 1972. An acid-base nomogram for clinical routine diagnosis (in German). Wien. Med. Wochenschr. 122:663–665.

Wahlund, H. 1948. Determination of physical working capacity. Acta Med. Scand. 132:1–78.

Wasmund, U., and R. Mocellin. 1972. Running in the second and third year at school. An investigation of training potential (in German). Sportwissenschaft 2: 258–272.

Aerobic Power, Lung Dimensions, Ventilatory Capacity, and Muscle Blood Flow in 12–16-Year-Old Boys with High Physical Activity

G. Koch

Information about the effect of intensive physical training on different circulatory and respiratory parameters during the years of rapid growth is scanty. Extensive studies dealing with the effect of physical training are limited to training periods of short duration (Von Döbeln and Eriksson, 1972; Eriksson and Koch, 1973; Koch and Eriksson, 1973a, 1973b). Most studies involving longer training periods (22 months—Daniels and Oldridge, 1971; and 32 months—Ekblom, 1969) were limited to the training effects on maximal oxygen uptake.

This investigation concerns a group of boys who were selected for a longitudinal study because of their high motivation for sports and exercise and the high intensity of physical activity they actually displayed. Because of lack of complete information, this study was initially focused on muscle blood flow (MBF), but, in addition to MBF, other cardiorespiratory parameters, both during submaximal and maximal exercise, and different lung dimensions and spirometric parameters were determined.

SUBJECTS

There were nine boys who participated (with parental consent) in this longitudinal study. At the initial study in 1973, these boys were 11.9 ± 0.2 years old (range 11.8–12.3). They were restudied exactly 1 (1974), 2 (1975), 3 (1976) and 4 (1977) years later. In 1975, however, two of the boys refused to participate in the annual examination; the total number after that was only seven. Some relevant anthropometric data are given in Table 1.

This study was supported by a grant from the Swedish First of May Flower Annual Campaign for Children's Health and from the Bundesinstitut für Sportwissenschaft (German Federal Republic Institute of Sport Science).

Table 1. Anthropometric data, blood volume, and total amount of hemoglobin (THb) at different ages (means and standard deviations)

		12 Years	13 Years	14 Years	15 Years	16 Years
Height (cm)	$\bar{x}$	150.0	156.2	164.1	174.0	179.8
	SD	4.3	5.0	5.5	4.5	4.5
Weight (kg)	$\bar{x}$	39.2	43.2	50.8	59.2	66.0
	SD	4.0	4.1	7.9	7.8	7.6
Blood Vol (l)	$\bar{x}$			5.1	5.8	5.9
	SD			0.8	0.9	0.9
THb (g)	$\bar{x}$			617.0	708.0	705.0
	SD			121.0	117.0	116.0

Prior to the initial study in 1973, all the boys were highly motivated by a strong interest in physical exercise and sports. They participated regularly in different sport activities such as soccer, running, badminton, and ice hockey, and could be considered well trained judging from their maximal oxygen uptake (mean = 59.5 ml/kg body wt). After the initial study, they were encouraged to continue at the same level or, preferably, even to increase their physical training. Training was supervised and coordinated by an experienced physical education instructor from the school with whom the boys were familiar. The boys were asked to specify and record their physical exercise every day. An evaluation of the average intensity of physical training performed during 40-week periods in the years 1973–1974, 1974–1975, and 1975–1976 is given in Table 2.

METHODS

On all occasions (April 1973, April 1974, April 1975, April 1976, and April 1977), the boys were studied with identical techniques and under

Table 2. Evaluation of intensity of physical training during 40-week periods (holidays excluded) in 1973–1974, 1974–1975, and 1975–1976

		1973–1974	1974–1975	1975–1976
Total number days/week[a] with physical exercise	$\bar{x}$(SD)	4.6 (0.6)	4.6 (0.5)	3.7 (1.0)
	Range	3.8–5.3	3.8–5.3	1.6–4.9
Number days/week[a] with running exercise (average 3.5 km per session, interval training)	$\bar{x}$(SD)	1.7 (1.2)	1.6 (1.7)	1.5 (1.3)
	Range	0.4–4.5	0.2–5.3	0.1–3.9
Number days/year reported sick at school	$\bar{x}$(SD)	16.1 (17.1)	17.5 (10.7)	26.5 (29.1)
	Range	0–50	6–42	2–80
In addition: 3 hr/week school gymnastics (mainly ball games)				

[a]Calculated according to the boys' own records.

identical conditions; the sequence of the different examination routines was exactly the same. The methods used are only briefly described here. Details have been reported elsewhere (Eriksson and Koch, 1973; Koch and Eriksson, 1973a; Koch, 1974).

Exercise Tests

The submaximal and maximal exercise tests were performed on two consecutive days in the sitting position on an electrodynamically braked bicycle ergometer (Elema). During the *submaximal test*, work was started at 250 kpm/min and loads were increased stepwise by 250 kpm/min until a pulse rate of at least 180 was reached. The boys exercised for 6 min at each work load; PWC_{170} was calculated by interpolation.

During the *maximal exercise test* the boys exercised for 3 min with a light load and for 6 min at a work load corresponding to 60% of their maximal capacity. They were then allowed to rest for about 30–60 sec sitting on the bicycle (the time required for injection of ^{133}Xe for measurement of MBF), and subsequently continued for about 2 min at a high submaximal (about 80% of maximal) and finally for 1–2 min at the maximal load that had been predicted from the pulse response during the previous submaximal exercise. In most cases, this test was repeated and the highest value of oxygen uptake obtained was used. Heart rate was obtained by continuous ECG recording, ventilation and oxygen uptake were measured by the Douglas bag technique, and blood pressures by the Riva Rocci cuff method. Oxygen and carbon dioxide were determined according to Scholander, and lactate in arterialized blood by an enzymatic method.

Muscle Blood Flow (MBF)

MBF was measured by determination of the clearance rate of ^{133}Xe after injection into the muscle to be studied (for details see Clausen and Lassen, 1971) in two different situations on two consecutive days:

1. After 2–3 min "ischemic" work in the tibialis anterior muscle; i.e., the subject flexed and extended his foot against a resistance with a pressure cuff, inflated to above 200 mm Hg, applied around the thigh. Maximal MBF occurs immediately after release of the cuff pressure, concomitant with the reactive hyperemia induced by tissue hypoxia and acidosis.
2. In the vastus lateralis muscle during successive submaximal and maximal bicycle ergometer exercise in the sitting position (for details see Koch, 1974).

Spirometry

A Bernstein spirometer was used for determination of the vital capacity and its subdivisions, and for tests of ventilatory capacity. The residual

Table 3. Means and standard deviations (in parenthesis) of some circulatory and respiratory data obtained during maximal exercise at different ages

Maximal work	12 Years		13 Years		14 Years		15 Years		16 Years	
Work load (kpm/min)	1015	(173)	1344[a]	(88)	1675[a]	(164)	1929[b]	(256)	2181[b]	(337)
Pulse rate (b.p.m.)	197	(6)	200	(6)	196	(5)	197	(11)	197	(11)
Respiratory rate	49	(9)	53	(8)	43[c]	(3)	56[c]	(9)	37[b]	(14)
Systemic BP (mm Hg)	160	(8)	172[b]	(8)	175	(14)	184[c]	(16)	199	(16)
Diastolic BP (mm Hg)	76	(3)	81	(3)	72	(3)	74	(4)		
Lactate (mM/l)	7.0	(1.4)	6.3	(1.3)	5.6[c]	(0.8)	5.1	(0.8)	6.0[c]	(0.7)
Lactate 4 min a w (mM/l)	9.3	(2.6)	8.8	(1.4)	9.4	(1.7)	5.8[b]	(0.8)	7.7[c]	(0.8)
$\dot{V}_E$ (l)	109.3	(16.8)	120.7[b]	(17.6)	87.4[a]	(9.2)	127.0[b]	(20.8)	112	(15.0)
$\dot{V}O_2$ (l)	2.33	(0.31)	2.46	(0.24)	2.92[c]	(0.40)	3.50[c]	(0.59)	4.72[b]	(0.50)
$\dot{V}O_2$/body weight (ml/kg)	59.5	(6.1)	56.8	(9.7)	58.5	(8.0)	61.8	(8.9)	72.6	(13.2)
$\dot{V}_E/\dot{V}O_2$	47.2	(6.5)	49.7	(4.0)	30.3[a]	(3.7)	37.1[c]	(3.9)	31.3[c]	(3.7)

Degree of statistical significance of changes from previous examination one year earlier: [a] $p < 0.001$; [b] $p < 0.01$; [c] $p < 0.05$.

Table 4. Muscle blood flow (average values of right and left leg, ml/min • 100 g) in the vastus lateralis muscle during bicycle ergometer exercise and in the anterior tibialis muscle in the supine position after ischemic work

Muscle blood flow		12 Years	13 Years	14 Years	15 Years	16 Years
M. vastus lateralis						
Submaximal work	$\bar{x}$ (SD)	64 (13)	79 (22)	61[a] (14)	60 (10)	55 (8)
Maximal work	$\bar{x}$ (SD)	77 (12)	71 (24)	63[a] (19)	60 (9)	52 (7)
After work	$\bar{x}$ (SD)	49 (20)		54 (19)	48 (17)	60 (18)
M. tibialis anterior						
Ischemic work	$\bar{x}$ (SD)	108 (32)	85[a] (35)	89 (18)	70[b] (15)	

Changes from previous examination one year earlier: [a] $p < 0.05$; [b] $p < 0.01$.

volume was determined by the closed helium method. Gas distribution and closed volume were evaluated by the nitrogen single breath test.

RESULTS

Submaximal and Maximal Exercise (Table 3)

PWC_{170} determined during submaximal exercise was unchanged from age 12 to 13, but showed a significant increase at reinvestigation at age 14; this increase was due to a significant decrease of exercise pulse rate. At age 14, there was also a significant decrease of ventilation and the ventilation equivalent; oxygen uptake was unchanged.

Maximal work load and maximal oxygen uptake (Table 3) showed a steady increase from 12–13 years ($\dot{V}_{O_2 \, max} = 2.4$ liters) to 16 years ($\dot{V}_{O_2 \, max} = 4.7$ liters); however, maximal oxygen uptake per kg of body weight and maximal heart rates did not reveal any significant change, although there was a clear tendency toward higher values of relative oxygen uptake at 16 as compared with previous years. Ventilation during maximal work remained at approximately the same level despite significantly higher work loads. The ventilation equivalent was significantly lower after the age of 14 years.

Muscle Blood Flow (Table 4)

Maximal MBF during both maximal bicycle and ischemic work showed a tendency toward lower values with increasing age, particularly with regard to MBF during maximal bicycle work between the ages of 13 and 14 years.

Lung Dimensions and Ventilation Capacity (Table 5)

Lung volumes (vital capacity, functional residual capacity [FRC], and total lung capacity [TLC]) and volume-dependent ventilatory capacity

Table 5. Means and standard deviations (in parentheses) of some spirometric data obtained at different ages

	13 Years	14 Years	15 Years	16 Years
VC	3.44 (0.36)	4.01^a (0.40)	4.98^b (0.01)	5.82^b (0.32)
VC/VC predicted	0.89 (0.08)	0.97 (0.07)	0.89 (0.11)	0.97 (0.03)
FRC	1.63 (0.27)	2.04 (0.47)	2.29^c (0.35)	2.81^b (0.42)
RV	0.57 (0.15)	0.94 (0.41)	0.87 (0.19)	0.92^c (0.28)
TLC	4.00 (0.46)	4.96^b (0.78)	5.67^b (0.82)	6.75^b (0.58)
FRC/TLC	0.41 (0.03)	0.41 (0.04)	0.41 (0.04)	0.42 (0.05)
RV/TLC	0.14 (0.03)	0.18 (0.05)	0.15 (0.02)	0.14 (0.03)
MVV	108 (15)	125^b (13)	156^b (18)	208^b (28)
FEV$_{1.0}$	3.02 (0.45)	3.40^b (0.62)	4.42^b (0.53)	5.47^b (0.20)
FEV/FEV predicted	1.03 (0.09)	0.98 (0.14)	0.92 (0.08)	1.08 (0.04)
FEV/VC	0.87 (0.07)	0.84 (0.09)	0.89^c (0.03)	0.94^a (0.03)
FIV$_{1.0}$	3.08 (0.33)	3.15 (0.67)	4.50^b (0.61)	5.64^a (0.43)
FIV/VC	0.90 (0.12)	0.88 (0.14)	0.91 (0.05)	0.97^c (0.03)
SBT (% N$_2$)	1.0 (0.4)	1.3 (0.9)	0.9 (0.9)	1.1 (0.5)
CLV/VC	9.4 (0.9)	6.3^b (2.2)	7.9 (1.7)	5.6 (1.8)

VC: vital capacity; FRC: functional residual capacity; RV: residual volume; TLC: total lung capacity; MVV: maximal voluntary ventilation; FEV$_{1.0}$: forced expiratory volume per second; FIV$_{1.0}$: forced inspiratory volume per second; SBT: single breath test; CLV/VC: closing volume in relation to vital capacity.

Changes from previous examination one year earlier: ^{a} $p < 0.001$; ^{b} $p < 0.01$; ^{c} $p < 0.05$.

(maximal voluntary ventilation, forced inspiratory and expiratory volumes per sec) showed steady and significant increases throughout the entire observation period. However, when corrected for body growth by dividing by height^3 (von Döbeln and Eriksson, 1972), these increases seemed to be entirely due to changes in body dimensions.

DISCUSSION

Cardiorespiratory Function

At the time that the boys were selected to enter the study, they had a high maximal oxygen uptake indicating a high level of physical training. The initial average maximal oxygen uptake of this group actually appears to be higher than any value reported for boys of corresponding age before engaging in a specific training program (Eriksson, 1972). In view of the level of the initial maximal $\dot{V}o_2$ (59.5 ± 6.1 ml/kg), it is not surprising that the relative maximal oxygen uptake did not show any further substantial increase during the three subsequent years despite continued high physical activity. This would imply that 60 ml/kg represents the average upper limit of trainability at the ages of 12 to 15 years. This, of course, does not mean that some individuals cannot reach higher values. Thus, the boy with the highest training intensity (5.3 days and 5.3 running sessions per week, Table 2) showed an increase in the maximal oxygen uptake from 55 ml/kg at age 12 to 75 ml/kg at 14 years. The value of 60 ml/kg is in good agreement with the results obtained in other specific training studies. Thus, the 11-year-old boys studied by Ekblom (1969) increased their relative maximal oxygen uptake from 53.9 to 59.4 ml/kg after 6 months of training; it was 58.1 ml/kg after 32 months. The group of 14 boys between ages 10 and 15 years studied by Daniels and Oldridge (1971) started with 59.5 ml/kg, and after 22 months of training (middle-distance runners training program) showed a maximal oxygen uptake of 58.3 ml/kg. Only at the age of 15 to 16 years did there appear to be a tendency toward higher maximal oxygen uptake, which obviously occurred concomitantly with the pubertal and postpubertal growth spurts.

During both submaximal and maximal exercise, the boys revealed, at the age of 14 years, a marked decrease in ventilation equivalent ($\dot{V}_E/\dot{V}o_2$) compared with the examinations at ages 13 and 12 years. This appears surprising in view of the higher $\dot{V}_E/\dot{V}o_2$ observed in a group of 11- to 12-year-old boys after 5 months of intensive physical training (Koch and Eriksson, 1973a). However, the present group had not only significantly higher $\dot{V}_E/\dot{V}o_2$ values, but also significantly higher maximal $\dot{V}o_2$ values, at both the ages of 12 and 13 years (59.5 and 56.8 ml/kg, respectively, versus 41.7 ml/kg). The difference in ventilation observed at the age of 12 to 13 years can probably be explained by the significant difference between the two groups with respect to aerobic power; after training, this difference was actually smaller. It is noteworthy that the significant decrease of $\dot{V}_E/\dot{V}_{O_2}$ in the present group at age 14 occurred simultaneously with a significant, apparently puberty-induced growth spurt reflected by height, weight, and lung dimension development (Tables 1 and 3). The increases in lung dimensions and ventilatory capacity could be entirely explained by normal maturation, as was the case in the training study previously mentioned (Koch and Eriksson, 1973a).

Muscle Blood Flow

MBF during both maximal and submaximal bicycle work in the vastus lateralis muscle showed a continuous tendency toward lower values from 12 to 16 years. The values obtained at the age of 14 years were practically identical with those reported for 25-year-old men of normal fitness (Nordenfelt, 1974). There was also a tendency toward lower MBF in the anterior tibialis muscle after ischemic work, especially from 12 to 13 and 14 to 15 years of age.

Prepubertal (Eriksson and Koch, 1973) and, to a lesser degree, pubertal boys (Eriksson et al., 1971) have been shown to have a slightly lower cardiac output as compared with young adults. They also tend to have a slightly higher arterial-mixed venous oxygen (AV_{O_2}) difference, at least at submaximal exercise levels. Higher MBF per unit of tissue at the ages of 12 and 13 years, together with a lower cardiac output and an identical or slightly higher AV_{O_2}, can most probably be explained by a different pattern of blood flow distribution. Because of a smaller effective muscle mass in the prepubertal boys, a smaller proportion of cardiac output is distributed to the working muscle, but blood flow in relation to muscle mass is higher. These differences apparently diminish greatly after the age of 14, when muscle development is accelerated because of the onset of puberty. At the age of 16 years, when muscle mass had markedly increased in all the subjects, relative muscle blood flows tended to be lower than in young men with normal physical activity and fitness (Nordenfelt, 1974). Most probably, this was due to the extensive physical training in which the boys continued to participate. It is well established that normally the blood flow required by the skeletal muscle during exercise at identical work loads decreases after training (Stenberg, 1971), while the density of mitochondria and the oxidative enzyme capacity increase (cf. Koch, 1978).

Blood lactate concentration during maximal work at the age of 12 to 13 years was identical with that observed in the 11- to 13-year-old boys after training (Eriksson and Koch, 1973). There was a tendency toward lower peak lactate values at the age of 14 and particularly 15 as compared with 13 and 12 years. This is in agreement with the observation of higher muscle but lower blood lactate concentrations during heavy exercise following physical training in boys ages 11 to 13 years (Eriksson et al., 1973). As an explanation those authors proposed that "this may have resulted from a greater extraction of lactate by other tissues or from a different rate of production and utilization by the different fiber types in the working muscle." Changes in the pattern of muscle fiber distribution and in muscle metabolism, mainly consisting of an enhanced glycolytic and oxidative capacity, have been shown to be induced by training in prepubertal boys (Eriksson et al., 1973), but probably occur, or continue to exist, even in older boys provided that vigorous training is continued. However, the changes in peak blood lactate can be explained by other mechanisms. Thus, the disproportionate expansion of plasma volume elicited by physical training (Koch and Röcker, 1977) would tend to lower lactate levels, in particular in the presence of a small muscle mass. The slight increase in peak lactate values observed at the age of 16 years as compared with 14 and 15 years (Table 3) should then be due to the marked increase of muscle mass observed during this period.

ACKNOWLEDGMENT

The important contribution made by Åke Mattisson, who supervised and evaluated the physical training, is gratefully acknowledged.

REFERENCES

Clausen, J. P., and N. A. Lassen. 1971. Muscle blood flow during exercise in normal man studied by the [133]-Xenon clearance method. Cardiovasc. Res. 5:245–251.
Daniels, J., and N. Oldridge. 1971. Changes in oxygen consumption of young boys during growth and running training. Med. Sci. Sports 3:161–165.
Ekblom, B. 1969. Effect of physical training in adolescent boys. J. Appl. Physiol. 27:350–355.
Eriksson, B. O. 1972. Physical training, oxygen supply and muscle metabolism in 11–13-year old boys. Acta Physiol. Scand. Suppl. 384.
Eriksson, B. O., P. D. Gollnick, and B. Saltin. 1973. Muscle metabolism and enzyme activities after training in boys 11–13 years old. Acta Physiol. Scand. 87:106–112.
Eriksson, B. O., G. Grimby, and B. Saltin. 1971. Cardiac output and arterial blood gases during exercise in pubertal boys. J. Appl. Physiol. 31:348–352.
Eriksson, B. O., and G. Koch. 1973. Effect of physical training on the hemodynamic response during submaximal and maximal exercise in 11–13 year old boys. Acta Physiol. Scand. 87:27–39.
Koch, G. 1974. Muscle blood flow after ischemic work and during bicycle ergometer work in boys aged 12 years. Acta Paediatr. Belg. 28 (Suppl.): 29–38.
Koch, G. 1978. Muscle blood flow in prepubertal boys. Effect of growth combined with intensive physical training. Med. Sport 11:39–46.
Koch, G., and B. O. Eriksson. 1973a. Effect of physical training on pulmonary ventilation and gas exchange during submaximal and maximal work in boys aged 11 to 13 years. Scand. J. Clin. Lab. Invest. 31:87–94.

Koch, G., and B. O. Eriksson. 1973b. Effect of physical training on anatomical R-L shunt at rest and pulmonary diffusing capacity during near-maximal exercise in boys 11–13 years old. Scand. J. Clin. Lab. Invest. 31:95–103.

Koch, G., and L. Röcker. 1977. Plasma volume and intravascular protein masses in trained boys and fit young men. J. Appl. Physiol. Respirat. Environ. Exercise Physiol. 43 (6):1085–1088.

Nordenfelt, I. 1974. Blood flow of working muscles during autonomic blockade of the heart. Cardiovasc. Res. 8:1227–1232.

Stenberg, J. 1971. Muscle blood flow during exercise. Effects of training. In: O. A. Larsen and R. O. Malmborg (eds.), Coronary Heart Disease and Physical Fitness, pp. 80–87. Munkgaard, Copenhagen.

von Döbeln, W., and B. O. Eriksson. 1972. Physical training, maximal oxygen uptake and dimensions of the oxygen transporting and metabolizing organs in boys 11–13 years of age. Acta Paediatr. Scand. 61:653–661.

Total Amount of Hemoglobin, Plasma and Blood Volumes, and Intravascular Protein Masses in Trained Boys

G. Koch and L. Röcker

Although metabolic adaptations and responses of the cardiovascular and respiratory systems to physical training in man have been extensively studied both in adults (Åstrand and Rodahl, 1970) and in children (von Döbeln and Eriksson, 1972; Eriksson and Koch, 1973; Koch and Eriksson, 1973a, b) during the last decade, there has only recently been evidence of increasing interest in the effects of training on intravascular proteins. A series of studies in sedentary and trained adults has shown that at least endurance training leads to an expansion of the plasma volume and a significant increase of intravascular masses of albumin and hepatogenic globulines (Röcker et al., 1976). Furthermore, it is well established that blood volume and total hemoglobin increase with physical exercise in the adult (Kjellberg et al., 1950). These responses of the blood and protein systems are rational adaptations of the organism to increase the availability of water for thermoregulation and the circulatory capacity for heavy exercise.

The purpose of this study was to provide some information on the response of the postpubertal growing organism to physical activity with respect to these adaptations. Plasma volume, total amount of hemoglobin, and plasma proteins were compared in postpubertal boys ages 14 to 15 years and in young men ages 17 to 20 years and 24 to 30 years, respectively. All subjects were highly trained. Further details of the study are given elsewhere (Koch and Röcker, 1977).

SUBJECTS

Boys

Eight boys volunteered (with their parents' consent) for the investigation. Seven of them formed a homogeneous age group and were studied at

Table 1. Means and standard deviations (in parentheses) of some anthropometric data, maximal oxygen uptake, plasma volume, and hemoglobin in experimental subjects

Variable	Boys, 14–15 years $(N=8)$		Men, 17–20 years $(N=10)$		Men, 24–30 years $(N=6)$	
Weight (kg)	52.4	(8.0)	69.6	(3.9)	61.7	(2.1)
Height (cm)	166	(8)	182	(6)	175	(4)
$\dot{V}O_2$ max (ml/min)	3.109[a]	(4.23)	4.312	(2.49)	3.922	(3.30)
$\dot{V}O_2$ max (ml/min per kg)	59.6	(6.5)	61.8	(3.4)	63.3	(4.1)
Plasma volume (liters)	3.10[b]	(0.61)	3.57	(0.32)	3.87	(0.54)
Plasma volume (ml/kg)	59.1	(12.0)	51.3	(4.0)	59.4	(5.9)
Hemoglobin (g/l)	134	(9)	144	(6)	137	(4)
THb (g)[c]	656[a]	(129)	907	(77)	885	(128)
THb (g/kg of body wt)	12.6	(1.9)	13.0	(1.0)	14.4	(2.0)

[a]$p < 0.001$.
[b]$p < 0.05$.
[c]Total amount of hemoglobin.

13.9 ± 0.2 (SD) and 14.9 ± 0.2 years of age. However, one of the boys was 14 months younger compared with the group's mean age. He was included because he did not differ significantly in any of the variables studied. All the data presented were calculated from the pooled data obtained at ages 14 and 15 years and are considered representative of the immediate postpubertal period.

All of the boys were highly motivated by a strong interest in physical exercise and regularly took part in different sporting activities such as soccer, running, and badminton in the summer, and ice hockey or cross-country skiing in the winter.

Men

Two groups of endurance-trained adult athletes were studied: 10 young men ages 17 to 20 years (mean 19.0 ± 0.9) and six men ages 24 to 30 years (mean 27.0 ± 1.8). They were all long-distance runners with a regular training schedule. Some relevant anthropometric and functional data are given in Table 1.

METHODS

The general procedures were identical for each of the three groups. All subjects were studied in the morning after fasting overnight. Plasma volume was determined by use of ^{125}I-tagged human serum albumin (RISA) with the 10-min distribution space taken as the plasma volume. Hemoglobin was measured by the spectrophotometric hemoglobin cyanide method and hematocrit by the microcapillary technique. Total serum protein concentrations were measured by the biuret method. The individual globulins (IgG, IgM, IgA, haptoglobin, macroglobulin,

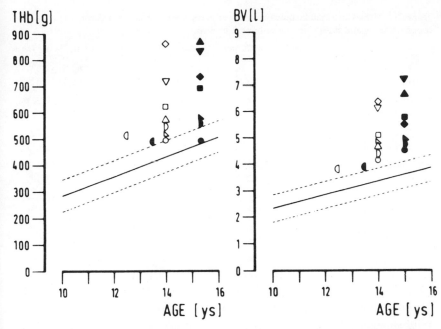

Figure 1.   Total amount of hemoglobin (THb) and blood volume (BV) of boys in relation to age at first (open symbol) and second (filled symbol) examination. Continuous line and dashed lines denote regression line ± 1 standard error of estimate for boys aged 5–16 years with normal physical activity (Koch, 1966).

transferrin) and albumin were determined according to the radial immunodiffusion principle. The intravascular protein masses (IPM) were obtained by multiplying the respective protein concentrations by the plasma volume. Details of analytical procedures and their reproducibility are given elsewhere (Röcker et al., 1976; Koch and Röcker, 1977). In none of the methods used did the coefficient of variation exceed 5%. Statistical analysis was performed using the nonparametric U test according to Wilcoxon.

RESULTS

The boys were within the mean ± 1 SD range according to the growth charts for height and weight development in Swedish children (Broman et al., 1942), but they had significantly larger plasma volumes, total amounts of hemoglobin, and blood volumes than children with normal physical activity (Figure 1). Data on IPM in children are extremely scanty; comparisons with the data available, however, indicate that the present group of trained boys had significantly larger masses in relation to body weight of all the plasma proteins that were determined (Koch and Röcker, 1977). Because of the smaller body dimensions, the boys had lower

Table 2. Means and standard deviations (in parenthesis) of plasma protein
concentrations and masses in experimental subjects

Variable	Boys, 13–15 years	Men, 17–20 years	Men, 24–30 years
Total protein (g/l)	65.6 (2.90)	68.1 (2.01)	68.5 (2.13)
Total protein mass (g/kg)	3.89 (0.63)	3.50 (0.29)	4.16 (0.32)
Albumin (g/l)	41.8[a] (1.69)	46.3 (1.75)	44.4 (2.32)
Albumin mass (g/kg)	2.50 (0.42)	2.38 (0.19)	2.70 (0.25)
IgG (g/l)	10.60 (2.06)	9.65 (1.81)	8.98 (1.29)
Total mass (mg/kg)	636 (207.8)	479 (98.9)	525 (96.1)
IgM (g/l)	1.07 (0.49)	1.22 (0.34)	1.20 (0.43)
Total mass (mg/kg)	62.6 (28.70)	62.7 (20.13)	70.4 (22.0)
IgA (g/l)	1.43 (0.57)	2.05 (1.03)	1.86 (0.56)
Total mass (mg/kg)	85.1 (35.57)	106.9 (63.9)	111 (38.4)
Haptoglobin (g/l)	0.75 (0.31)	0.73 (0.36)	0.69 (0.41)
Total mass (mg/kg)	45 (20.9)	35.7 (19.8)	41 (22.7)
α_x-Macroglobulin (g/l)	4.60[a] (0.80)	3.44 (0.59)	2.89 (0.47)
Total mass (mg/kg)	277 (79.3)	182 (27.8)	176 (34.4)
α_1-Antitrypsin (g/l)	3.3 (0.9)		
Total mass (mg/kg)	207.0 (103.4)		
Transferrin (g/l)	3.76[b] (0.28)	2.06 (0.27)	2.16 (0.25)
Total mass (mg/kg)	227[b] (56.4)	104 (14.8)	132 (26.8)

[a] $p < 0.05$, boys versus adults.
[b] $p < 0.001$, boys versus adults.

($p < 0.005$) maximal oxygen uptakes and lower ($p < 0.05$) plasma volumes
in terms of absolute values than the two adult groups. However, these differences vanished when maximal oxygen uptake and plasma volume were
related to body weight (Table 1). There were no statistically significant
differences in any of the anthropometric variables, maximal oxygen uptake, plasma volume, or plasma proteins between the two adult groups.
Among the plasma constituents determined (Table 2), only α_2-macroglo-
bulin and transferrin differed significantly ($p < 0.01$) from the respective
values in the adults, with both protein fractions roughly 80% higher in the
boys when expressed as total mass in relation to kg of body weight. The
weight-corrected masses of total protein, albumin, immunoglobins, and
haptoglobin were virtually identical in the three groups. No values of
α_1-antitrypsin were available in the adult athletes.

DISCUSSION

In the adult, physical training, and in particular endurance training, have
been shown to induce an expansion of plasma and blood volumes and an
increase in total hemoglobin and intravascular protein masses (Kjellberg
et al., 1950; Röcker et al., 1976). However, because of disproportionate

Table 3. Electrophoretic mobility and main biological
functions of plasma proteins determined

Protein fraction	Electrophoretic mobility	Biological function
Albumin	albumin	Maintenance of osmotic pressure. Vehicle for hormones, free fatty acids, drugs.
IgG IgA IgM	γ = globulin	Main constituents of the humoral antibody system.
α_2 = macroglobulin	α_2 = globulin	Binding of hormones, e.g., insulin. Proteinase inhibitor, complement factor.
α_1 = antitrypsin	α_1 = globulin	Trypsin and chemotrypsin inhibitor, acute phase reactant protein.
Transferrin	β_1 = globulin	Binding and transport of iron; antibacterial and antiviral properties.
Haptoglobin	α_2 = globulin	Binding free hemoglobin preventing iron loss. Peroxydase-like activity; acute phase reactant protein.

Modified from Simmons et al. (1969).

increases in plasma volume, total protein and, in particular, albumin concentrations, hemoglobin concentration, and hematocrit were lower; therefore the trained individuals tended to have lower blood viscosity and colloid-osmotic pressures than their untrained counterparts (Röcker et al., 1976). These changes would tend to increase physical work capacity as well as implying a definite advantage for thermoregulation and perfusion in terminal vascular beds. Because of the specific biological functions (Table 3) of the globulins, an increase in their total mass appears to be an additional advantage.

Compared with children following normal physical activity routines, the boys in this study had considerably larger plasma and blood volumes and increased masses of hemoglobin and of the quantitatively most important proteins, particularly albumin. Furthermore, plasma volumes and masses of most of the intravascular proteins were practically identical in the boys and in the adult athletes when compared on a body weight basis. Thus, it appears that the hematological response and the adaptation of the plasma protein system to endurance training is not specific for, or confined to, the adult organism, but occurs in a similar manner in children at least at or after pubertal age.

However, the boys had roughly 80% higher relative IPMs of α_2-macroglobulin and transferrin. It is well established that children, at least during the period of rapid growth, have higher concentrations of both macroglobulin and transferrin (Koch and Röcker, 1977); this growth-correlated characteristic probably explains the differences found in this study between boys and adults. It has further been shown that adult athletes have higher relative amounts of both α_2-macroglobulin and transferrin than nonathletes (Röcker et al., 1976). It appears that this is also true for trained as compared to untrained children, although comparable values are extremely scanty.

This study confirms earlier reports (Röcker et al., 1976) that the trained individual tends to have lower hemoglobin and hematocrit values than his untrained counterpart. Since the total amount of hemoglobin is elevated, however, the lower hemoglobin concentration of the trained individual is due to the disproportionate expansion of the plasma volume rather than being indicative of anemia.

CONCLUSIONS

Physically highly active boys at postpubertal age (13 to 15 years) showed the same pattern of adaptive increase in plasma volume, total amount of hemoglobin, and plasma proteins as endurance-trained adult athletes. These changes tend to increase the water-binding capacity of the plasma and to improve the circulatory system's ability to sustain heavy exercise.

Endurance training apparently elicits the same response of the plasma protein system regardless of age, at least after pubertal age has been reached.

REFERENCES

Åstrand, P.-O., and K. Rodahl. 1970. Textbook of Work Physiology. McGraw-Hill Book Co., New York.

Broman, B., G. Dahlberg, and A. Lichtenstein. 1942. Height and weight during growth. Acta Paediatr. Scand. 30:1–66.

Eriksson, B. O., and G. Koch. 1973. Effect of physical training on the hemodynamic response during submaximal and maximal exercise in 11–13 year old boys. Acta Physiol. Scand. 87:27–39.

Kjellberg, S. R., U. Rudhe, and T. Sjöstrand. 1950. Increase of the amount of hemoglobin and blood volume in connection with physical training. Acta Physiol. Scand. 19:146–151.

Koch, G. 1966. Determination of total amount of hemoglobin, blood volume and red cell volume. In: H. Opitz and F. Schmid (eds.), Handbook of Pediatrics (in German), pp. 261–265. Springer Verlag, Berlin.

Koch, G., and B. O. Eriksson. 1973a. Effect of physical training on pulmonary ventilation and gas exchange during submaximal and maximal work in boys 11–13 years. Scand. J. Clin. Lab. Invest. 31:87–94.

Koch, G., and B. O. Eriksson. 1973b. Effect of physical training on anatomical R-L shunt at rest and pulmonary diffusing capacity during near-maximal exercise in boys 11–13 years old. Scand. J. Clin. Lab. Invest. 31:95–105.

Koch, G., and L. Röcker, 1977. Plasma volume and intravascular protein masses in trained boys and fit young men. J. Appl. Physiol. Respirat. Environ. Exercise Physiol. 43 (6):1085–1088.

Röcker, L., K. A. Kirsch, and H. Stoboy. 1976. Plasma volume, albumin and globulin concentrations and their intravascular masses. Eur. J. Appl. Physiol. Occup. Physiol. 36:57–64.

Simmons, P., P. Ronald, and I. Goller. 1969. Plasma proteins: A review. Med. J. Aust. 2:494–506.

von Döbeln, W., and B. O. Eriksson. 1972. Physical training, maximal oxygen uptake and dimensions of the oxygen transporting and metabolizing organs in boys 11–13 years of age. Acta Paediatr. Scand. 61:653–661.

Effect of Physical Training in Former Female Top Athletes in Swimming

B. O. Eriksson, U. Freychuss, A. Lundin, and C. A. R. Thorén

Top athletes in endurance sports are characterized by a high aerobic capacity (for references, see Åstrand and Rodahl, 1970). This high aerobic capacity is achieved by means of intensive physical training over many years. It is obvious, however, that not every subject can reach a position as a top athlete in spite of very intensive training. Thus, top athletes must be the result of a natural selection; only those individuals who respond to physical training with a marked increase in aerobic power will become top athletes. It is not known which underlying mechanism constitutes this capability to achieve increased aerobic power. Neither is it known whether this characteristic will be maintained once the period of intensive physical training is over. However, it is attractive to assume that a former top athlete will have a more pronounced capability to increase his aerobic power with physical training than an ordinary, sedentary person.

This hypothesis was the basis for a retraining study of former girl swimmers (Eriksson et al., 1975). The women studied had had very high values for maximal oxygen uptake; this was achieved by means of a very intensive and time consuming swim-training (Åstrand et al., 1963). After cessation of swim-training, their maximal oxygen uptake had decreased markedly (Eriksson et al., 1967; Eriksson et al., 1971; Eriksson et al., 1975; Eriksson et al., 1978). Ten years after the first examination it had been reduced from 2.80 liters/min to 2.18 liters/min and from 51.4 ml/kg•min to 36.4 ml/kg•min (Eriksson et al., 1978). Thus, these women seemed to be appropriate for the testing of the hypothesis of a super-capacity to increase aerobic power in former top athletes. However, it was not possible to fully answer the question. The former girl swimmers did not increase their aerobic power more than sedentary subjects had in the earlier study (Eriksson et al., 1975). On the other hand, the participation in the training performed was not as good as expected. Furthermore, the

Table 1. Physical characteristics of four former elite girl swimmers
and four sedentary healthy controls before training (mean values ± SE are given)

	Former girl swimmers	Controls	Difference
Age (years)	29.8 ± 0.43	30.8 ± 0.83	N.S.
Height (cm)	173.0 ± 2.28	168.0 ± 1.49	a
Weight (kg)	64.8 ± 2.61	58.5 ± 3.80	a
Triceps skinfold (mm)	13.2 ± 1.02	14.7 ± 2.74	N.S.

Levels of significance between the former girl swimmers and the controls: N.S. = no significant difference; $a = p < 0.05$.

16 women studied were not the very top athletes in the 1961 study (Åstrand et al., 1963). Finally, in that training study, no control group was included and the women did not train entirely by swimming (Eriksson et al., 1975).

It was therefore felt to be of interest to repeat the retraining study and only include the real top athletes from the 1961 study. Furthermore, it was decided that a matching control group of young women at the same age, and who had been mainly sedentary, should be included. The main topic of the study was to evaluate whether former top athletes in swimming had a greater capability to increase their aerobic power in comparison with sedentary subjects.

SUBJECTS

From the 30 girls studied in 1961 (Åstrand et al., 1963) only the nine girls from club B, the dominant swim club in Sweden at that time, were asked to participate in the present study. They had had the highest values for $\dot{V}_{O_2\ max}$, with a mean of 3.18 liters/min in 1961, corresponding to 55.1 ml/kg•min. Three of the nine women had moved abroad and were thus unable to participate in the study. Another woman could not join the study because of her occupation. In fact, she joined the study in the beginning but had to leave it because she could not fulfill the training program. Of the remaining five women, four volunteered for the study. They were nos. 10, 15, 27, and 28 in the "Girl Swimmers" study (Åstrand et al., 1963). Their ages were 29, 31, 29, and 29 years, respectively; their mean body height and body weight were 173 cm and 64.8 kg, respectively (Table 1). For each woman an age-matched control woman was selected who, for practical reasons, had to live in the neighborhood of the former girl swimmer and not have had any former intensive physical training. The characteristics of the control group are included in Table 1.

METHODS

Body height and body weight were carefully measured. Skinfold measurements were performed at three different places: right triceps, biceps, and subiliac. Lung volumes were measured with the closed helium circuit method and by Bernstein spirometry (Comroe et al., 1967). Heart volume was measured in the lying prone position according to the method of Kjellberg et al. (1949). Blood volume was measured with the ^{131}I-labeled albumin method (Williams and Fine, 1961); plasma volume was derived from blood volume and hematocrit determinations. Thoracic impedance data were obtained using four aluminized Mylar tape electrodes (3M Company, Minnesota) attached circumferentially to the patient. The inner electrodes were placed around the base of the neck and at the xiphisternal joint, respectively. The outer two electrodes were placed at least 3 cm from the inner electrodes. The electrodes were attached to an IFM and Minnesota Impedance Cardiograph, Model 304 A, which supplies a constant sinusoidal alternating current of 4 mA at a frequency of 100 kHz that is transmitted between the outer electrodes. From the two inner electrodes the standing impedance (i.e., basal impedance [Z_0]) was read on a digital display. A crystal microphone was placed over the second left intercostal space in order to record a phonocardiogram, thus facilitating proper timing of the second heart sound. Three output signals were recorded on the multichannel graphic recorder (Mingograph, Siemens-Elema, Sweden): 1) electrocardiogram, 2) phonocardiogram, and 3) the first derivative of the diminution of Z_0 (dZ/dt) occurring with the heart cycle. The stroke volume was calculated according to the formula given by Kubicek et al. (1966):

$$P \cdot \left(\frac{L}{Z_0} \right)^2 \cdot T \cdot \frac{dZ}{dt}$$

where P = resistivity of blood (taken as 135 ohm-cm); L = distance (cm) between electrodes two and three; Z_0 = basal impedance (ohm); T = ventricular ejection time (sec); and dZ/dt = first derivative of the diminution of Z_0 (ohm/sec). In each subject the average of 5 beats was used to calculate the stroke volume. The cardiac output was calculated by multiplying the stroke volume by the heart rate that was obtained from ECG recording.

Exercise was performed on an electrically braked ergometer (Elema) at 60 rpm. Oxygen uptake was determined with the Douglas bag method, the volume of the bags being measured in a balanced Tissot spirometer. Gas fractions of oxygen and carbon dioxide were determined with the micro-Scholander technique (Scholander, 1947). Heart rate was obtained from ECG recordings, and respiratory rate by auscultation for 30 sec. Blood lactate was measured by a sample from a prewarmed finger tip and analyzed with an enzymatic method (Scholz et al., 1950). Perceived exertion was rated according to the method of Borg and Linderholm (1967).

Table 2. Pulse rate determinations in b.p.m. during a swim-training session in four former elite girl swimmers and their four healthy control women counterparts

Subject	10 min with distance training	10 min with interval-training	10 min with distance training
Former girl swim-mers			
#10	192	180	—
#15	170	—	175
#27	170	175	170
#28	165	170	170
Controls			
Control to #10	170	170	165
Control to #15	160	170	—
Control to #27	165	165	168
Control to #28	160	165	155

PROCEDURE

The study was performed from December, 1975, until May, 1976. The former girl swimmers and their controls were examined before and after the period of physical training. All women passed the whole examination program. Maximal oxygen uptake was determined on a bicycle ergometer with stepwise increases in the work loads each 6 min. Maximal oxygen uptake was defined using the leveling-off criterion (Åstrand, 1952). Further criteria were a ventilatory equivalent exceeding 30, a respiratory quotient exceeding 1.00, and a blood lactate concentration exceeding 8.0 mmol/liter. All women fulfilled these criteria. The former girl swimmers became rather well acquainted with this procedure during the 14 years they had been followed. Lung volume, blood volume, heart volume, and cardiac output were determined before the exercise tests.

PHYSICAL TRAINING

The women performed all physical training by swimming. Each former girl swimmer and her control trained together and at the same time. Because of the obvious differences in swimming technique and efficiency, the former girl swimmers covered considerably longer distances. A total of three training sessions a week over 16 weeks were performed. The training period ended with a week-long training camp in Madeira, where swim-training was performed twice a day.

Training efficiency was checked by manual pulse rate determination by one of us (A.L.—Table 2). The pulse rate was determined during swimming. The individual mean values are given in Table 3. The average pulse rate for the former girl swimmers was 169 b.p.m., compared

Table 3.   Mean values for pulse rate at the swim-training sessions in four former girl elite swimmers and in their four healthy control women counterparts

Subject	Pulse rate (b.p.m.)	Number of estimations	Maximum pulse rate at swimming
Former girl swimmers			
# 10	165	21	184
# 15	172	30	183
# 27	169	31	183
# 28	170	17	175
Controls			
Control to # 10	165	37	178
Control to # 15	169	32	185
Control to # 27	161	30	175
Control to # 28	159	35	170

to 163.5 b.p.m. for the controls. The maximal heart rate at swimming was 181.3 b.p.m. for the former girl swimmers and 177.8 b.p.m. for the controls.

RESULTS

Pretraining Values

The four former girl swimmers were about the same age as the controls, but they were 5 cm taller and 6.3 kg heavier (both $p < 0.05$). Skinfold values were comparable (Table 1). The values for heart volume ($p < 0.01$), blood volume ($p < 0.01$), and vital capacity and MVV_{free} (both $p < 0.001$) were significantly higher in the group of former girl swimmers (Table 4). Aerobic power was higher—2.32 versus 1.91 liters/min ($p < 0.01$). This last difference, however, was not significant when the values for $\dot{V}O_{2\,max}$ per kg of body weight were compared (Table 4). Thus the former girl swimmers had a mean value of 36.0, as compared to the mean value for the control group of 33.3 ml/kg·min. No significant differences between the former girl swimmers and the control group were found for the maximal values for $\dot{V}_E$, $\dot{V}_E/\dot{V}O_2$, blood lactate concentration, heart rate, and respiratory quotient (Table 4).

The mean values for the stroke volume in the supine position were 78 ml both in the former girl swimmers and in the control group. However, the recordings for cardiac output and thus stroke volume in two of the former girl swimmers were not satisfactory; the values obtained were too low. After omitting these two women, the remaining two former girl swimmers had higher values for stroke volume than the controls (Figure 1).

The estimation of perceived exertion did not differ between the two groups. In fact training did not change the estimation, either (Figure 2).

Table 4. Some physiological and functional data of four former elite girl swimmers and four sedentary healthy controls before (B) and after (A) four months of swim training (mean values ±SE are given)

	Former girl swimmers		Controls	
	B	A	B	A
Heart volume (ml)	697 ±39	740 ±40	598 ±15	626 ±32
Blood volume (l)	4.69± 0.23	4.50± 0.12	3.59± 0.29	3.73± 0.14
Vital capacity (l)	4.69± 0.142	4.82± 0.173	3.77± 0.143	3.90± 0.044
MVV_{free} (l)	155 ± 6.5	166 ±12.2	110 ± 6.0	123 ± 9.9
$\dot{V}O_{2\,max}$ (l/min)	2.32± 0.160	2.76± 0.164[a]	1.91± 0.078	2.15± 0.35[b]
$\dot{V}O_{2\,max}$/weight (ml/kg·min)	36.0 ± 1.08	42.8 ± 2.56[b]	33.3 ± 2.63	36.5 ± 1.94
$\dot{V}_{E\,max}$ (l/min)	81.0 ± 8.66	106.0 ± 5.71[a]	76.5 ± 4.34	103.0 ± 4.76[b]
$\dot{V}_E / \dot{V}O_{2\,max}$	36.0 ± 2.95	38.7 ± 2.66	38.7 ± 2.65	48.5 ± 3.64[b]
Heart rate$_{max}$ (b.p.m.)	196 ± 3.1	190 ± 3.7[a]	188.8 ± 4.3	183 ± 4.3[a]
Blood lactate$_{max}$ (mmol/l)	11.0 ± 0.68	11.8 ± 0.40	12.3 ± 0.60	128 ± 1.90
Respiratory quotient$_{max}$	1.04± 0.026	1.07± 0.027	1.11± 0.32	1.15± 0.044

Levels of significance between values before and after training: [a] $p < 0.01$; [b] $p < 0.05$.

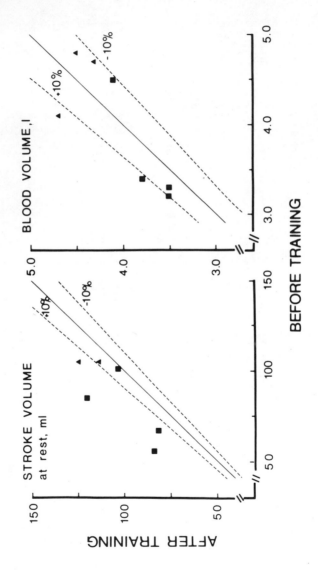

Figure 1.   Individual values for stroke volume and blood volume in four former girl swimmers (triangles) and in a control group of four sedentary women (squares) before and after a 16-week period of swim-training. The 45° line of identity with ± 10% are drawn.

PERCEIVED EXERTION

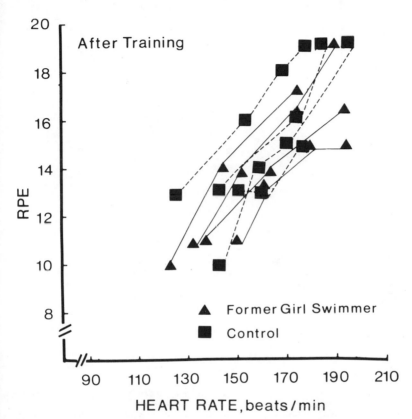

Figure 2. Individual scores of perceived exertion, according to Borg and Linderholm (1967), in relation to heart rate in the former girl swimmers and in a control group.

Posttraining Values

The spirometric data and blood and heart volumes were not significantly changed by training (Table 4). Maximal oxygen uptake increased significantly in both groups, from 2.32 to 2.76 liters/min and from 1.91 to 2.15 liters/min in the former girl swimmers and in the control group, respectively. Thus, the former girl swimmers had a 19% increase while the control group had a 12.5% increase. This difference is more marked when comparing the data of $\dot{V}o_{2\,max}$ per kg of body weight (Table 4). The 19% increase in the former girl swimmers should be compared with a 10% increase in the control group. In fact the former girl swimmers had an unchanged body weight, in contrast to some of the women in the control group (Figure 3).

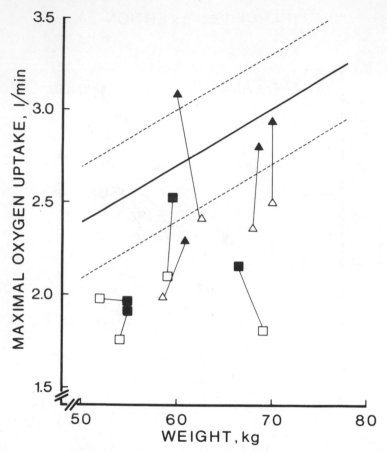

Figure 3.   Individual values for $\dot{V}_{O_2 \, max}$ in relation to body weight in former girl swimmers and in a control group before and after a 16-week-long period of swim-training. The solid line is the regression line with $\pm$ 2 SD for normal Swedish women as given in Åstrand et al. (1963). Open symbols denote values obtained before training and filled symbols values obtained after training. The triangles denote the former girl swimmers and the squares the controls.

The stroke volume of the heart increased significantly in both groups; in the former girl swimmers this increase was 33%, to a mean value of 105 ml, and in the control group 26%, to a mean value of 97 ml (Figure 1).

DISCUSSION

It has been discussed earlier whether or not these former girl swimmers can be looked on as normal individuals (Eriksson et al., 1971; Eriksson et al., 1975; Eriksson et al., 1978). The sizes of their lungs (Table 4) and their hearts (Figure 4) do exceed what is supposed to be normal, whereas those of the controls were fairly normal. It has also been discussed whether or

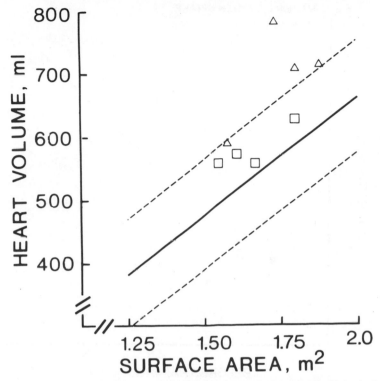

Figure 4.   Individual values for heart volume in the supine position in relation to body surface area (Kjellberg et al., 1949). For explanation of the symbols, see Figure 1.

not a large heart volume per se constitutes a greater potential for increasing aerobic power (Ekblom, 1969). If this is true, these former girl swimmers would have a greater potential to increase aerobic power. On the other hand, their aerobic power was also higher in comparison with the control groups. It has been speculated that the higher the pretraining value of the $\dot{V}_{O_2 \, max}$, the lower the percentage of increase that will be obtained (Saltin et al., 1969).

In spite of these circumstances, a rather large increase of the $\dot{V}_{O_2 \, max}$ was achieved, 19% as compared to 12.5% for the control group. This increase for the former girl swimmers was better than that achieved in the former training study (Eriksson et al., 1975). It can therefore be summarized, with some cautiousness, that a former female top athlete in swimming has a greater potential to increase her aerobic power.

When looking at the individual response to training, it is interesting to note that one of the women in the control group did not show any increase in $\dot{V}_{O_2 \, max}$ in spite of 16 weeks of physical training (Figure 5). This phenomenon is interesting. It can be questioned whether or not she really trained hard enough. However, the pulse rate controls revealed that she really had trained hard (Table 1). Thus, there must be constitutional dif-

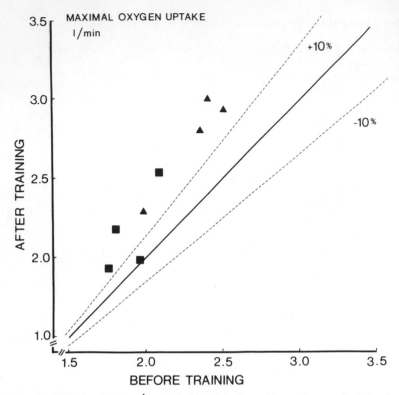

Figure 5.   Individual values for $\dot{V}_{O_2\ max}$ before and after a 16-week-long period of swim-training in four former girls swimmers (triangles) and in four controls (squares). The 45° line of identity with ± 10% is drawn.

ferences in the ability to increase $\dot{V}_{O_2\ max}$. Although some subjects can reach very high values for $\dot{V}_{O_2\ max}$ with training, other subjects may respond very poorly.

As can be seen in Figure 5, the three other women in the control group showed an increase in $\dot{V}_{O_2\ max}$ similar to that of the former girl swimmers. Thus, the difference in response to this period of swim-training is mainly due to the lack of increase in one of the subjects in the control group. This finding really emphasizes the importance of having a matching and properly selected control group that also contains a sufficient number of subjects.

This study has given some support to the hypothesis that a former top athlete has a greater capability to increase her aerobic power with training. However, a further study including more subjects must be done before this statement can be made with certainty.

REFERENCES

Åstrand, P.-O. 1952. Experimental Studies of Physical Working Capacity in Relation to Age and Sex. Munksgaard, Copenhagen.

Åstrand, P.-O., L. Engström, B. O. Eriksson, P. Karlberg, B. Saltin, and C. Thorén. 1963. Girl swimmers. Acta Paediatr. Scand. 52(Suppl. 147): 1–75.

Åstrand, P.-O., and K. Rodahl. 1970. Textbook of Work Physiology. McGraw-Hill Book Co., New York.

Borg, G., and H. Linderholm. 1967. Perceived exertion and pulse rate during graded exercise in various age groups. Acta Med. Scand. (Suppl. 472):194–206.

Comroe, J. H., Jr., R. E. Forster, A. B. Dubois, W. A. Brisscoe, and E. Carlsen. 1967. The Lung. Clinical Physiology and Pulmonary Function Tests. 2nd Ed. Year Book Medical Publications, Chicago.

Ekblom, B. 1969. Effect of physical training in adolescent boys. J. Appl. Physiol. 27:350–355.

Eriksson, B. O., I. Engström, P. Karlberg, B. Saltin, and C. Thorén. 1971. A physiological analysis of former girl swimmers. Acta Paediatr. Scand. 60(Suppl. 217):68–72.

Eriksson, B. O., I. Engström, P. Karlberg, B. Saltin, and C. Thorén, 1978. Long-term effect of previous swimtraining in girls. A 10-year follow-up of the "girl swimmers." Acta Paediatr. Scand. 67:285–292.

Eriksson, B. O., A. Lundin, and B. Saltin. 1975. Cardiopulmonary function in former girl swimmers and the effects of physical training. Scand. J. Clin. Lab. Invest. 35:135–145.

Eriksson, B. O., C. Thorén, I. Engström, and P. Karlberg. 1967. Influence of physical training on growth. A study of girl swimmers. Acta Paediatr. Scand. 56(Suppl. 177):84–85.

Kjellberg, S. R., U. Rudhe, and T. Sjöstrand. 1949. The relation of cardiac volume to the weight and surface of the body, the blood volume and the physical capacity for work. Acta Radiol. 31:113–122.

Kubicek, W. G., J. N. Karnegis, R. P. Pattersson, D. A. Witsoe, and R. H. Mattson. 1966. Development and evaluation of an impedance cardiac output system. Aerosp. Med. 37:1208–1221.

Saltin, B., L. H. Hartley, Å. Kilbom, and I. Åstrand. 1969. Physical training in sedentary middle-aged and older men. II. Oxygen uptake, heart rate and blood lactate concentration at submaximal and maximal exercise. Scand. J. Clin. Lab. Invest. 24:323–334.

Scholander, P. F. 1947. Analyzer for accurate estimation of respiratory gases in one-half cubic centimeter samples. J. Biol. Chem. 167:235–250.

Scholz, R., H. Schmitz, T. Bücher, and J. O. Lampen. 1950. Concerning the effect of Nystatin on yeast (in German). Biochem. Z. 331:71–86.

Williams, J. A., and J. Fine. 1961. Measurement of blood volume with a new apparatus. N. Engl. J. Med. 264:842–848.

Experience of Pulse-conducted Ergometry in Trained, Normal, and Physically Inactive Schoolchildren

M.-L. Hursti, L. Pihlakoski, K. Antila, L. Halkola, and I. Välimäki

The pulse-conducted exercise ECG test (PCXT) was originally designed by Arstila (1972) as a general-purpose clinical ergometric test. In a recent review by Arstila et al. (1977) concerning more than 10,000 test procedures in five laboratories, the PCXT appeared feasible for the great majority of test subjects above the age of 7 years, as well as for disabled, untrained, unmotivated, and aged individuals. We think that this follows from the basic principle of the PCXT, commencing at a zero load and individually increasing the load up to the subjective maximum tolerance of the patient, as well as from the noninvasive nature of the test. The automated test procedure (Välimäki et al., 1978) was developed for mass screening and epidemiological purposes, but so far our experience in pediatric field studies is limited.

Recently plans were made for an epidemiological study to investigate various determinants of the physical condition of Finnish schoolchildren (Härkönen et al., 1977). The purposes of the present pilot study were 1) to evaluate whether or not the automated PCXT could be utilized as a practical and sensitive ergometric technique in a large project such as this, and 2) to determine the discrimination power of noninvasive techniques in the estimation of cardiac pump function under exercise conditions in preselected small groups of physically inactive, normal, and well trained schoolchildren.

TEST SUBJECTS

A total of 37 schoolchildren was studied: physically well trained (9 boys and 7 girls), normal physical activity (6 boys and 6 girls), and physically

This project has been supported by the Finnish Research Council for Physical Education and Sports, and the Juho Vainio Foundation, Finland.

inactive (6 boys and 3 girls). The ages of the subjects were from 11 to 13 years. The well trained children regularly participated in track and field training and competitions, having been systematically trained for at least 1 year. The normally active and inactive children were selected from the pupils of a primary school in the city of Turku by means of interviewing the children themselves, their classmates, and their teachers. The children represented all social classes. All children were healthy and of average stature; none of them was obese. Their heights and weights are given in Table 1.

METHODS

Each subject performed a multiparametric exercise test (PCXT) on a bicycle ergometer (Elema-Schönander). A continuous triangular loading profile was generated, increasing the heart rate by a 8 b.p.m.[2] by the automatic control unit (Välimäki et al., 1978) of the ergometer (Figure 1). The duration of the test was 9–12 min. In addition to the ergometric parameters (total work, PWC_{170}), the systolic time intervals (STI), pre-ejection period (PEP), and left ventricular ejection time (LVET) were estimated by recording the carotid pulse, ECG, and phonocardiogram prior to and immediately after the exercise. Impedance cardiographic records were also taken simultaneously with the carotid pulse and phonocardiogram. This technique proved useful for continuous monitoring of the LVET, but was unreliable for estimation of the cardiac output [see also Betz (1978)]. Therefore, the impedance signal was used as a supplementary signal for STI only (Äärimaa and Ylitalo, 1977; Balasubramanian et al., 1978).

The student's t test was used to test the statistical significance of the intergroup differences of the output of the ergometric procedures. Linear regression/correlation analysis was applied to relate the STI to the corresponding heart rate.

RESULTS

A typical example of the ergometric output is depicted in Figure 1. The test could be carried out under automatic control in all subjects. The maximal heart rates (Table 1) indicate that the maximal level of exercise intensity was reasonably well achieved. No significant intergroup differences were found between the heart rates and blood pressures of the three groups of subjects (Table 1).

ERGOMETRIC OUTPUT

The ergometric parameters of the subjects (PWC_{170} as graphically estimated from the loading curve of the PCXT and the total work as a time

130

Table 1. Heights, weights, and values of heart rate (HR) and blood pressure (BP) at rest and during maximal exercise in 37 children, ages 11 to 13 years

Group		Girls			Boys		
		Active (N=7)	Normal (N=6)	Inactive (N=3)	Active (N=9)	Normal (N=6)	Inactive (N=6)
Height (cm)	$\bar{x}$	151.1	149.1	156.6	153.6	157.1	148.3
	range	139.2–168.0	145.4–157.1	139.6–166.6	144.5–166.5	147.0–166.5	140.5–159.1
Weight (kg)	$\bar{x}$	35.4	38.6	54.0	38.2	48.2	38.3
	range	29.4–41.4	35.6–46.0	46.0–67.2	29.6–46.0	39.0–56.5	28.8–55.0
HR at rest (b.p.m.)	$\bar{x}$	61	77	71	64	71	71
	range	50–75	65–90	66–73	60–75	48–87	62–92
HR_{max} (b.p.m.)	$\bar{x}$	200	196	177	203	178	189
	range	192–207	185–204	168–190	183–220	152–198	175–203
BP_{syst} (mm Hg)	$\bar{x}$	103	118	117	119	118	100
	range	90–120	110–130	110–120	110–130	110–140	85–125
BP_{diast} (mm Hg)	$\bar{x}$	71	78	80	77	77	74
	range	65–80	65–90	70–90	60–90	60–90	65–90
$BP_{syst\ max}$ (mm Hg)	$\bar{x}$	156	150	153	164	165	142
	range	140–180	140–170	140–160	150–180	150–180	130–160
$BP_{diast\ max}$ (mm Hg)	$\bar{x}$	63	69	70	62	78	72
	range	50–80	60–80	60–80	50–80	60–110	60–90

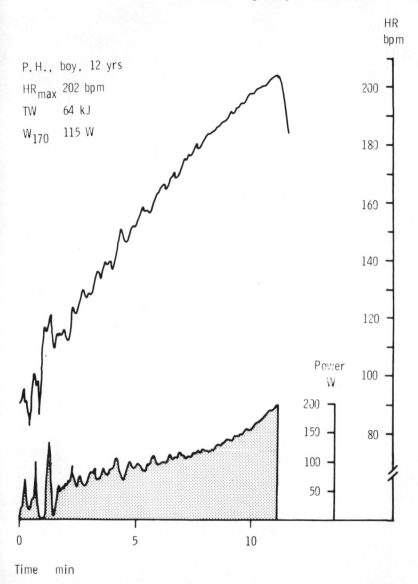

Figure 1.   Typical patterns of the simultaneous plots of the heart rate and ergometric braking power during PCXT (acceleration 8 b.p.m.²). The hatched area indicates the total work.

integral of the load), computed per kg of body weight, are shown in Figure 2 and Table 2. The means of PWC_{170} for active, normal, and inactive boys (Figure 2a, Table 2) were 3.44, 3.37, and 3.09 W/kg, respectively. The corresponding figures for girls were 3.38, 2.91, and 2.47 W/kg, respectively. The intergroup differences were almost significant ($p < 0.05$) only between the active and inactive girls (Table 2). The respec-

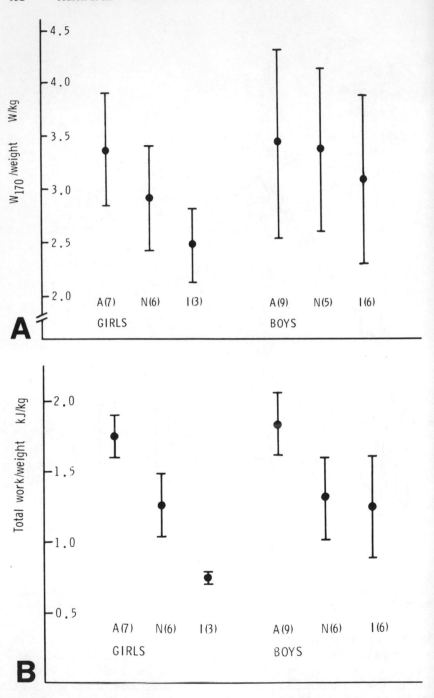

Figure 2.   A) W_{170} in relation to body weight in 36 schoolchildren. B) Total work in relation to body weight in 37 schoolchildren. A = active, N = normal, and I = inactive children. Circles indicate the mean, bars indicate ± 1 SD.

Table 2. Relative values of PWC_{170} and total work in 37 children, ages 11 to 13 years

		Boys			Girls		
		Active	Normal	Inactive	Active	Normal	Inactive
N		9	5[a]	6	7	6	3
PWC_{170}/kg (W/kg)	$\bar{x}$	3.44	3.37	3.09	3.38[b]	2.91	2.47[b]
	SD	0.88	0.75	0.78	0.51	0.84	0.35
N		9	6	6	7	6	3
Total work/kg (kJ/kg)	$\bar{x}$	1.84[c]	1.31[c]	1.25[c]	1.74[d]	1.26[c,d]	0.76[c,d]
	SD	0.22	0.28	0.36	0.16	0.22	0.03

[a]One case with HR_{max} of 152 b.p.m. was rejected.
[b]$p < 0.05$ between active and inactive girls.
[c]$p < 0.01$ between active and normal and between active and inactive boys; between normal and inactive girls.
[d]$p < 0.001$ between active and normal and between active and inactive girls.

Table 3. Correlation between the systolic time intervals and heart rate in 37 children, ages 11 to 13 years

Linear regression equation			Standard error of the estimate	Correlation coefficient
At rest	LVET	= -2.19 HR + 451 msec	13.1	-0.86
	PEP	= -0.03 HR + 96.6 msec	17.2	-0.20
	QS$_2$[a]	= -2.23 HR + 548 msec	17.0	-0.79
Postexercise	LVET	= -1.71 HR + 433 msec	17.8	-0.74
	PEP	= -0.30 HR + 118 msec	14.9	-0.23
	QS$_2$	= -2.00 HR + 550 msec	16.7	-0.81

[a]Time from onset of Q wave to onset of second heart sound.

tive corresponding data of the total work (Figure 2b, Table 2) were 1.84, 1.32, and 1.25 kJ/kg for the three groups of boys; and 1.74, 1.26, and 0.76 kJ/kg for the girls. These intergroup differences between the active, normal, and inactive children proved to be significant ($p < 0.01$) except between normal and inactive boys (Table 2).

The ergometric data were also computed using the new formula for body surface area (Haycock et al., 1978) where both height and weight were considered, and nearly identical results were obtained.

HEMODYNAMIC OUTPUT (STI)

The values of STI were used to compute the regression of LVET and PEP in relation to heart rate (Table 3). For the regression analysis, all three subgroups were combined because no significant differences could be detected between the clusters of LVET of inactive, normal, and active children. However, the active group appeared to show larger LVET and lower heart rate, particularly at rest. We therefore amplified this effect by combining the influence of the LVET and PEP and computed the PEP:LVET ratios for the individual groups at rest and after exercise (Figure 3). The PEP:LVET ratio was lowest in the active children and highest in the inactive ones, indicating a better pump function in the active subjects. Although the difference between the active and inactive groups indicated the same trend in both sexes—both at rest and after exercise—it proved almost significant ($p < 0.05$) only in the boys after exercise.

DISCUSSION

Several ergometric methods currently in use were recently reviewed by Thorén (1978). It is often questionable to introduce a new principle or technique for a laboratory test if a set of standardized, validated, and reliable procedures already exists. However, the triangular test offers certain advantages for automation of the procedure and for studies of car-

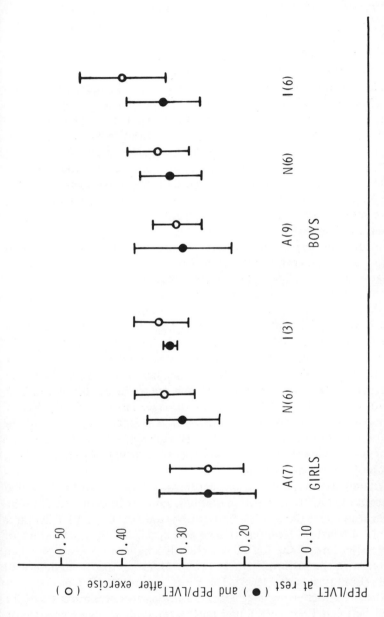

Figure 3.   Systolic time intervals PEP:LVET at rest and after exercise in 37 schoolchildren. A = active, N = normal, and I = inactive children. Circles indicate the mean, bars indicate ± 1 SD.

diac control, in adults as well as children (Arstila, 1972; Petäjoki et al., 1974; Antila et al., 1978; Välimäki et al., 1978). The present pilot study clearly demonstrated the discrimination power of the PCXT as a means of estimating the work capacity of children with different physical activity levels.

The ergometric output of the PCXT, total work, proved to be superior to the submaximal PWC_{170}, the latter having been previously used by several investigators [see Thorén (1978) and Petäjoki et al. (1974)].

Details of the influences of physical training on children at the ages of 11–13 years have been previously described in long range studies (Eriksson and Koch, 1973; Thorén et al., 1973). The increased physical performance has been attributed to the elevation of maximal oxygen uptake due to increased cardiac stroke volume (Eriksson and Koch, 1973). On the basis of this, it is understandable that a difference could be clearly detected in the relative values of total work of the well trained group versus the other groups in the present study. It is often presumed that children are spontaneously physically active and they are fitter than adults. However, as indicated in this study, a group of healthy, nonobese inactive children could be selected in a normal school population whose physical capacity was considerably lower than that of the other children of the same age and/or size. The mean relative values of total work were lower in this inactive group than in a corresponding group of obese schoolchildren in our city (Ylitalo, 1978, personal communication). Therefore, this inactive group appears interesting from the points of view of both physical education and public health.

The systolic time intervals have been considered a convenient noninvasive method for the estimation of cardiac hemodynamics. The LVET has a high correlation to the heart rate, but not to the age of the child; on the contrary, the PEP correlates better with age. The ratio PEP:LVET is independent of both (Spitaels et al., 1974). The linear regression of the LVET in our group at rest was steeper (LVET = 451.5 − 2.19 heart rate) than the ones reviewed by Spitaels et al. (1974), probably because of our inclusion of the trained group.

Dynamic exercise caused considerable abbreviation of the PEP and LVET in our subjects, as has been found in adults (Lindqvist et al., 1973). The heart rate–targeted test has been found to abbreviate LVET in adults more than a constant load test (Lance and Spodick, 1975). The slope of the regression line of the LVET was slightly smaller after exercise when compared with the resting situation (Table 3), as has also been described in adults (Lindqvist et al., 1973). The abbreviation of LVET has been attributed to the increasing afterload; however, no correlation could be detected between PEP:LVET and the corresponding blood pressure in our study, as could be found in an earlier study of adults (Lindqvist et al., 1973). The regression line of the PEP was steeper in the postexercise phase than at rest (Table 3). However, the slope changed considerably less (-0.03 at rest, -0.30 postexercise) in our study than in adults (-0.44 at rest, -0.91 postexercise) in the study of Lindqvist et al. (1973).

Our values of the PEP:LVET ratio for the normals were of the same magnitude as in the study of Spitaels et al. (1974). The boys tended to show higher PEP:LVET ratios than the girls. The ratio PEP:LVET increased in all groups as a response to exercise (Figure 3). This is at variance with the corresponding result of Lindqvist et al. (1973) in adults. The difference between these studies may be attributed to the different behavior of the PEP. In children, the PEP has been found much less heart rate dependent than in adults (Spitaels et al., 1974). In the present study, the correlation between the heart rate and PEP was also very low (Table 3). The active groups had the lowest and the inactive groups the highest mean PEP:LVET ratios, both at rest and after exercise, although the intergroup difference was almost significant only between the inactive and active boys after exercise. The results demonstrated that the hemodynamic responses of the three activity groups to the exercise test were similar but the level of function of the heart varied with each group.

REFERENCES

Äärimaa, T., and V. Ylitalo. 1977. Feasibility of impedance cardiography in estimation of left ventricular ejection time (LVET) in neonates. Proceedings of the XVth International Congress of Pediatrics, New Delhi, Abstract 107/03, p. 13.

Antila, K., M.-L. Petäjoki, M. Arstila, and I. Välimäki. 1978. Tape recording of electrocardiogram during exercise testing in children and adolescents. In: S. Stern, (ed.), Ambulatory ECG Monitoring, pp. 69–75. Year Book Medical Publishers, Inc., Chicago.

Arstila, M. 1972. Pulse-conducted triangular exercise-ECG test. A feedback system regulating work during exercise. Acta Med. Scand. 529 (Suppl. 529).

Arstila, M., H. Wendelin, I. Vuori, and I. Välimäki. 1977. Pulse-conducted exercise test. A review (in Finnish). Duodecim 93:568–579.

Balasubramanian, V., O. P., Mathew, A. Behl, S. C. Tewari, and R. S. Hoon. 1978. Electrical impedance cardiogram in derivation of systolic time intervals. Br. Heart J. 40:268–275.

Betz, R. 1978. Analysis of impedance cardiography as a method for the determination of stroke volume (in German). M.D. Dissertation, Ludwig Maximilians-Universität, München.

Eriksson, B. O., and G. Koch. 1973. Effect of physical training on hemodynamic response during submaximal and maximal exercise in 11–13 year old boys. Acta Physiol. 87:27–39.

Härkönen, M., R. Telama, O. Wasz-Höckert, and I. Välimäki. 1977. Physically active child. A project plan for a multicenter study on the physical activity of Finnish school children. Unpublished paper.

Haycock, G. B., G. J. Schwartz, and D. H. Wisotsky. 1978. Geometric method for measuring body surface area: A height-weight formula validated in infants, children and adults J. Pediatr. 93:62–66.

Lance, V., and D. Spodick. 1975. Constant-load versus heart-rate targeted exercise: Responses of systolic time intervals. J. Appl. Physiol. 38:794–800.

Lindqvist, V., R. Spangler, and S. G. Blount. 1973. A comparison between the effects of dynamic and isometric exercise as evaluated by the systolic time intervals in normal man. Am. Heart J. 85:227–236.

Petäjoki, M.-L., M. Arstila, and I. Välimäki. 1974. Pulse-conducted exercise test in children. Acta Paediatr. Belg. 28(Suppl.):40–47.

Spitaels, S., R. Arbogast, J. C. Fouron, and A. Davignon. 1974. The influence of heart rate and age on the systolic and diastolic time intervals in children. Circulation 49:1107–1115.

Thorén, C. 1978. Exercise testing in children. Paediatrician 7:100–115.

Thorén, C., U. Seliger, M. Mácek, J. Vavra, and J. Rutenfranz. 1973. The influence of training on physical fitness in healthy children and children with chronic diseases. In: F. Linneweh (ed.), Current Aspects of Perinatology and Physiology in Children, pp. 81–112. Springer Verlag, Berlin.

Välimäki, I., M.-L. Petäjoki, M. Arstila, P. Viherä, and H. Wendelin. 1978. Automatically controlled ergometer for pulse-conducted exercise test. Med. Sport 11:47.

Training Effect on the Anaerobic Performance of Children as Measured by the Wingate Anaerobic Test

A. Grodjinovsky, O. Inbar, R. Dotan, and O. Bar-Or

Some drawbacks of existing laboratory tests of anaerobic performance in humans are cost, invasive nature, relative complexity, and unclear validity. An effort has been directed in recent years toward the development of simpler, yet accurate, reliable, and valid tests (Margaria et al., 1966; Cumming, 1972; Szögy and Cherebetiu, 1974). In our laboratory, a 30-sec all-out pedaling test (Wingate Anaerobic Test, WAnT) was developed and found reliable (Ayalon et al., 1974; Bar-Or et al., 1977), valid (Inbar et al., 1976; Inbar and Bar-Or, 1977; Bar-Or and Inbar, 1978; Bar-Or, 1979), simple, and feasible (Bar-Or et al., 1977). Performance in this test was found related to preponderance of fast twitch muscle fibers (Inbar et al., 1979; Bar-Or et al., 1980).

The purpose of this study was to determine whether or not the WAnT is sensitive in detecting changes in anaerobic performance induced by a short and moderately intense anaerobic training program in children 11–13 years old.

SUBJECTS AND METHODS

Fifty boys enrolled in the sixth grade of an elementary school located in Natanya, Israel, participated in this study. They represented the full male population of their respective classes. The study comprised a 6-week training period preceded and followed by the WAnT.

This study was performed, in part, by a grant from the Sports and Physical Education Authority, Ministry of Education and Culture, Israel.

The Wingate Anaerobic Test

Following a 12-min warm-up on a bicycle ergometer (heart rate reaching some 150 b.p.m.), the child rested for 4–5 min and then performed the WAnT. The Fleisch ergometer was used, in which one pedal revolution causes a 10-m advance at the flywheel. Resistance was relative to the subject's body weight (45 g/kg). To the command "start," the child began to pedal as fast as he could. To overcome inertia, the initial resistance was very low, but it quickly increased, and within 2–3 sec reached the prescribed level. At that stage, the electrically triggered counter and the stopwatch were activated and measurements began. The number of revolutions was recorded at 5-sec intervals for a total of 30-sec. Mechanical output every 5 sec was calculated in absolute terms (kgm/min) and relative to body weight (kgm/kg•min). Total mechanical work in 30 sec and the peak 5-sec power output were taken as indices of "anaerobic capacity" and "anaerobic power," respectively (Margaria, 1966, 1967). The difference between the peak 5-sec output and the lowest 5-sec output, divided by the time elapsed between the two points, was calculated. The value thus obtained was taken as an index of fatigue.

Training

The subjects were randomly divided into two training groups and one control group (C) that did not train. The training lasted 6 weeks, and was carried out 3 times per week (total of 18 sessions). One group trained using only a bicycle ergometer (B) and the other performed only sprint running (S). The S group initially ran three all-out 40-m runs followed by three all-out 150-m runs in each training session. Times were recorded to motivate the children. The number of runs was progressively increased every 2 weeks in order to maintain adequate training intensity. A training session of the B group consisted initially of pedaling three 8-sec all-out riding bouts followed by three 30-sec all-out rides. The number of rides was subsequently increased as described above. The quantity of the two training regimens was equated by the duration of the respective activities. Their quality was equated by having the subjects perform each effort maximally.

Data Analysis

To evaluate the training effect within each group, a student t test was used. For the between-groups comparisons, an analysis of covariance was used, posttraining values being the dependent variable and the pretraining values the covariate.

RESULTS

Power output at 5-sec intervals during the anaerobic test is demonstrated in Figure 1. A trend toward an increase in output during the posttraining

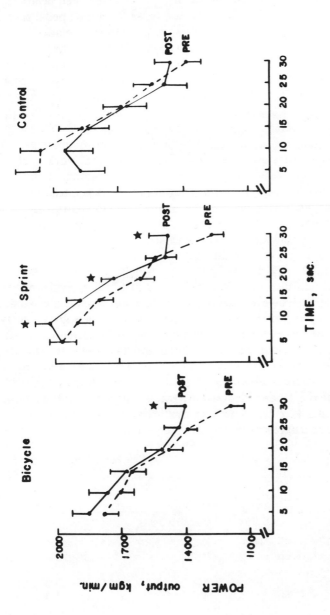

Figure 1.   Number of pedal revolutions during the WAnT. Values are mean ± 1 SD. * denotes $p < 0.05$.

Table 1.   Anaerobic capacity of the three groups prior to and following training

| | | Total anaerobic capacity | | | | | |
| | | kgm/min | | | kgm/min·kg | | |
Group		Pre	Post	% Change	Pre	Post	% Change
Bicycle ($N = 17$)	$\bar{x}$	1534.3	1607.4	+ 4.8[a]	43.7	45.2	+ 3.4[b]
	SE	57.6	65.2		1.0	1.2	
Sprint ($N = 19$)	$\bar{x}$	1678.2	1760.9	+ 4.9[b]	43.6	45.2	+ 3.7[b]
	SE	55.6	53.6		1.3	1.3	
Control ($N = 14$)	$\bar{x}$	1765.3	1710.4	− 3.1	45.2	43.0	− 4.9
	SE	94.0	89.6		1.2	1.7	

[a]Significant at the 1% level (between pre- and posttraining).
[b]Significant at the 5% level (between pre- and posttraining).

test compared with output of the pretraining test was evident at almost every stage of the test in both training groups, but not among the controls. Anaerobic capacity in absolute values, as well as per kg of body weight, prior to and at the end of the training period are presented in Table 1. The two training groups, but not the control group, improved their anaerobic capacity (total as well as per kg of body weight) by some 3.5%–5%. A similar trend was also evident in the effect of training on the anaerobic power (Table 2). However, the training effect was statistically significant only in the bicycle group. Individual performance (anaerobic capacity) of all participants before and after training is plotted in Figure 2. When the slope representing fatigue was calculated and a comparison between the pre- and posttraining slopes made, no significant differences were found in any of the groups studied. However, a small reduction in power output during the final 5 sec is evident in both training groups, but not among the controls (Figure 1). F ratios between the three groups for anaerobic capacity and for anaerobic power are summarized in Table 3.

Table 2.   Peak anaerobic power output during 5 sec prior to and following training ($\bar{x} \pm$ SE)

| | | Peak anaerobic power | | | | | |
| | | kgm/min | | | kgm/kg·min | | |
Group		Pre	Post	% Change	Pre	Post	% Change
Bicycle ($N = 17$)	$\bar{x}$	1806.1	1902.0	+ 5.3[a]	51.4	53.4	+ 3.9[a]
	SE	65.9	85.0		1.0	1.4	
Sprint ($N = 19$)	$\bar{x}$	1985.7	2075.8	+ 4.5	51.4	53.0	+ 3.1
	SE	78.0	69.3		1.4	1.3	
Control ($N = 14$)	$\bar{x}$	2123.9	2063.5	− 2.8	54.4	51.7	− 5.0
	SE	114.7	113.9		1.3	2.0	

[a]Significant at the 5% level (between pre- and posttraining).

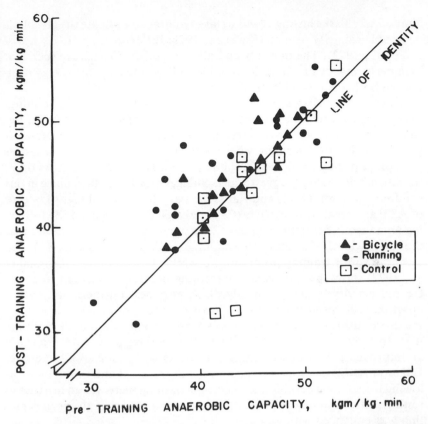

Figure 2.   Individual data of the anaerobic capacity by groups. Comparison between pre- and posttraining.

DISCUSSION

The ability to perform short supramaximal tasks is dependent on, among other factors, anaerobic power (the alactacid component of the oxygen deficit) and anaerobic capacity (the lactacid component) (Margaria, 1966; Houston and Thomson, 1977). A performance test to evaluate the alactacid component should represent the top effort of the subject and last

Table 3.   Differences between adjusted mean improvements—F values (analysis of covariance)

Group	Anaerobic capacity	Anaerobic power
Sprint vs. control	7.54[a]	1.22
Bicycle vs. control	4.77[b]	1.97
Bicycle vs. sprint	0.61	0.09

[a]Significant at 1% level.
[b]Significant at 5% level.

about 6 sec. Tasks lasting 20–60 sec are required to evaluate the glycolytic anaerobic capacity of man (Karlsson, 1971; Eriksson et al., 1972; Karlsson et al., 1972). The intensity and duration of the WAnT are such that high performance on this task probably reflects a fast rate of energy turnover in both alactic and lactic components.

The results of this study indicate a mild, but significant, training-related improvement in performance of the WAnT among children. Because no measurements were taken in this study at the muscle cell level, it is not possible to determine what histological and biochemical changes took place during the 6-week training period. However, data from other training studies would suggest which changes may have taken place in our children. Karlsson (1971) and Karlsson et al. (1972) found that the stores of ATP and creatine phosphate (CP) increased by as much as 25% following an anaerobic training regimen. Thorstensson et al. (1975) found that the activity level of creatine phosphokinase (CPK) increased by 36% following a sprint training program of 8 weeks. Other studies (Karlsson et al., 1972) show that an anaerobic training program will result in an increased activity level of some glycolytic enzymes. Furthermore, such a program will speed up the breakdown of glycogen to lactic acid and, therefore, using this pathway, supply larger quantities of ATP per time unit. In some cases (Fox, 1975), such changes have been shown to cause an improved performance during aerobic as well as anaerobic exercise. Eriksson (1972) investigated children 11–13 years old and found that following a combined aerobic and anaerobic training there was an increase in resting value of muscle ATP, CP, and glycogen, and that glycogen depletion was enhanced with exercise.

Assuming that similar training-related changes have taken place in the muscle cells of our subjects who belonged to the two training groups, the results of this study indicate that the WAnT is sensitive in reflecting changes in the anaerobic capacity of children, as produced by a moderate training program. This is indicated by the significant improvement of the anaerobic capacity of the two training groups, but not of the control group. One can assume that more intense training programs would have caused even greater improvement in performance in the WAnT. To determine whether a causative relationship exists between improved performance in the Wingate Anaerobic Test and muscle cell histological and biochemical changes, a longitudinal study should be performed in which all variables are periodically measured and correlated.

ACKNOWLEDGMENTS

The authors express their appreciation to Hinda Anenberg, Sara Erez, Dinah Figenbaum, Ira Jacobs, and Uri Goldbourt for their devotion and valuable assistance.

REFERENCES

Ayalon, A., O. Inbar, and O. Bar-Or. 1974. Relationship among measurements of explosive strength and anaerobic power. In: R. C. Nelson and C. A. Morehouse (eds.), Biomechanics IV. International Series on Sport Sciences. Vol. 1, pp. 527–577. University Park Press, Baltimore.

Bar-Or, O. 1979. A new anaerobic capacity test—characteristics and applications. Proceedings of the 21st World Congress on Sport Medicine. In press.

Bar-Or, O., R. Dotan, O. Inbar, A. Rothstein, J. Karlsson, and P. Tesch. 1980. Anaerobic capacity and fiber type distribution in man. Int. J. Sports Med. In press.

Bar-Or, O., and O. Inbar. 1978. Relationship among anaerobic capacity sprint and middle distance running of school children. In: R. J. Shephard and H. Lavallée (eds.), Physical Fitness Assessment—Principles, Practice, and Application, pp. 142–147. Charles C Thomas, Springfield, Ill.

Bar-Or, O., O. Inbar, and R. Dotan. 1977. A 30-sec all-out ergometric test: Its reliability and validity for anaerobic capacity. Isr. J. Med. Sci. 13(Abstr.):326.

Cumming, G. R. 1972. Correlation of athletic performance and aerobic power in 12 to 17 year-old children with bone age, calf muscle, total body potassium, heart volume and two indices of anaerobic power. In: O. Bar-Or (ed.), Proceedings of the Fourth International Symposium on Pediatric Work Physiology, pp. 109–134. Wingate Institute, Israel.

Eriksson, B. O. 1972. Physical training, oxygen supply and muscle metabolism in 11–13 year-old boys. Acta Physiol. Scand. Suppl. 384:1–48.

Eriksson, B. O., P. Gollnick, and B. Saltin. 1973. Muscle metabolism and enzyme activities after training in boys 11–13 years old. Acta Physiol. Scand. 87:485–497.

Fox, E. L. 1975. Differences in metabolic alterations with sprint versus endurance interval training. In: H. Howald and J. Poortmans (eds.), Metabolic Adaptation to Prolonged Physical Exercise, pp. 119–126. Birkhauser Verlag, Basel.

Houston, M. E., and J. A. Thomson. 1977. The response of endurance-adapted adults to intense anaerobic training. Eur. J. Appl. Physiol. 36:207–213.

Inbar, O., and O. Bar-Or. 1977. Anaerobic capacity and running performance of children. Isr. J. Med. Sci. 13:1141. Abstract.

Inbar, O., R. Dotan, and O. Bar-Or. 1976. Aerobic and anaerobic components of a 30 second supermaximal cycling test. Med. Sci. Sports 8:51. Abstract.

Inbar, O., P. Kaiser, R. Dotan, O. Bar-Or, R. Schéle, and J. Karlsson. 1979. Indices of the Wingate Anaerobic Test, fiber-type distribution and running performance in man. Med. Sci. Sports. 11:89.

Karlsson, J. 1971. Lactate and phosphagen concentration in working muscle of man. Acta Physiol. Scand. Suppl. 358.

Karlsson, J., L. Nordesjö, L. Jorfeldt, and B. Saltin. 1972. Muscle lactate, ATP and CP levels during exercise after physical training in man. J. Appl. Physiol. 33:199–203.

Margaria, R. 1966. Assessment of physical activity in oxidative and aerobic maximal exercise. Int. Z. Angew. Physiol. Arbeitsphysiol. 22:115–124.

Margaria, R. 1967. Anaerobic metabolism in muscle. Can. Med. Assoc. J. 96:770–774.

Margaria, R., P. Aghemo, and E. Rovelli. 1966. Measurement of muscular power (anaerobic) in man. J. Appl. Physiol. 21:1662–1664.

Szögy, A., and G. A. Cherebetiu. 1974. One minute bicycle ergometer test for determination of anaerobic capacity. Eur. J. Appl. Physiol. 33:171–176.

Thorstensson, A., B. Sjödin, and J. Karlsson. 1975. Enzyme activities and muscle strength after "sprint training" in man. Acta Physiol. Scand. 94:313–318.

Habitual Physical Activity

Longitudinal Studies of the Changes in Habitual Physical Activity of Schoolchildren and Working Adolescents

J. Ilmarinen and J. Rutenfranz

The physical work capacity of adults is known to be associated with the level of habitual physical activity. At school age, however, this relationship seems to be less clear (Watson and O'Donovan, 1977). It can be assumed that, up to the age of 12 years, the effects of extra training are rather limited. Between the ages of 12 and 16 years training may increase the functional capacities of the heart and the lungs, but with detraining the changes soon disappear (Eriksson et al., 1978). After the age of 15, the negative effects of a lack of regular training are obvious (Rutenfranz et al., 1978).

After the age of 16, lifestyle appears to change, and the possibilities for participation in sports and other physical activities seem to diminish. In the Federal Republic of Germany, boys and girls in secondary school are required to attend physical education classes, but the pupils in vocational schools or in vocational training are not. In fact, Rutenfranz and Lederle-Schenk (1968) found that the majority of such adolescents in Dortmund had no leisure-time physical activity.

This transition period from school to work, and its effects on young adults, has been incompletely studied with respect to physical activity. Therefore, a longitudinal investigation was undertaken to determine the possible changes that occur in leisure-time physical activity and physical work capacity during this period.

A side-effect of the fact that the study was longitudinal should have been a greater interest in leisure-time sport activities. This was also found in a small group of schoolchildren who improved the $\dot{V}_{O_2 \, max}$ about 8.5% by cross-country running two times a week after school hours for 3 months (Ilmarinen et al., 1979).

The present report is a part of this longitudinal study and concerns the data of four retrospective questionnaires, which were completed annually, concerning habitual physical activity and maximal aerobic power ($\dot{V}_{O_2 \, max}$) at the ages of 16 and 17 years.

SUBJECTS

The subjects were 25 girls and 26 boys living in a rural inland community in the Federal Republic of Germany. They were all 14 years of age at the beginning of the study and had agreed to participate in a longitudinal and cross-sectional investigation of the physical activity and physical work capacity of youth.

At the age of 16, the children in the rural areas choose between school and vocational training, or looking for a job. Of the boys only 7 (27%) continued in school, and 19 (73%) either began vocational training or found work. About half of the girls (48%) stayed at school (school group) and the other half (occupational group) went to work.

METHODS

Habitual physical activity was assessed in four annual retrospective interviews with a standardized questionnaire. The subjects were asked about their physical activities during the previous year.

The quality, quantity, and intensity of the physical activities were assessed as follows:

1. Quality: type of sport activities.
2. Quantity: average hours per month and number of months per year.
3. Intensity: average MET (multiple of basal metabolic rate) value of individual sport events, calculated according to standardized tables.

From all sports activities listed, the following two scores were calculated:

1. Yearly sports activity score: Σ hours per month•MET•months.
2. Monthly sports activity score: Σ hours per month•MET.

The $\dot{V}_{O_2 \, max}$ of the subjects at the ages of 16 and 17 was measured directly on a bicycle ergometer according to the method of the International Biological Program.

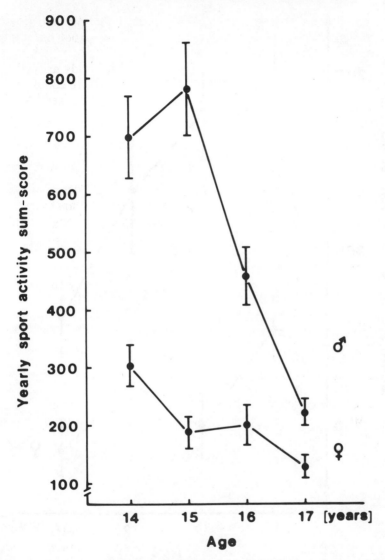

Figure 1.   The yearly sport activity score ($\bar{x} \pm$ SE) of the subjects between the ages of 14 and 17.

RESULTS

Sport Activity Scores between the Ages of 14 and 17

Figure 1 shows the variation in the yearly sport activity scores of the boys and girls during the 4 years of the study. For both sexes, the scores tended to decrease with age. A clear decrease was seen among the boys after the

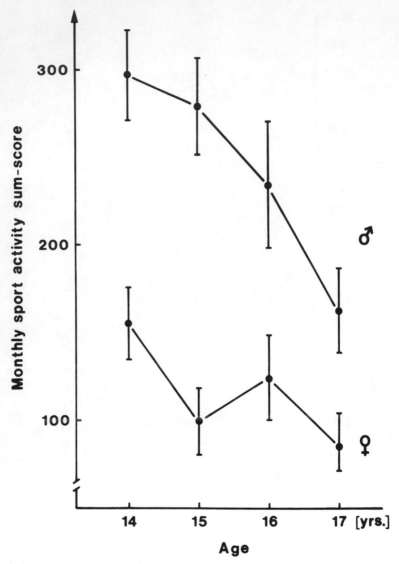

Figure 2.   The monthly sport activity score ($\bar{x} \pm$ SE) of the subjects between the ages of 14 and 17.

age of 15; i.e., by about 70% between the ages of 15 and 17. The yearly sport activity of the girls decreased between the ages of 14 and 17 by 57%. At the age of 15, the total sport activity score of the boys was about 4 times higher than that of the girls, but by the age of 17 the difference was only twofold.

The variation in the monthly activity scores is demonstrated in Figure 2. The same decreasing tendency that occurred in the yearly activity score can be seen. Although the scores of the boys steadily decreased between

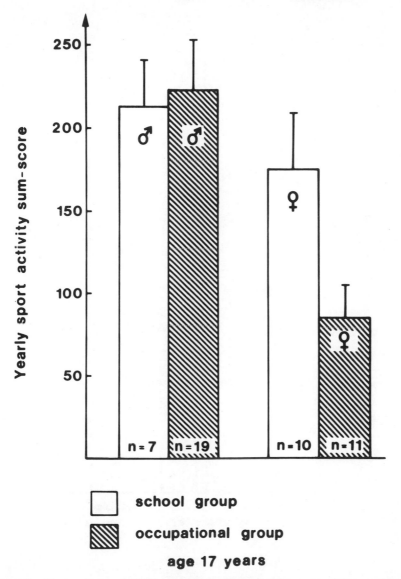

Figure 3.   The yearly sport activity scores of the school and occupational groups of boys and girls at the age of 17. The school girls were more active than the occupational girls ($p < 0.05$).

the ages of 14 and 17, those of the girls showed the clearest decrease between the ages of 14 and 15 years. The total decrease during the four years was 45% for both boys and girls.

Comparison of the School Group and the Occupational Group

Figure 3 shows the yearly activity scores of the boys and girls in the school group, and in the occupational group. Among the boys no difference was

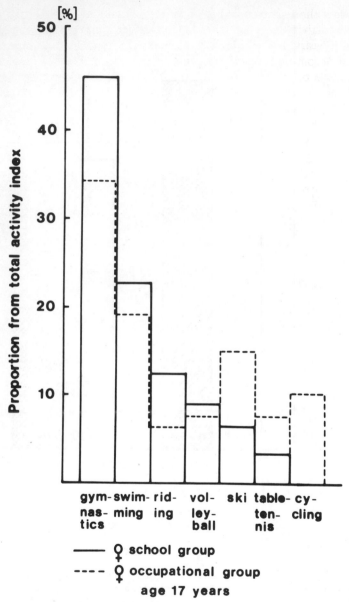

Figure 4.   Proportion of different sports in the total sport activity scores of school and occupational groups of girls at the age of 17.

found between the groups. However, the score of the school girls was 2
times higher than that of the girls in the occupational group. This difference was statistically significant ($p < 0.05$).

Figure 4 shows the contribution of individual activities to the total yearly sport activity score in the school and occupational groups of girls at the age of 17 years. Gymnastics was the most common, and swimming the second most common activity in both groups. Gymnastics represented 46% and 34% of the total sports score of the school and occupational groups, respectively. In aerobic endurance sport activities like swimming, the school group was more active, but in skiing and cycling the occupational group showed greater activity.

In the last year of the study, the $\dot{V}_{O_2 max}$ decreased by about 13% in both groups of girls (Figure 5). The occupational group showed about 5% higher absolute (liter/min) and 3% higher relative (ml/min•kg) values of $\dot{V}_{O_2 max}$ than the school group, but the differences were not statistically significant.

The proportions of the individual sports activities in the yearly score are shown in Figure 6 for the boys. Soccer accounted for the highest proportion in both groups. Although the $\dot{V}_{O_2 max}$ of the girls showed a decreasing tendency, the school group of boys maintained their absolute $\dot{V}_{O_2 max}$ (+2.0%), and only a small decrease in the relative value was found (−3.8%), as is shown in Figure 7. In the occupational group, both values decreased (−6.5% and −13.2%, respectively). The difference in $\dot{V}_{O_2 max}$ change between the occupational and school groups was significant ($p < 0.05$).

DISCUSSION

The main observation in this study was the decrease of sport activities with age. The decrease was more significant for the boys than for the girls, and, as Figures 1 and 2 show, the difference in physical activity level between the boys and girls lessens with age. This result agrees with those reported for more than 4000 Finnish school children (Telama, 1971).

It was further observed that the transition from the school environment to work life accelerated the decrease in participation in sport activities. This was particularly apparent for the occupational group of girls and may have been caused by many factors, e.g., an increase in other interests, as is often mentioned with girls, or tiredness resulting from the new daily occupational duties. We hope to know more about the different causes after the more detailed time-budget studies and the data on the continuous 24-hr recording of heart rate made annually for these adolescents have been analyzed. The $\dot{V}_{O_2 max}$ or its change between the ages of 16 and 17 was the same for both the school and occupational groups of girls, although the yearly sport activity scores differed significantly. One explanation may be that girls generally choose sport activities that are not aerobic in nature.

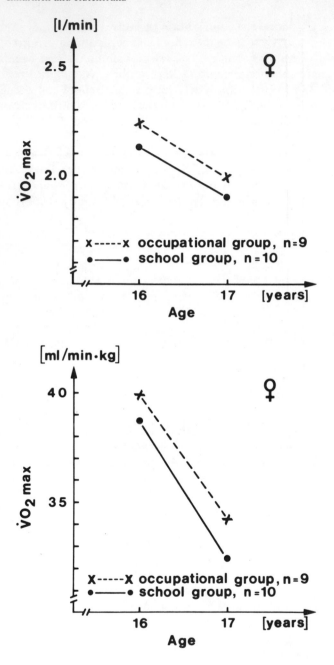

Figure 5.   The change in maximal aerobic power ($\dot{V}_{O_2\,max}$) of the school and occupational groups of girls between the ages of 16 and 17.

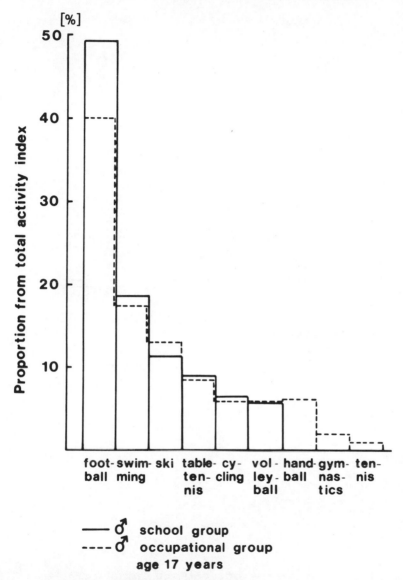

Figure 6.   Proportion of different sports in the total sport activity scores of the school and occupational groups of boys at the age of 17.

Summarized from the point of view of occupational work physiology, work capacity and leisure time physical activity tend to decrease, especially among girls, as adolescents leave the school environment and enter work life. If this decreasing tendency continues after the age of 17, the demands of work could overload working adolescents and young adults and lead to occupational health problems later in life.

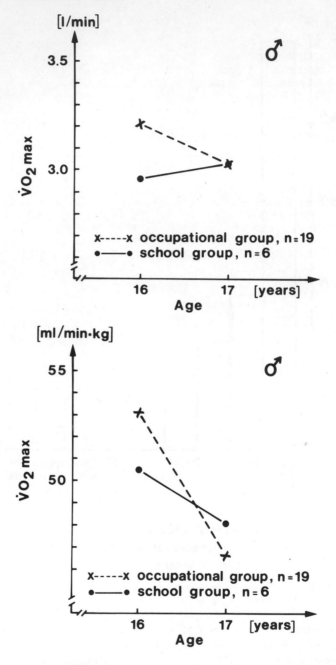

Figure 7.   The change in maximal aerobic power ($\dot{V}O_{2\,max}$) of the school and occupational groups of boys between the age of 16 and 17. The change in $\dot{V}O_{2\,max}$ (liters/min) between occupational and school boys was significant ($p < 0.05$).

REFERENCES

Eriksson, B. O., I. Engström, P. Karlberg, A. Lundin, B. Saltin, and C. Thorén. 1978. Long-term effect of previous swim training in girls. A 10-year follow-up of the "girl swimmers." Acta Pediatr. Scand. 67:285–292.

Ilmarinen, J., J. Rutenfranz, and M. Achenbach. 1979. Some problems of assessing the maximal aerobic power and the daily physical activity of school children in longitudinal and intervention studies. International Congress of Physical Education Evaluation, Jyväskylä, Finland, June 28–July 3, 1976. Report of the Finnish Society for Research in Sport and Physical Education 64:165–176.

Rutenfranz, J., J. Ilmarinen, and R. Ilmarinen. 1978. Aspects of work physiology for special youth positions (in German). Der Kinderarzt 2:193–201; 3:329–333.

Rutenfranz, J., and U. Lederle-Schenk. 1968. School sport and sporting interests upon growing up (in German). Die Berliner Ärztekammer, pp. 408–410.

Telama, R. 1971. Secondary School Pupils' Physical Activity and Leisure-time Sports. III: Age and Sports Activities (in Finnish). Institute for Educational Research, Report No. 107. University of Jyväskylä, Finland.

Watson, A. W. S., and D. J. O'Donovan. 1977. Influence of level of habitual activity on physical working capacity and body composition of post-pubertal school boys. Q. J. Exp. Physiol. 62:325–332.

The Influence of Sport Activity on the Development of Physical Performance Capacities of 15–17-Year-Old Boys

J. Rutenfranz and R. Singer

In general, it is well accepted that training may increase the physical performance capacity. Most of us believe that sport activities in youth can improve the state of health and may raise the physical performance capacities of children. Therefore, parents and teachers try to motivate children to participate in activities of sport clubs, and often membership in such clubs is used as an indicator of high levels of daily physical activity.

On the other hand, it is well known that only a small group of children can be motivated for higher levels of daily physical activities, and we know nearly nothing about the causes of these interindividual differences. To explain these differences two hypotheses are conceivable:

1. The levels of daily physical activity of children who participate in sports are higher because they are more highly motivated.
2. The levels of daily physical activity of children who participate in sports are higher because they have a higher physical performance capacity than the other children, which may be genetically caused.

To resolve the issue, the data from a former longitudinal study that was directed toward the development of physical performance capacity in youth have been reanalyzed. In this study we were only interested in the status of physical performance capacity and did not want to stimulate the adolescents to increase their daily physical activity, especially their sport activities. Therefore, the children's choice of activities could be observed and in the same way the nearly undisturbed development of the physical performance capacity of these children could be followed up.

PROCEDURES

There were 403 boys who participated for 3 years in the longitudinal study. The boys were in the ninth grade of high school or in vocational education schools. At the beginning of the study in 1965, the mean age of the boys was 14.95 years. All boys were unpaid volunteers; they worked in different professions with different levels of energy expenditure.

The main goals of the former study were the study of the development of the physical performance capacity, the development of vocational interests, and the development of sensorimotoric skills. The main results have been published elsewhere (Lederle-Schenk, 1972; Rutenfranz et al., 1972).

In the study each boy completed a vocational interest test every year. In and after the second year of the study, the questionnaire included some items about sport activities during school time and during leisure time. Furthermore, the physical performance capacity of all boys was assessed by the PWC_{170} method. These procedures were repeated every year for 4 years, but after the third year the number of participants decreased markedly because vocational education was completed. Therefore, only the first 3 years of the study were included in this reanalysis. For the statistical analysis of the original data, variance analysis and covariance analysis were used.

RESULTS

In Figure 1 the results of the study are presented as values relative to the physical performance capacity of the first year. Moreover, the data are grouped depending on the physical activity or inactivity in the second and third years of investigation. Of the 403 boys, 198 were nonactive in both years and 144 were active in both years; 25 boys were active in the second year but inactive in the third year; and 36 boys were inactive in the second year and active in the third year. Because no information about the sport activities of the children in the first year was available, it was assumed that their levels of activity were identical.

As it can be seen in Figure 1, all children increased their physical performance capacity during the study. However, there was—as expected—a clear dependency of the physical performance capacity on the engagement of the boys in sport activities. The highest level of physical performance capacity was reached by children active over all the years of the study, and the lowest by children inactive over all the years. Children who changed their level of activity during the study reached a lower or higher physical performance capacity than the year before. These observed differences between the groups are statistically significant ($p < 0.001$) in the second

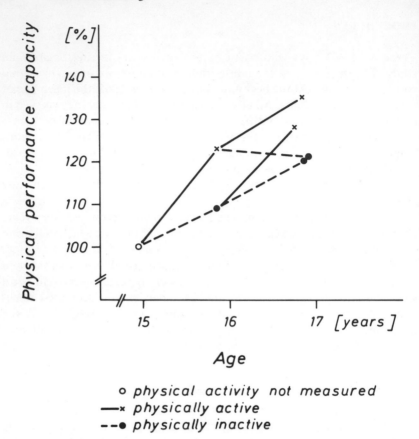

Figure 1.   Physical performance capacity during a 3-year longitudinal study relative to the inactive boys in the initial year of the investigation.

and the third years. The interpretation of this result is difficult, because it is not known whether the data for each year were influenced by the data from the previous year. Therefore, the data on the activity of the boys in the second year were sorted out and expressed relative to the physical performance capacity of inactive boys in the first year of the investigation. As can be seen in Figure 2, the 234 inactive boys had a lower physical performance capacity than the 169 active boys not only during the second year but also during the first year of investigation.

The result of the covariance analysis of these data showed that the difference between these two groups was highly significant ($p < 0.001$) even in the first year of the investigation. Furthermore, the two groups were even significantly different ($p < 0.01$) in the second year of investigation, when the covariate "physical performance capacity in the first year of investigation" was statistically excluded. Therefore, these data seem to be in accordance with the general accepted hypothesis previously mentioned.

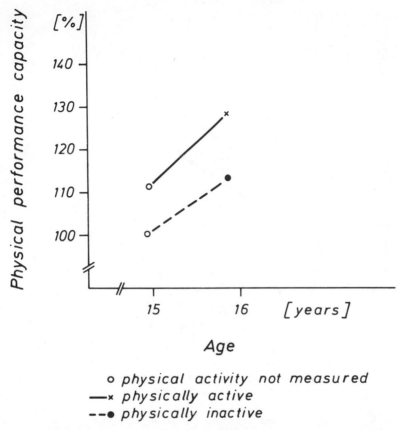

o *physical activity not measured*
—× *physically active*
--● *physically inactive*

Figure 2.   Physical performance capacities of active boys in the second year of a longitudinal study relative to inactive boys in the first year of investigation.

Because, in the first year of investigation, the variable "sport activity" had not been measured, in Figure 3 the physical performance capacity of the four groups is shown; in regard to the sport activity within the second and third years it shows a different pattern. The data in Figure 3 are presented as relative values with regard to the physical performance capacity of the inactive group (inactive in the second and third year) in the first year of investigation. As can be seen in Figure 3, the differences that occurred among the four groups concerning the physical performance capacity in the third year of investigation already existed in the second year, to such an extent that within these four groups there existed a nearly parallel development of the physical performance capacity. This result is clearly in contradiction to the hypothesis that the development of the physical performance capacity among juveniles is influenced by their sport activity. Thus, the physical performance capacity from the second to the third year of investigation within those groups that had been physically active during the time apparently did not increase more than within

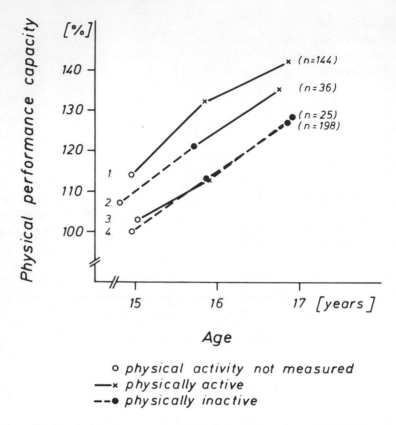

Figure 3. Physical performance capacities of physically active and inactive boys over 3 years, expressed as relative values to physical performance capacities of inactive boys during the initial year of investigation.

those groups that had been physically inactive during this time interval. The analysis of covariance among the mean of these four groups in the third year of investigation—with the covariate "physical performance capacity in the second year of investigation"—resulted in a nonsignificant ($p > 0.05$) main effect. A significant ($p < 0.01$) main effect in the second year of investigation (see Figure 2) is contrasted with a nonsignificant ($p > 0.05$) main effect in the third year of investigation (see Figure 3).

DISCUSSION

The influence of sport activity on the development of physical performance capacity within the 15- to 17-year-old boys investigated could not be shown. Fleiss (1974) obtained a similar result. He observed the performance development of 12-year-old pupils in sport classes, who had 8 sport lessons a week, and of pupils in normal classes, who had 4 sport lessons a week, over 2 years and found no effect of the more intensive training on development in the area of motor abilities. Because in both investigations the extent of physical load has not been recorded exactly, this finding may be due to the fact that the training was not intense enough to result in a discrete course of development.

However, it is not explained why juveniles who are regularly engaged in sports or start sport activities, apparently from the beginning show higher values of physical performance capacity than juveniles who are not engaged in sports or who quit sports. In order to explain this, one could propose the hypothesis that for juveniles of this age a high level of physical performance capacity may not only be a result of sport activity, but also may be a prerequisite to sport activity. Therefore, juveniles who are engaged more intensively in sports may represent not only a group of especially motivated youngsters but, even more, a self-selected group that reinforces its higher physical performance capacity by participating in sport activities.

From an epidemiological point of view the most important groups are, however, the groups with low physical performance capacity at the beginning of puberty, who have only limited interests in sport activities and all other forms of daily physical activity. It seems to be difficult to motivate them to a minimal level of daily physical activity without a prior improvement in their physical performance capacity. This can only be achieved during the school time by physical educators who are especially interested in these groups of children and not only in the more gifted children.

REFERENCES

Fleiss, O. 1974. The motor abilities of sport and normal classes (in German). In: G. Bernhard (ed.), Schulversuche—Schulsport in Österreich, pp. 99–115. Selbstverlag Karl Frauteus Universität, Graz.

Lederle-Schenk, U. 1972. The development of interests of youth and pupils in masculine professions. Dissertation Rer. Nat., University of Köln.

Rutenfranz, J., U. Lederle-Schenk, and A. Iskander. 1972. Performance changes during the beginning procedure of an assembly task and their dependence on beginning performance (in German). Int. Z. Angew. Physiol. 30:217–231.

The Relationship between Working Performance, Daily Physical Activity, Fatness, Blood Lipids, and Nutrition in Schoolchildren

W. H. M. Saris, R. A. Binkhorst, A. B. Cramwinckel,
F. van Waesberghe, and A. M. van der Veen-Hezemans

Interest in the relationship of physical fitness and daily physical activity to general health is increasing among physiologists, epidemiologists, and those who deal with primary prevention of coronary heart disease. This article presents the results of a pilot study that was part of a longitudinal intervention study of the effects of a school health program on general health and health habits among primary schoolchildren.

The first purpose of the pilot study was to obtain normative data on physical fitness, daily physical activity, body composition, nutrition, and blood lipids among the children as a basis for the health program evaluation. The second purpose was to study the relationship between physical performance capacity (PPC) and the above variables. The notion that PPC contributes to a better state of health is generally accepted. However, there is very little research concerning the factors that can affect PPC in children. The relative influence of certain high risk habits (such as a fatty diet) on PPC is currently unclear, and it is not known whether these habits affect the amount of body fat and blood lipids, traditionally considered to have a negative influence on health. Rather than focusing on one or two factors influencing general health maintenance, we chose to combine several variables in the areas of daily habits and physical constitution.

Health information and education project (G.V.O. Project), supported by grants from the Dutch Preventive Fund.

METHODS

Subjects

We studied 171 kindergarten children (ages 4–6) and 54 primary school-children (ages 8–12) from three schools in the Nijmegen area of The Netherlands. The children came from middle and lower socioeconomic level families. The data were collected in February, March, and April, thus excluding any seasonal variation. All of the data were collected during school time.

Physical Performance Capacity (PPC)

Physical performance capacity was measured by the PWC_{170} method using a treadmill (Quinton, U.S.A.). The 4–6-year-old children walked at a controlled speed of 4.0 km/hr; the 8–12-year-old children walked at a controlled speed of 4.5 km/hr. The treadmill was horizontal at the beginning of the walk. Every 2 min the treadmill gradient was increased by 5%. The heart rate was recorded during the last 10 sec of each minute using an electrocardiogram. The test period ended when the child's heart rate reached approximately 170 b.p.m. The PPC was expressed as the treadmill gradient at which a heart rate of 170 (PWC_{170}) was reached.

Daily Physical Activity

Daily physical activity was determined from questionnaires and heart rate recordings over an entire day. Three questionnaires were used to calculate three physical activity (PA) indexes. The first questionnaire (PA1) measured the mother's attitude toward her child's daily physical activity; a second questionnaire (PA2) asked the teacher to rate the child's degree of physical activity during selected school activities (such as playing, or paying attention); and the third questionnaire (PA3) asked the mother to recall her child's activities of the previous day.

The first two questionnaires (PA1 and PA2) used a 5-point scale. A score of 1 or 2 represented low physical activity; a score of 4 or 5 represented a high degree of activity. The third questionnaire (PA3) asked the mother to recall the activities of the child during each of 114 10-min periods during the previous nonschool day hours. The level of activity during each 10-min period had to be filled in according to the scoring system of Passmore and Durnin (1967). The 10-min periods covered only the child's free time activities—school time was not taken into account.

Activities were categorized into seven levels ranging from sleeping (low) to running (high). The energy expenditure during sleeping and lying down was calculated for the 4–6-year-old children based on the individual predicted basal metabolic rate (BMR) (Lewis et al., 1937), and for the 8–12-year-old children based on the table from Talbot (1938). The energy expenditure of the other five levels was calculated from the tables constructed after Passmore and Durnin (1967). The total energy output from all 10-min periods was calculated. From these results the PA3 score in percentage was calculated. A minimal energy output of sleeping 24 hr corresponds with 0% of the PA3 score. An average score of 7 (heavily active) corresponds with a 100% PA3 score.

The heart rate over a chosen school day was recorded with an eight-level heart rate integrator (Saris et al., 1977). The total number of minutes in each heart rate range was tabulated. Only the children in the least active group (lowest quartile) and those in the most active group, as determined by the teacher's questionnaire (PA2), were measured.

Body Composition

Body composition was determined from weight and the sum of four skinfold thicknesses: biceps, triceps, subscapular, and crista iliacal (Durnin and Womersley, 1974). The skinfold measurements were taken with an electronic Holtain caliper.

Blood Lipids

Blood lipids were analyzed in a venous blood sample collected in a non-fasting state during the morning school hours. Total cholesterol and high density lipoprotein cholesterol were determined by the modified Huang method (Huang et al., 1961) and calibrated using the Abell method (Abell et al., 1952). The Soloni method (1971) was used to measure the total serum triglycerides.

Food Intake

Data on food intake were collected using the dietary 24-hr recall method. The nutritional composition of the food intake was calculated by computer (Commissie, 1975). Both food intake and physical activity questionnaire data were collected by trained dietitians visiting the families at home.

RESULTS

The results are presented for each age group, boys and girls together. The children were divided into three subgroups according to their PWC_{170} scores: the high PPC group, the upper quartile of the PWC_{170}; a middle performance group, the middle two quartiles of the PWC_{170}; and low PPC children, the lower quartile of the PWC_{170}. Student t tests for significant differences were only applied between the upper and lower groups.

The results of the physical performance capacity (PWC_{170}), physical activity indexes, and heart rate are presented in Table 1. The PWC_{170} scores were significantly different between the high and low PWC_{170} quar-

Table 1. Daily physical activity indices and heart rate results of children with different physical performance capacity scores $(PWC_{170})^a$

Group (PWC_{170})	N	PWC_{170}^b	Activity questionnaires			Heart rate method		
			PA1	PA2	PA3	Heart rate	Minutes at 125–176 b.p.m.	Minutes over 176 b.p.m.
4–6 years								
High	45	$(20.8)^{c,d}$	63.2^c	70.2^c	63.4	96^e	126^c	4^e
Middle	82	(16.6)	56.4	51.1	64.0	f	—	—
Low	44	$(12.4)^c$	53.3^c	40.1^c	64.3	101^e	202^c	15^e
8–12 years								
High	15	$(18.2)^c$	62.5^c	64.7^e	58.3	87^e	113^g	4
Middle	25	(12.4)	56.8	59.2	60.2	—	—	—
Low	14	$(07.9)^c$	47.6^c	54.6^e	60.6	94^e	197^g	6

aPhysical activity indexes are represented as percentile scores on each of the three questionnaires, PA1, PA2, and PA3.
bTreadmill speed was 4 km/hr for 4–6-year-old children; and 4.5 km/hr for 8–12-year-old children.
cp<0.001.
dt test between lowest (<25%) and highest (>75%) PWC_{170} quartiles.
ep<0.05.
fMiddle PWC_{170} quartiles were not measured.
gp<0.01.

tiles. Significant differences were also found between low and high PWC_{170} quartiles for PA1, PA2, mean heart rates over 24 hr, and time with a heart rate of 125–176 b.p.m. for both age groups. The number of minutes with a heart rate over 176 b.p.m. was significantly different only for the 4–6-year-old age group. No significant differences were found in the energy expenditures during nonschool hours (PA3) between the low and high qualities for both age groups.

Data on body composition and blood lipids are presented in Table 2. No significant differences were found among any of the variables in the 4–6-year-old age group. In the 8–12-year-old group, body weight and the sum of the four skinfolds were significantly different between the low and high PWC_{170} quartiles. The low PWC_{170} quartile was heavier and had a higher total skinfold thickness than the high PWC_{170} quartile.

Data on daily nutritional intake are shown in Table 3. In the 4–6-year-old age group, a significant difference was found between high and low PWC_{170} quartiles in total daily energy intake and cholesterol intake. No significant differences were found between the PWC_{170} groups for different sources of energy intake. Among the 8–12-year-old children, on the other hand, no significant difference in total energy intake was found between high and low PWC_{170} quartiles. However unlike the 4–6-year-old group, significant differences were found between high and low PWC_{170} quartiles for the percentage of calories obtained from fat and saturated fat, and in the amount of cholesterol intake. The younger children differed from one another in the amount, but not the source, of energy intake. The older children, on the other hand, did not differ in the amount of energy intake, but they did differ on the source.

DISCUSSION

Since the number of children per age group (4–6 and 8–12 years) was small, the results were not divided into boys and girls, which would be relevant in a more detailed analysis on a larger group (especially in the older age group). Thus, some of the data should be interpreted as preliminary and tentative. (The results of another study we just completed with a group of about 700 5–7-year-old children showed the same tendencies as were shown in this pilot study.)

The higher PWC_{170} scores in the younger age group may be due to differences in the treadmill speed. The younger age group walked at a lower speed (4.0 km/hr) than the older group (4.5 km/hr). The results of the PA1 and PA2 questionnaires showed a significant relationship between physical performance capacity (PWC_{170}) and daily physical activity for both age groups. The PA3 questionnaire, which used the 24-hr recall method showed no such relationship. This was contrary to the findings of Pařízková (1972) and Rutenfranz et al. (1974), who found a significant re-

Table 2. Body composition and blood lipids of children with different physical performance capacity scores (PWC_{170})

Group (PWC_{170})	Body composition			Blood lipids		
	Weight (kg)	Length (cm)	Sum 4 skinfolds (mm)	Total cholesterol (mg/100 ml)	HDL cholesterol (mg/100 ml)	Triglycerides
4-6 years						
High	19.3	112.6	26.9	169	52	69
Middle	19.2	111.6	28.1	171	54	62
Low	19.7	110.9	28.8	172	51	66
8-12 years						
High	30.8[a,b]	139.2	26.6[c]	182	53	86
Middle	31.5	139.2	34.8	192	53	72
Low	34.0[b]	141.1	48.8[c]	186	52	68

[a] t test between lowest (<25%) and highest (>75%) PWC_{170} quartiles.
[b] $p < 0.05$.
[c] $p < 0.001$.

Table 3.   Daily energy intake from different sources among children with different physical performance capacity scores (PWC$_{170}$)

Group (PWC$_{170}$)	Total energy intake	Source of energy intake (% calories)					Cholesterol (mg)	Fiber (g)
		Protein	Fat	Saturated fat	Polyunsaturated fatty acid	Carbohydrates		
4-6 years								
High	1835[a,b]	12.1	40.1	17.4	4.1	47.3	220[c]	4.8
Middle	1759	11.8	39.1	17.6	4.4	48.4	195	4.8
Low	1610[b]	12.8	40.9	18.9	4.1	46.6	129[c]	4.3
8-12 years								
High	2114	11.9	43.0[c]	18.7[c]	5.6	44.3	283[b]	5.7
Middle	2094	12.5	37.2	15.5	4.7	49.5	202	6.1
Low	1935	13.9	35.9[c]	13.5[c]	5.1	49.5	193[b]	5.5

[a] t test between lowest (<25%) and highest (>75%) PWC$_{170}$ quartiles.
[b] $p < 0.05$.
[c] $p < 0.01$.

lationship between PPC and daily physical activity using a 24-hr record method. Whereas Pařízková and Rutenfranz et al. gave the 24-hr questionnaire to the subjects themselves (subjects were mostly older) and used 1-min periods, in this study the questionnaires were administered to the parents. This discrepancy suggests that the latter method is unreliable for at least one of the groups. For younger children, the PA1 and PA2 questionnaires seemed to be more suitable, because they cannot answer the questionnaire themselves.

Contrary to what was expected, children with a high physical performance capacity who were also highly active had a lower mean heart rate and, consequently, spent longer periods with a lower heart rate than did the low PPC–low activity group. These results may be explained by the well known observation that a better state of fitness coincides with a greater heart stroke volume and, therefore, a lower mean heart rate (Åstrand and Rodahl, 1970). The state of fitness of the children seems to have more effect on the daily mean heart rate than does the amount of daily activity.

The relationship between daily activity, total daily energy intake, and body composition was different for the two age groups. In the younger age group, children with a low physical activity also had a lower daily energy intake than the high physical activity group. Therefore, it was not surprising that body weight and skinfold thickness were the same for both groups. The older children, on the contrary, exhibited significant differences in body weight and skinfold thickness; this was probably due to the same amount of energy intake despite significant differences in total daily physical activities. The less active children tended to weigh more and have more body fat.

No relationship was found between PWC_{170} quartile groups and blood lipids, nor was there such a relationship between skinfolds and blood lipids, as was found in several studies with adults (Albrink and Meigs, 1971; Montoye, 1975), suggesting that this relationship probably appears only after several years of obesity.

From an analysis of the sources of energy intake, there was no relationship between body fat, blood lipids, and intake of fatty foods. In the younger age group, the highly active children tended to eat more high quality foods to obtain the extra calories; whereas the highly active children in the 8–12-year-old age group had a significantly higher intake of fatty foods than the lesser active children of the same age group. The differences between the age groups were probably due to more parental control of a child's diet at an early age. However, the higher intake of saturated fats and cholesterol did not lead to higher blood lipids among the more active children. These findings support the idea that saturated fatty acids and cholesterol in the diet are not harmful as long as one is physically active.

REFERENCES

Abell, L. L., B. B. Levy, B. B. Brodic, and F. E. Kendall. 1952. A simplified method for the estimation of total cholesterol in serum and demonstration of its specificity. J. Biol. Chem. 195:357–366.

Albrink, M. J., and J. W. Meigs. 1971. Serum lipids, skinfolds thickness, body bulk and body weight of native Cape Verdeans, New England and United States factory workers. Am. J. Clin. Nutr. 24:344–352.

Åstrand, P. O., and K. Rodahl. 1970. Textbook of Work Physiology. McGraw-Hill Book Co., New York.

Commissie, U. C. V. 1975. Development of a system to calculate data of dietary questionnaires with the aid of the computer (in Dutch). Voeding 36:356–360.

Durnin, J. V. G. A., and J. Womersley. 1974. Body fat assessed from total body density and its estimation from skinfolds thickness: Measurements on 481 men and women. Br. J. Nutr. 32:77–97.

Huang, T. C., C. P. Chen, V. Weifer, and A. Raferty. 1961. A stable reagent for the Lieberman Burchard reaction. Anal. Chem. 33:1405–1409.

Lewis, R. C., G. M. Kinsman, and A. Iliff. 1937. The basal metabolism of normal boys and girls from two to twelve years old. Am. J. Dis. Child. 53:348–428.

Montoye, H. J. 1975. Physical Activity and Health: An Epidemiologic Study of an Entire Community. Prentice-Hall, Inc., Englewood Cliffs, N.J.

Pařízková, J. 1972. Obesity and physical activity. In: J. de Wijn and R. A. Binkhurst (eds.), Nutritional Aspects of Physical Performance. Nutricia Zoetermeer, The Netherlands.

Passmore, R., and J. V. G. A. Durnin. 1967. Energy, Work and Leisure. Heinemann Educational Books, Ltd., London.

Rutenfranz, J., I. Berndt, and P. Knauth. 1974. Daily physical activity investigated by time budget studies and physical performance capacity of school boys. Acta Paediatrica Belgica 28: Suppl. 1.

Saris, W. H. M., P. Snel, and R. A. Binkhorst. 1977. A portable heart rate distribution recorder for studying daily physical activity. Eur. J. Appl. Physiol. 37: 17–25.

Soloni, F. G. 1971. Simplified manual micromethod for determination of serum triglycerides. Clin. Chem. 17:529–533.

Talbot, F. B. 1938. Basal metabolism standards for children. Am. J. Dis. Child. 55:455–459.

Functional Demands of Physical Education Lessons

V. Seliger,* J. Heller, V. Zelenka, V. Sobolová,
M. Pauer, Z. Bartůněk, and S. Bartůňková

The lower physical activity in contemporary civilized society brings about a decrease in physical fitness, which above all is related to impaired efficiency of the circulatory and respiratory systems (Åstrand, 1974). The reduced movement reflects unfavorably on the functional state of the organism, especially during the period of growth and development. On the other hand, increased motor activity, in the form of different exercises, is regarded as a preventative factor for some diseases of civilization (Cassel et al., 1971; Morris et al., 1973).

The school physical education program presents the most suitable area for influencing the motor regimens of youth. It should be noted that it is necessary to modernize the process of physical education in a number of different ways. The main physiological problem is to determine a sufficient intensity for physical education lessons, their frequency, utilization of time for exercising, and the effectiveness of exercises (Dietrich, 1967).

It was decided to estimate, from the physiological point of view, the functional and energy demands of some models of intensified lessons for school physical education for different age groups and to compare them with a currently used physical education lesson.

METHODS

The energy metabolism of the subjects in this study during exercise was determined by means of indirect calorimetry, using suitable half-masks (Seliger, 1968) and telemetered heart rates. The experiment was designed so that the variables were measured during the entire time of the experi-

---

*Prof. Seliger died on December 31, 1979.

ment and during a recovery period lasting 20 min. The teacher prepared and carried out with the pupils a typical model of a common physical education lesson lasting 25 to 36 min and also followed a model of the intensified exercises. The ages of the boys ranged from 4.9 to 16.1 years. A total of 34 children and youths were involved in the investigation, 14 for the nonintensified exercises and 20 for the intensified exercises.

RESULTS

Characteristics of the Sample

The sample was selected in order to secure boys attending the last class of kindergarten, the first, fourth, sixth, and eighth classes of the Basic Nine-Year School, and the first grade of secondary school. Comparing the children's weight, height, and percentage of body fat with the norms of the Czechoslovakian population (Seliger and Bartůněk, 1976), it was confirmed that the children in this investigation belonged to the mean of the Czechoslovakian population. There were no significant differences in the main somatometric indices between the pupils exercising in the intensified model and those exercising in the nonintensified model.

Functional Load

From the point of view of the three age groups involved (ages 6, 12, and 15 years), it was found that the mean *pulse rate* increased with age in both the nonintensified and the intensified groups (Table 1). The differences in the exercise load on the organism in both types of exercises were significant at the 5% level with 12- and 15-year-old boys. The mean pulse rate in exercise increased during nonintensified exercises nearly linearly with age (from 119 to 142 b.p.m.), whereas in intensified exercises it increased exponentially (from 130 to 170 b.p.m.). *Pulmonary ventilation* showed a similar change, but statistical significance between both models was found only in the 15-year-old boys ($p < 0.01$). The values rose exponentially with age, in nonintensified lessons from approximately 11 to 33 liters/min, and in intensified lessons from 12 to 55 liters/min. *Oxygen consumption* also rose exponentially with age. Significant differences were found in the 6-year-old boys ($p < .05$) and in the 15-year-old boys ($p < .05$ and $.01$). The value of oxygen consumption rose in nonintensified lessons from 11 to 17 ml/min•kg and in intensified lessons from 15 to 24 ml/min•kg. The *oxygen pulse* also increased with age, but there was no statistically significant difference between the two exercise groups (from 2.7 to 8.6 ml). In general, in the group of 15-year-old youths functional indices approached two-thirds of the population norm in the intensified lessons and one-third in the nonintensified lessons.

Table 1. Selected functional indices and indices of energy metabolism of three age groups (6, 12, and 15 years) in the models of nonintensified and intensified exercises[a]

Variable	6 years			12 years			15 years		
	$\bar{x}$	SD	$p <$	$\bar{x}$	SD	$p <$	$\bar{x}$	SD	$p <$
HR (b.p.m.)	129.6	11.37	N.S.	148.2	9.00	0.05	170.2	11.96	0.05
	119.2	9.98		124.5	10.81		141.8	19.66	
$\dot{V}$ (l/min)	12.23	1.42	N.S.	23.57	6.29	N.S.	54.81	8.53	0.01
	10.95	0.39		17.19	2.20		32.93	6.35	
$\dot{V}O_2$ (l/min)	0.37	0.03	0.05	0.73	0.16	N.S.	1.47	0.27	0.05
	0.32	0.03		0.51	0.14		1.13	0.18	
$\dot{V}O_2$ (ml/min·kg)	15.17	0.61	0.05	16.58	2.48	N.S.	24.01	4.33	0.01
	11.06	2.32		14.24	3.26		17.44	2.35	
$\dot{V}O_2$ HR (ml)	2.85	0.43	N.S.	4.83	0.85	N.S.	8.61	1.74	N.S.
	2.66	0.21		4.04	0.91		8.01	1.07	
O_2 debt (l)	0.40	0.26	N.S.	0.65	0.53	N.S.	2.97	1.20	N.S.
	0.78	0.50		0.79	0.99		1.92	1.25	
$\dot{V}O_2$ work (%)	94.38	3.41	N.S.	96.21	2.80	N.S.	92.52	3.11	N.S.
	89.48	5.85		95.49	5.99		93.78	3.00	
Energy output (kcal/min)	1.17	0.11	N.S.	2.72	0.71	0.05	7.01	1.50	0.01
	1.29	0.54		1.77	0.81		4.55	1.18	
Energy output (kcal/min·kg)	0.048	0.001	N.S.	0.06	0.01	N.S.	0.11	0.02	0.01
	0.05	0.03		0.05	0.02		0.07	0.01	
Energy output (% BMR)	254.83	6.29	N.S.	365.52	59.68	N.S.	658.20	90.95	0.01
	264.33	85.09		292.79	86.26		447.56	78.12	

[a]The first value for each variable is for the intensified exercises; the second value is for the nonintensified excrcises.

Table 2. Selected functional indices at maximal load on the bicycle ergometer and during differently intensified exercise lessons in absolute values and in the percentage maximal value in two 15-year-old boys participating in the nonintensified and intensified physical education lessons[a]

Variable	Nonintensified			Intensified		
	BE	M	%	BE	M	%
HR (b.p.m.)	206	134	65	206	181	88
$\dot{V}$ (l/min)	115	33	29	82	48	59
$\dot{V}$/kg (l/min)	1.79	0.51	29	1.58	0.93	59
$\dot{V}O_2$ (l/min)	3.47	1.11	32	2.89	1.35	47
$\dot{V}O_2$ (ml/min·kg)	53.9	17.3	32	55.9	26.0	47
PWC_{170} (W)	136	—	—	87	—	—
PWC_{170}/kg (W)	2.87	—	—	1.69	—	—
Energy output (kcal/min)	—	4.8	—	—	6.3	—

[a]BE = bicycle ergometer; M = differently intensified exercise lessons; % = percentage maximal value.

Energy Metabolism

Almost all the exercises were performed on aerobic metabolism (see Table 1), which means that the oxygen consumption during work attained 93%–96% of the total oxygen consumption. Oxygen debt was relatively low, at 0.4 and 0.7 liters in the 6- and 12-year-olds, and 3.0 liters in the 15-year-olds. In both indices the differences between the two exercise intensity groups were not statistically significant. Energy output in the given model of exercises, expressed in kcal/min, in kcal/min·kg, or in percentage of basal metabolic rate (BMR) also rose exponentially with age, but statistical significance was obtained only in the group of 15-year-olds ($p < 0.1$).

Individual differences in the nonintensified or intensified physical education programs may be quite considerable relative to the functional and energy indices. For example, the functional indices attained in riding a bicycle ergometer to maximum and the functional indices obtained in differently intensified exercise lessons were compared in two 15-year-old boys. These data are presented in Table 2 and Figures 1 and 2. The exercises in the nonintensified lesson caused the functional indices to increase to about 30% of the population norm; the pulse rate had several peaks, but these exercises were not very intensive and there was a total fall of pulse rate during the progress of the exercises. The intensified exercises increased the functional indices to 47%–59% of the population norm; the pulse rate repeatedly reached maximum, and during the short intervals it seldom fell below 150 b.p.m.

DISCUSSION

In general, the results of the measurements of functional and energy indices indicate that functional demands of exercises increased with age

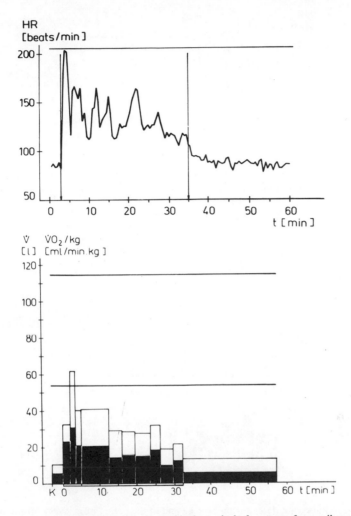

Figure 1.   Pulse rate (HR) during exercise and in the period of recovery for pupil no. 9, who participated in the nonintensified model of physical education lessons. A) Vertical lines indicate the beginning and end of exercises; horizontal line traces maximum pulse rates. B) The black columns in the graph indicate oxygen consumption ($\dot{V}_{O_2}$/kg) and the white columns indicate pulmonary ventilation ($\dot{V}$); horizontal lines show maximal values of these indices. The first column (k) shows rest values, the columns showing exercise values are underscored, and the last column shows recovery values.

more slowly in nonintensified physical education when the subjects participated in the intensified lessons. In special exercises, such as running, relay races, jumping, circuit training, and soccer, the pulse rate attained even higher values (170–200 b.p.m. or more). Such exercises can be included in the program only for a short period, of course, and they must be followed by less intensive exercises. Missiuro and Perlberg (1937) identified three peaks in a physical education lesson. Today, however, it is more

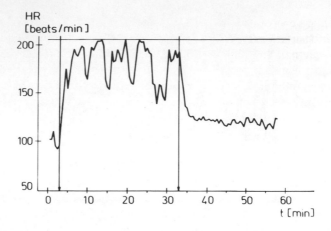

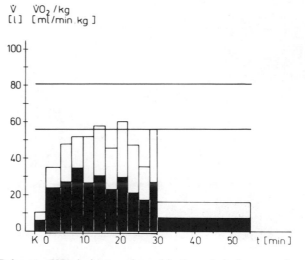

Figure 2.   Pulse rate (HR) during exercise and in the period of recovery for pupil no. 17, who participated in the intensified model of physical education lessons. A) Vertical lines indicate the beginning and end of exercises; horizontal line traces maximum pulse rates. B) The black columns in the graph indicate oxygen consumption ($\dot{V}O_2/kg$) and the white columns indicate pulmonary ventilation ($\dot{V}$); horizontal lines show maximal values of these indices. The first column (k) shows rest values, the columns showing exercise values are underscored, and the last column shows recovery values.

probable that such peaks are more numerous. In older pupils (secondary school) the peaks were more frequent and higher even in the nonintensified lessons.

The teacher's personality constitutes another important factor influencing the progress of the exercises. It is very possible that the teachers of younger age groups (6 and 12 years) were not able to motivate their pupils to sufficient exertion. However, it is also possible that the reason for the lower intensity of exercises in younger age groups is the predominance of exercises demanding high coordination, which require much more time-consuming learning processes. The modern school physical education program is, of course, a result of a combination of intensity of motor activity, quality of the movement, and education.

If we want to improve physical fitness—and this should be the aim of physical education lessons—on the average, a pulse rate higher than 140 b.p.m. should be attained; many programs have not fulfilled this condition. We are of the opinion that the total mean pulse rate (140 b.p.m.) is not as important as the need for a few short (1–5 min.) high loads to be imposed on the organism in order to induce maximal or near maximal intensity in metabolism. As far as the number of highly intensive exercises, it is better to include several periods of high intensity, as in the interval training of athletes. However, Bar-Or and Zwiren (1973) have found no functional changes either after intensive special training or after a more frequent load in a greater number of training sessions. They are of the opinion that the range of activities in school physical education programs may not be sufficient in comparison with the activities done out of school.

In conclusion, it is possible to say that an attractive and intensive school physical education program may help to create a life-long positive attitude toward physical activities in general, and it may create a desire for physical activity even into old age.

REFERENCES

Åstrand, P.-O. 1974. Effects of sport on the cardiovascular system and repercussions of the practice on the health of the masses. Schweiz. Med. Wochenschr. 104:1538–1542.

Bar-Or, O., and L. D. Zwiren. 1973. Physiological effect of increased frequency of physical education classes of endurance conditioning on 9- to 10-year-old girls and boys. In: O. Bar-Or (ed.), Pediatric Work Physiology, pp. 183–189. Proceedings of the 4th International Symposium. Wingate Institute, Natanya.

Cassel, J., S. Heyden, A. G. Bartel, B. M. Kaplan, H. A. Tyroler, J. C. Cornoni, and C. G. Hames. 1971. Occupation and coronary heart disease. Arch. Intern. Med. 128:920–928.

Dietrich, W. 1967. On some changes in sport education in the German Democratic Republic (in German). In: The IInd International Congress on the Physical Fitness of Youth, pp. 335–339. Olympia, Praha.

Missiuro, W., and A. Perlberg. 1937. Investigation of the effects of a lesson in gymnastics on the gas metabolism (in German). Arbeitsphysiol. 9:514–527.

Morris, J. N., C. Adam, C. S. Chave, C. Sirey, L. Epstein, and D. J. Sheehan. 1973. Vigorous exercise in leisure time and the incidence of coronary heart disease. Lancet 2:333–339.

Seliger, V. 1968. Energy metabolism in selected physical exercises. Int. Z. Angew. Physiol. 25:104–120.

Seliger, V., and Z. Bartůněk. 1976. Mean value of various indices of physical fitness in the investigation of the Czechoslovak population aged 12–55 years. Czechoslovak Union of Physical Education, Praha.

Automatic Analysis of Electrocardiogram Long-Term Recordings During Training and Daily Activity with Reference to Physical Activity Events Analysis

M. Rieu, J. P. Fouillot, J. Devars, and J. P. Cocquerez

The heart rate has been used for a long time to indirectly estimate energy consumption, even though linearity of the oxygen consumption/heart rate relationship is questionable. However, heart rate provides us with good information on daily physical activity.

Telemetry enabled the patient to be free of any connection with encumbering equipment and it was of considerable interest to study a patient's ECG in real time to discover when it is absolutely necessary to modulate his physical activity in reference to the received signal. However, it is not possible with telemetry to easily measure the effect of physical exercises on the patient's heart rate with respect to his behavior in normal life because the receiver has to remain somewhere near the subject. This obstacle was minimized by ambulatory monitoring. The development of tape-recording technology has made it feasible to acquire and store data on an unrestricted subject for periods of 24 hr or more. The first practical application was made by Holter (1961); ten years later, a number of two- and four-channel minitape recorders were developed for general purposes. However, the complete autonomy provided by such systems, weighing between 500 and 800 g, has not eliminated all obstacles impeding the study of heart rate or the detection of ECG anomalies.

The generous support given to this work by the Délégation Générale à la Recherche Scientifique et Technique (Grant No. 76.7.1078) is hereby acknowledged.

When examining long term recordings, inevitably one must face the problem of the generation of nearly overwhelming quantities of data. A 6-day ECG recording will contain from 20 to 50,000 complexes. Automatic signal processing is justified and essential when the tape reading speed is 60 times higher than the recording speed. In such a case, correspondence between the frequencies of the analyzed signal and the physical activity, or modifications in the subject's environment, creates a new problem. Most of the recording systems have a signal marker that can be operated by the subject. This binary-type coding process is sufficient in pathology when it can be shown that the subject is able to perceive a symptom or event. In work physiology, the event marker can be used to synchronize the recording of bioelectrical signals and the observation of any type of activity and its duration. Then, it is possible to carry out a sequential study of signals with the observations made by means of a grid. However, when sequences of physical activity are brief and follow one another rapidly, it can be very tiresome to code observations in this manner without a risk of error. Therefore, an attempt was made to automate not only the heart rate and ECG processing, but also the collection of the coded observations of the subject's physical activity. It would have been possible to record observations on a magnetic recorder similar to that carried by the subject and to code the events with a combination frequency or with amplitude modulated pulses. This was disadvantageous because the cost of another recorder, additional time for tape reading, and analog-digital conversion would have been necessary for data processing. Therefore, we preferred to design a digital, autonomous, and portable scratch pad to measure the duration of each activity sequence and characterize it by a four-digit code. The cumulative recording of the duration and codes of all physical activity sequences was synchronized initially and the bioelectrical signals were recorded to enable a synchronous automatic and combined processing of two types of information.

EQUIPMENT AND METHOD (Figure 1)

Digital Scratch Pad

It is possible with this unit to acquire and to chronologically memorize observation codes. It assumes three functions:

1. Time counting of each sequence observed, the start being synchronized with the recording of parameters.
2. Entry of observation codes of physical activity or any other event by use of a keyboard.
3. Storage of the time-observation code couple.

This unit is made from a CMOS technology microprocessor system **characterized by** its very low energy consumption. In fact, this system has

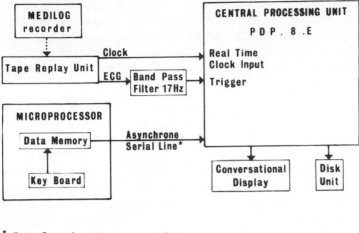

*:Data Format : n(⎵⎵⎵⎵ ⎵⎵⎵⎵)
              code   time

Figure 1.   Processing system configuration.

an autonomy of at least 72 hr of continuous operation, so that it is truly portable. It comprises an eight-digit display, a 12-key keyboard, a read-only memory in which a program is inserted, data storage, and a serial input-output module. All five of these subsystems have the following functions:

1. The eight-digit display makes possible the display of:
    a. the subject's identification number;
    b. the recording date; and
    c. a time-observation code couple—four digits are assigned to the observation code and four other ones to the time.
2. The unit can measure to the hundredth or to the tenth of a second or to the second.
3. It is possible with the 12-key keyboard to select the following functions:
    a. entry of derived codes into the memory from ten digit keys;
    b. recording control of the identification numbers and date;
    c. recording control of time-observation code couples;
    d. data-reading control, enabling the operator to sequentially display the bulk of data stored during the whole physical activity; and
    e. control of data-stored transfer to the PDP8 laboratory processor.
4. The read-only memory where the program is inserted is divided into modules relating to one specific function. It is organized in such a way that it is possible to add one module corresponding to another function without major modification.

5. It is possible with this data memory to record 220 time-observation code couples. This memory is autonomous and battery fed, which provides additional protection against any loss of information.
6. The input-output unit is of the asynchronous serial line type. It is needed to arrange transfer of data from the recording system to the PDP8 processor.

After starting up the program, the entry of the subject's identification number, time and date of recording, and the choice of the time unit, the observer initiates the time counting in synchronism and the event marking on the magnetic recorder carried by the subject. When time is displayed on half the digital display, the observer displays the four-digit code of the physical activity on the other half. As soon as the sequential time counting has stopped, the displayed data are stored, and the chronometer is put to zero to measure the time of the following sequence. Observations stored chronologically and by accumulation can be transferred by interface onto the processor where they are stored on a disc.

ECG Recording and Heart Rate Processing

Technical Recording   The Medilog cassette recorder was used to register the ECG at 2 mm/sec on standard C120 cassettes. Although four channels could be recorded, only two were used: an ECG channel and an event marker. The event marker channel was also permanently used for a 60-Hz timing pulse given by a crystal controlled oscillator, from which output was placed directly on the tape. This provided accurate real time for analyses, especially with regard to recording and playback tape speeds, which could be in an independent position. The electrodes were applied to the manubrium of the sternum in the V5 position. A third electrode served as a ground. After the ECG signals were checked with an oscilloscope, the subjects were sent back to their daily activity or physical training.

At the beginning of the observation, the initiation of the time counting with the digital scratch pad was carried out in synchronism with the event marker.

Processing Speed   The tapes were played back on a standard Oxford Instruments recorder at 60 times real time.

Primary Processing   The ECG signal was passed through an adjustable bandpass filter with a response equivalent to 10 to 30 Hz in real time. A trigger pulse was formed from this filtered signal and then transmitted through an interface to the central processing unit, a PDP8-E computer.

The 60-Hz signal recorded simultaneously on the tape with the ECG was multiplied by eight in order to obtain a 2.083 msec accuracy in real time, taking into account RR intervals by counting time between two detection pulses in two heartbeat complexes. The duration of these RR intervals was recorded and stored on a disc cartridge.

Analysis of Data

The heart rate was subjected to two kinds of processing for each sequence of physical activity identified by the digital scratch pad as well as for the whole recording:

1. Numeric or graphic print-out of the heart rate calculated on a whole number of systoles for periods of 5, 10, 15, 30, or 60 sec in the course of all physical activity sequences.
2. RR interval histogram that was an effective means of condensing the heart rate data of a long recording into a simple diagram (Cashman, 1976). RR interval difference histogram was also simultaneously generated. Statistical analyses could also be performed on physical activity data to determine means, standard deviations, and so on.

RESULTS

The following examples show how the data were arranged. However, this was not the main interest of the method. Its purpose was not so much to get the heart rate represented in a graphical form by a curve or histogram as to condense the ECG data corresponding to a physical activity sequence and to develop a model of the physical activity and of the corresponding biological responses.

This method, originally applied to the study of training in an adult athlete, is now being used to study spontaneous physical activity in a child. The print-out of the physical activity sequences (Figure 2) recorded for a 12-year-old boy while he was cycling shows a progressive decrease of the successive high-speed sequences duration (code 0011). During these periods, the heart rate reached 200 b.p.m. for a short time, as shown by the RR interval histogram (Figure 3). This boy displayed low arrythmia when making moderate efforts (Figure 4); but this arrythmia increased considerably at rest, especially in a sequence where he was playing the piano (Figure 5). This appeared totally different in an 8-year-old boy who, for the same activity, showed 81% of the complexes in which the difference between intervals was not higher than ± 15 msec.

DISCUSSION

With ambulatory monitoring it is possible to easily study a subject in his environment; with regard to the weight and size, this equipment is less cumbersome for a boy who is over 6 years old. With this technique, a great deal of data had to be analyzed, but, with regard to the heart rate,

```
RUN RKR1 TRAING SY

FICHIER CHRONO  RKA100  SCHM03

    DEB      FIN      CODE
     0    0     6    40  0001
     6   40    10    45  0010
    10   45    11    30  0011
    11   30    12    30  0010
    12   30    13     0  0011
    13    0    18    20  0010
    18   20    18    35  0011
    18   35    22    15  0010
    22   15    22    55  0011


*** TRAITEMENT DE RR ***

FICHIER SIGNAL  RKA100  SCHL03
TRAITEMENT SUR     6. MN 40. S    608 SYSTOLES
ORIGINE :  0 H  0 M  0 S   CODE  0001
```

Figure 2. Physical activity analysis print-out of a spontaneous "interval training" exercise on a bicycle with the time intervals and code of sequence of a 12-year-old boy.

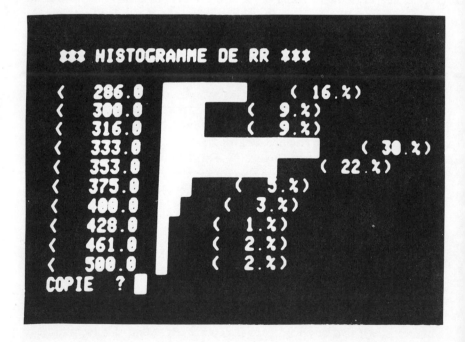

Figure 3. RR interval histogram of sprint sequence of 30 sec on a bicycle for a 12-year-old boy.

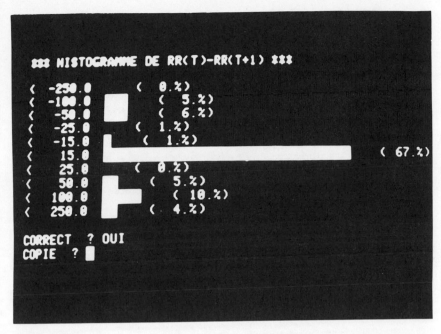

Figure 4.   RR interval difference histogram of a slow speed sequence on a bicycle for a 12-year-old boy.

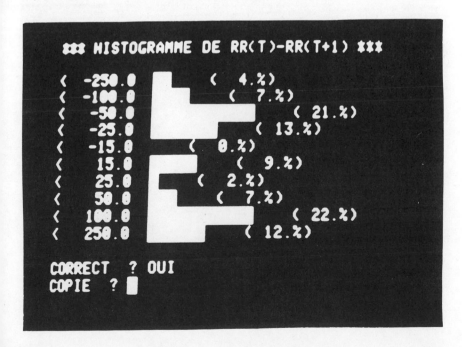

Figure 5.   RR interval difference histogram of the same 12-year-old boy playing the piano.

this was not much of a disadvantage if the data were only plotted in graphical form. This observation was a global approach to the phenomenon and it did not make possible an easy comparison of heart rates obtained during the different physical activities.

The condensation of data in the form of RR interval histograms provided interesting information on patterns of the ventricular rhythm. The study of correspondences between these ventricular rhythm patterns and the physical activity (or any other data of the child's behavior or environment) by factorial analysis procedures led to the study of several hundred sequences. Such a study was made easier by complete automatic data processing, including not only bioelectrical signals but also data observed and coded by the digital scratch pad. The data were related to the subject's physical activity, general behavior, and environment.

REFERENCES

Cashman, P. M. 1976. Methods for tape analysis. Postgrad. Med. J. 52(Suppl. 7): 19–23.
Holter, N. J. 1961. New method for heart studies. Science 134:1214.

Muscle Development, Structure, and Function

Skeletal Muscle Development in the Human Fetus and during Childhood

A.-S. Colling-Saltin

Studies describing the structure of muscle tissue are published quite frequently; therefore, there exists detailed knowledge of development as well as of differentiation and growth of the muscles. There are three main reasons why the muscles have been so thoroughly studied. Muscle tissue attains remarkable differentiation and has a great capacity to grow. Thus, it is a perfect tissue for studying cell differentiation and growth. The muscles are also the site of various diseases that might either originate from the muscle cell or be secondary to pathological conditions in other organs or tissues. Knowledge of what affects and controls the structure of the muscle is critical to the prevention and treatment of such diseases and in rehabilitation after their occurrence. A third factor contributing to the many studies of the growth of the skeletal muscles, in particular, is the fact that for certain populations in the world muscles are an important source of protein.

Information on the differentiation and growth of muscles can be found in many survey articles and books (Guth, 1968; Bourne, 1972; Dubowitz and Brooke, 1973). Fischman, Bourne and Bourne, and Goldspink, in three different chapters of a book on the structure and function of muscles (Bourne, 1972) have thoroughly discussed the early development of skeletal muscles. These surveys show that most studies are made using animals other than man; therefore, although there are great similarities in the development and growth of muscles, there are differences in the time course for development and differentiation rates.

Economic support for the author's studies cited in this article was obtained from Stiftelsen Allmänna Barnbördshuset and Segerfalkska fonden, Helsingborg Hospital.

However, these problems have also been the object of several studies in man since Wohlfart's (1937) detailed studies of the skeletal muscle fiber development. In this article, an attempt has been made to summarize results from studies on muscle fiber development in the human fetus. To a large extent I depend on my own work, but comparisons are made with other studies that have appeared during the last two decades.

MYOGENESIS

From the 13th fetal week, promyoblasts, myoblasts, and myotubes are found in the muscles in different developing stages (Cuajunco, 1942; Fenichel, 1963; Dubowitz, 1965, Ringqvist et al., 1977; Colling-Saltin, 1978a). Thereafter, the plasma membrane is usually identifiable and satellite cells can be identified with more certainty (Tomanek and Colling-Saltin, 1977). These cells occur frequently during the rest of the fetal period and are also found in the muscle of the newborn and the adult (Schmalbruch and Hellhammer, 1976). After the 16th fetal week, more and more muscle cells with myofibrils and peripherally localized nuclei are seen; i.e., the first muscle fibers can be identified (Fenichel, 1963; Dubowitz, 1965; Colling-Saltin, 1978a). From the 20th to the 22nd fetal week, the number of muscle fibers are dominant (Colling-Saltin, 1978b). Solitary myoblasts can still be seen, and there are myotubes in decreasing numbers up to birth (Dubowitz, 1965; Colling-Saltin, 1978a).

In the periphery of early myotubes—close to the cell wall—the thin filaments are observed asymmetrically, and nearby there are accumulations of thick filaments seen in the extension of their associated ribosomes. When actin (thin) and myosin (thick) filaments can be identified, "lattice" and Z lines are also seen centrally. In the continuous sarcomere formation, the thin and thick filaments seem to synthesize in different sites of the cell with the myosin farthest from the cell wall. The Z line synthesis appears to take place in the center of the cell where actin filaments are formed. Signs of continuous synthesis of contractile filaments are seen in areas of the muscle cell with little or no formation of myofibrils. In these areas, microtubules are frequently seen in the extension of developing sarcomeres. The protein content of the muscle tissue increases gradually during the fetal period and has at birth reached a level very near that found in adults (Figure 1). The water content of the muscle tissue also decreases and a negative relation between the protein and the water content of the muscle can be noted (Figure 1). The protein storage mainly takes place intracellularly, but the extent of intra- or extracellular water decrease has not been studied.

MITOCHONDRIAL ENZYMES

The ultrastructural picture indicates few and small mitochondria without pronounced crista formation during the fetal period up to the last month,

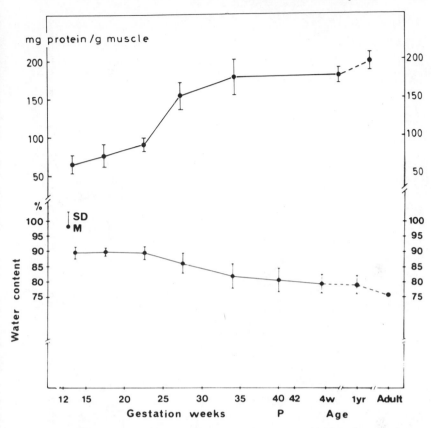

Figure 1.   Mean water and mean protein content for muscle samples obtained from extremity and abdominal muscles of fetuses of different gestation and from infants. For comparison, the mean value found in adult muscle is included (Karlsson, 1971). (Adapted from Colling-Saltin, 1978b.)

at which time a certain increase of mitochondria as well as development of the intramitochondrial structure can be noted (Tomanek and Colling-Saltin, 1977). The oxidative potential, measured as succinate dehydrogenase (SDH) activity, is very low during the whole fetal period, although a stepwise increase is seen at the 25th week of gestation (Figure 2).

During the neonatal period the SDH activity gradually increases, but does not reach the level seen in adult muscles. The staining for NADH-diaphorase (NADH-DH) is very slight during the fetal period. Along with the arising differentiation into different fiber types, it is found that the type I fibers are somewhat more stained (Colling-Saltin, 1978b). This is particularly valid for the large type I fibers. However, they are so few in number that they can play only a minor role in the fetal oxidative potential. The obvious difference in oxidative potential between the two main types of fibers that exist in the human adult muscle is very insignificant at birth, but a differentiation into a chessboard pattern develops rather

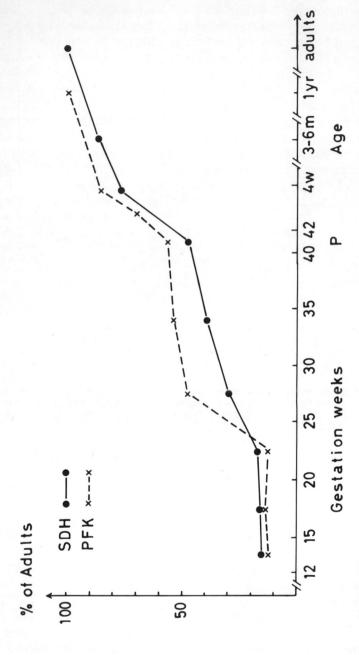

Figure 2. Mean values for the activity of SDH and PFK at different gestations in percentage of adults. Correction for water content has been made. (Adapted from Colling-Saltin, 1978b).

rapidly during the first year of life. Differentiation in staining intensity for NADH-DH between subgroups of the type II fibers is not seen either at birth or during the first year of life (Colling-Saltin, 1978b).

Goldspink (1969) has stated that this difference in color intensity related to the different contents of the mitochondria in the fiber is not only a function of metabolic differentiation but can also be secondary to a more pronounced growth of the cross section of the fiber. By following the growth in fiber size and total amount of mitochondria in mice during their rapid development immediately after birth, Goldspink showed that the gradual loss of staining for mitochondrial enzyme in the type II fibers was not an expression of a decrease of the total content of mitochondria in the fiber, but rather a consequence of the pronounced increase in the contractile filament. A dilution of the mitochondria takes place and, therefore, the type II fibers get pale when stained for succinate dehydrogenase; it is the same in adults. Muscle contractions with high tension development lead to an increase of the area of the type II fibers, especially, without an increase in the capacity for aerobic energy liberation (Gordon et al., 1967; Edström and Ekblom, 1972). In extremely well trained persons, the type II fibers can be twice the size of the fibers in physically inactive persons, but staining for NADH-DH is slight. The activity for SDH in these individuals is only 50% of the activity observed in sedentary people (Gollnick et al., 1972; Costill et al., 1976). These findings indicate that there are different stimuli for growth of contractile filaments in the muscle cell and mitochondrial enzyme, a fact that seems to be similar in different animals.

GLYCOLYTIC ENZYMES

The glycolytic potential evaluated from the activity for phosphofructokinase (PFK) is very low during the first 6 months of the fetal period. The increase then takes place rather fast. At the end of the neonatal period, a level close to the one seen in muscles of adults is reached (Figure 2).

The differentiation in metabolic characteristics between fiber types in fetuses is poor at birth, but appears more clearly after the first year of life. The growth in diameter of types I and II fibers is similar during this period (Figure 3). The increase in staining for NADH in the type I fiber and for α-glycerophosphate dehydrogenase in the type II fiber thus appears as a direct expression of a metabolic differentiation of the fibers.

SUBSTRATE METABOLITES

The periodic acid–Schiff reaction is not pronounced during the first 6 months of the fetal period, but later a certain increase in intensity is noted. However, any distinct differences between fiber types are not

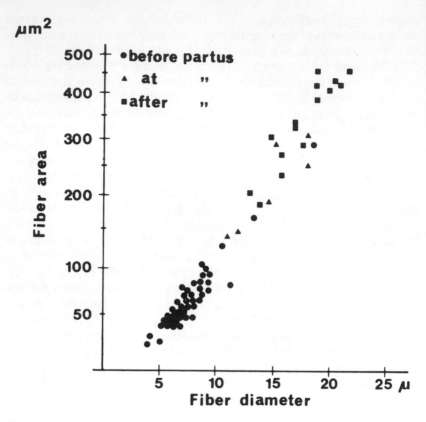

Figure 3.   Mean fiber area in relation to mean fiber diameter. Note the logarithmic scale (Colling-Saltin, 1978a).

observed. The discovery of the rare appearance of glycogen granules in the ultrastructural analysis corresponds with the histochemical picture. A richer appearance of glycogen granules is not noted until the last trimester of the fetal period. Also notable is the fact that most of the glycogen granules found during the fetal period are found in vacuoles. The quantitative determination of glycogen does not show low values, and at the end of the fetal period is similar to that found in adults. Measured dry weight of the glycogen content per kg of fetal muscle is considerably high early during fetal life. It is likely that there is a certain difference between the quantitative and the more indirect method for evaluating the glycogen content.

DIFFERENTIATION OF FIBER TYPES AND FIBER SIZES

Up to the 20th fetal week, all fetal muscle cells are pH stable; i.e., irrespective of pH incubation, a strong staining for myofibrillar ATPase is

Table 1.   Mean values in percent for the number of large-size type I fibers found in three muscles from fetuses at different gestations (upper values indicate percentage of type I fibers found in muscles with large-size type I fibers; lower values represent the percentage of muscles where large-size type I fibers were found) (Colling-Saltin, 1978a)

	Weeks of gestation					
	12–15	16–20	21–25	26–30	31–37	38–42
M. quadriceps femoris	0	0[a]	1.4	1.0	1.4	0.3
(vastus lateralis)	0	0	77	83	87	52
M. deltoideus biceps	0	0	2.1	2.0	2.3	0.5
branchii	0	0	50	75	77	50
M. rectus abdominis	0	0[a]	2.4	4.7	1.9	1.5
	0	0	75	75	75	75

[a]A very few large-size type I fibers were found in one sample from the vastus lateralis and one sample from the rectus abdominus out of 40 samples studied. The muscle samples came from two fetuses at 20 weeks of gestation, fetal length being 23 cm in both cases.

obtained. A small number of the cells are still in the myoblast stage, but after the 19th to 20th fetal week, when a small percentage of the cells are still myoblasts, they are no longer found. Instead, solitary ATPase-negative (type I) fibers are identified. At first these fibers are found in about 50% of the three muscles tested (Table 1). It has not been proven that certain muscles contain more of this type I fiber or that the fiber occurs more frequently in certain muscles. Never during the fetal period does a muscle contain more than 4%–5% of this type I fiber, nor is it common to find this fiber type in all muscles examined in a fetus. This fiber may seem more predominant because it is easily identified, since it is larger than other fibers, and it has a tendency to exhibit stronger staining intensity for NADH-DH.

Around the 30th fetal week, more ATPase-negative (type I) fibers are found. They increase rapidly, and at birth they constitute 50% of all fibers. This fiber type is also easily identified. It differs from the type II and undifferentiated fibers in that it is ATPase negative after alcalic preincubation. It also differs from the above-mentioned type I fibers by not diverging in size from the majority of fibers and thus being smaller than the first solitary type I fibers.

After the 30th fetal week the first ATPase-negative (type II) fibers (after acid preincubation) can be identified. Most of these are type II A fibers (Colling-Saltin, 1978a). At birth only a few percent of the type II B fibers are found, whereas the type II A fibers have increased in relative frequency up to 20%. Therefore, at birth five types of fibers are seen: large-size type I (0%–2%), normal-size type I (50%–60%), type II A (20%), type II B (3%–5%), and as yet histochemically undifferentiated (15%–20%). In adult muscles few or no undifferentiated fibers are found, nor are any type I fibers found that differ in size from other fibers.

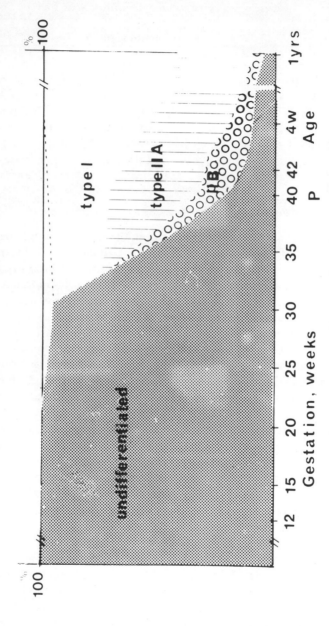

Figure 4.   A schematic description of fiber distribution at different gestations in the neonatal period and in childhood. The dashed line at the top divides the type I fibers into two groups related to size. Those that appear first are the largest size. (Adapted from Colling-Saltin, 1978a).

Ultrastructural examinations also indicate a differentiation within fiber types. Up to the 25th–30th fetal week, the thickness of the Z lines is relatively homogeneous in all fibers, but later a wider spread is found. This is most pronounced in the abdominal and extremity muscles. In the soleus muscle thick Z lines with little variation are found. At the end of the fetal period, the sarcoplasmatic reticulum is less well developed in the soleus muscle than in other muscles.

The size of the fibers (as indicated by the smallest diameter) is 6 μm in the 14th–15th fetal week. The first type I fibers are 12–13 μm; at the same stage of development, the other fibers have a diameter of 6–7 μm (Colling-Saltin, 1978b). The growth in size then gradually increases, and the diameter at birth is 15 μm for undifferentiated, types II A and B, and normal-size type I fibers. At the same time a few type I fibers have a mean diameter of 23 μm (Colling-Saltin, 1978b). Adult muscle has a fiber diameter of 50–60 μm (Dubowitz and Brooke, 1973). At the age of 1 year, only 30% of that size is reached, and at the age of 5 years approximately 50% is reached (Brooke and Engel, 1969).

The above statement of results (illustrated in Figures 4, 5, and 6) might indicate that the differentiation in fiber types and the growth in size should appear very similar in all muscles and in all fetuses. This is not the case. The variation in fetuses of the same age can be quite significant, like the variation found in comparisons of different muscles from the same fetus. The relationship between fetal length and fiber differentiation and size is the same as that for fetal age and fiber differentiation and size. It is to be noted, however, that a slight uncertainty in the exact data concerning the fetal age must be considered.

Significant differences between upper and lower extremities or abdominal muscles are not found; this is also true when comparing proximal and distal muscles. There is also no difference between sexes. It should be noted, however, that the biceps muscle of the arm may be differentiated earlier than other skeletal muscles (Kamieniecka, 1968; Ringqvist et al., 1977).

Dubowitz (1965), after studying the differentiation in the skeletal muscles of different animals, has suggested that differentiation is related to the length of the fetal period. His own findings in human fetuses indicate an early differentiation in fiber types, which results at birth in a variation similar to that found in adults. The present study does not prove that the differentiation into various fiber types is completed at birth. The finding of 15%–20% undifferentiated [type II C (Brooke and Kaiser, 1970)] fibers in the skeletal muscle at birth supports this assumption. The apparent difference between Dubowitz's and this author's results does not necessarily exist. The explanation could be that a combination of staining for myofibrillar ATPase after alcalic preincubation is not sufficiently sensitive to discriminate between the subgroups of the type II fibers nor to

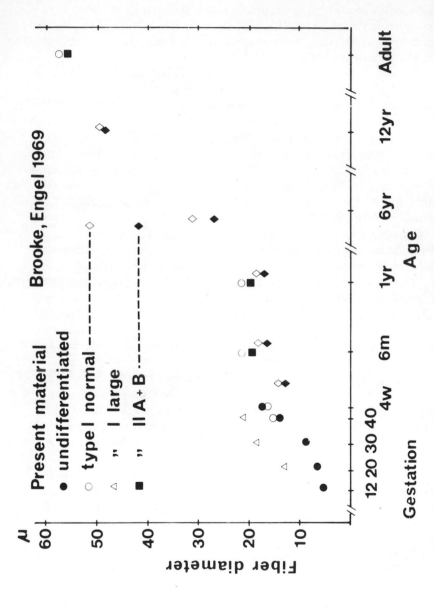

Figure 5. Mean values for the size of different fiber types during different phases of development. The type I fibers have been divided into two groups. Muscle fibers from a group of children of different age are also added (Brooke and Engel, 1969).

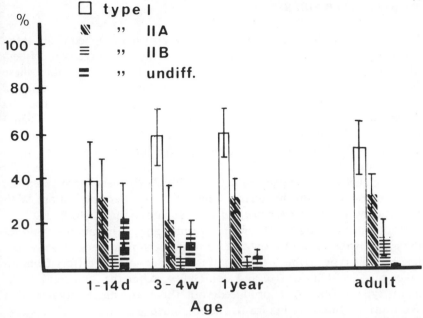

Figure 6.   Fiber distribution in early childhood and adulthood. The bars denote means and the vertical lines SD. During the first weeks of infancy, up to 1% of the type I fibers are of the large size. Values in adults are from the work of Hedberg and Jansson (1976). They studied the lateral portion of a quadriceps femoris. Because the majority of the muscle samples from the infants are from the rectus abdominis muscle, 10 samples (8 female and 2 male) were obtained during surgery and analyzed for relative frequency of fiber types. Mean values ± SD with range were as follows: type I 51 ± 1.6 (37%–65%), type II A 36 ± 12.0 (12%–47%), type II B 12 ± 10 (1%–31%), and undifferentiated 1 ± 1.6 (0%–4%). The abdominal and the thigh muscles were then quite similar in fiber composition in the adults (Colling-Saltin, 1978a).

determine which fibers are undifferentiated. There are two main reasons why the sensitivity of the fibers for low pH before the staining for myosin ATPase is necessary for a more detailed differentiation of fiber types. During the fetal period and at birth, the metabolic development and differentiation are only slight and this limits the possibility for classification. During the first year of life, the differentiation between fiber types increases, thus providing a better possibility to subgroup the two main groups of fibers (Sjögaard et al., 1978). However, neither in neonatal nor in adult muscles are the differences large enough to give clearcut boundaries between the subgroups of fibers. The fact is that the variation in glycolytic and oxidative enzyme contents are overlapping (Essén et al., 1975). The substrate contents of the fibers do not offer any possibility for differentiation because the glycogen is homogeneous in all fiber types (Dubowitz, 1965; Edström and Nyström, 1969; Essén and Henriksson, 1974). The lipid content differs in type I and type II fibers (Schmalbruch and Kamieniecka, 1974) and is probably not very large when comparing the subgroups of the type II fibers (Essén, 1978).

WOHLFART'S B FIBERS

One of the most dramatic things that can be proven histochemically at the onset of fiber differentiation is the debut of the very large type I fibers after the 19th to 20th fetal week (see Figure 4). Wohlfart called these fibers "B-faser" as distinguished from the A-faser, which were small in size and stained for ATPase. These B fibers differ remarkably from the other fibers of the muscle, especially up to the 30th fetal week, when a continued pronounced differentiation is noted. Due to the uniqueness of Wohlfart's B fibers, their development and function have been thoroughly studied.

Fenichel (1963) suggested that Wohlfart's B fibers represented the upper extreme within the normal range of fiber types in question. With time the rest of the fibers grow and differentiate so that the B fibers "disappear" into a more homogeneous normal range. This author's studies (like Dubowitz's study) show that up to the 30th fetal week there is only one type of type I fiber—the Wohlfart B fiber—which differs from all other muscle fibers in size and stainability. After the 30th fetal week, many type I fibers are produced, but these are much smaller than Wohlfart's B fiber (see Figure 4). The continued growth up to birth occurs at the same rate for all fiber types; and, thus, at birth Wohlfart's B fiber is (almost) twice as large as the other fibers. During the neonatal period, very large type I fibers disappear, but it takes an additional 6 months before the mean diameter of the muscle fiber is as large as Wohlfart's B fiber was at birth. Like Fenichel, this author came to the conclusion that Wohlfart's B fiber is not a specific fiber type. This is based on the fact that the histochemical staining for Wohlfart's B fiber totally corresponds to that one seen normally in type I fibers (Dubowitz and Brooke, 1973). On the other hand, the difference in size is obvious between Wohlfart's B fibers and other type I fibers. It is of interest that no definite function could be ascribed to these early large type I fibers; nor is it mentioned in the literature that they exist in other animals.

WHAT CONTROLS THE DEVELOPMENT
AND DIFFERENTIATION OF THE MUSCLE?

There are many hypotheses concerning how the differentiation and growth of muscles take place. A genetic coding is decisive. The importance of a nervous influence is supported by many studies (Gutmann, 1976); evidence for the importance of an intact sensible afferent inflow has also been presented (McArdle and Sansone, 1977), as well as the need for mechanical loading (Gutmann et al., 1976).

The question of whether the nerve has any influence during the fetal period is particularly interesting. Cuajunco (1942), using histochemical techniques, studied the motor nerve development in human skeletal muscle. He determined that a contact between nerve and muscle cell was established from the 13th fetal week. Although Cuajunco has shown this early innervation, he disclaimed that the nerve has a decisive role in early muscle movements and development. He based these conclusions on the fact that both phenomena started before any nerve contact was established. Kamieniecka (1968) has presented the opposite hypothesis. In her study, the parallel in time of the functional contact between motor nerve and muscle fiber are the reason for ascribing importance to the motor nerve. What makes it difficult to ascribe an important role to the motor nerve is the fact that human muscle fiber up to birth is innervated by several different motor nerves, as is the case in many other animals. The fact that the muscle at birth has achieved a content of protein, glycogen, and triglycerides almost of the same amount as is found in adult muscles—while the oxidative and, partly, the glycolytical potential between fiber types is still developing—contradicts a nervous control during this period. If a nervous control does exist, it must be extremely complex, having selective stimuli for the metabolic characters already discussed.

If the muscle after birth has no intact motor innervation, the growth of the fiber is limited and potentially slow fiber muscles could not develop their special contraction abilities. The nervous effect is ascribed to a so-called trophic factor (Gutmann, 1976). According to this theory, still unidentified material is transported through the axon of the motor nerve and affects the muscle fiber. The other possibility is that the muscle activity itself is decisive for maintenance and development of the contractile abilities (Brown, 1973). Brown denervated the lower extremity of rabbits at birth and directly stimulated electrically the tibialis anterior muscle and the extensor digitorum longus muscle during a long period of time with a frequency pattern of impulses typical for phasic nerves. Denervated but electrically stimulated muscles had somewhat longer contraction times than the control muscle and were significantly faster than denervated muscles. In later experiments with longer continuous periods of stimulation, the denervation effects could be avoided totally (Sréter et al., 1973). There is thus a possibility that the influence of the nerve is only a consequence of the motor activity it initiates. If this possibility is combined with the fact that the muscle fiber itself can perhaps influence what type of nerve is establishing functional contact (Purves, 1976), it must then be concluded that the control of the development and differentiation of the muscle cell, both during the fetal period and in the neonatal period, is inherited and genetically coded in the nucleus of the muscle cell.

REFERENCES

Bourne, G. 1972. The Structure and Function of Muscle. 2nd Ed. Vol. I. Academic Press, Inc., New York.

Brooke, M., and W. Engel. 1969. The histograph analysis of human muscle biopsies with regard to fiber types. Neurology (Minneap.) 19:591–605.

Brooke, M. H., and K. K. Kaiser. 1970. Muscle fiber types: How many and what kind? Arch. Neurol. 23:178–179.

Brown, M. 1973. Role of activity in the differentiation of slow and fast muscles. Nature 244:178–179.

Christensen, E. 1959. Topography of terminal motor innervation in striated muscles from stillborn infants. Am. J. Phys. Med. 38:65–78.

Colling-Saltin, A.-S. 1978a. Enzyme histochemistry on skeletal muscle of the human foetus. J. Neurol. Sci., Vol. 39.

Colling-Saltin, A.-S. 1978b. Some quantitative biochemical evaluations of developing skeletal muscles from the foetus. J. Neurol. Sci., Vol. 39.

Costill, D. L., J. Daniels, W. Evans, W. Fink, G. Krahenbuhn, and B. Saltin. 1976. Skeletal muscle enzymes and fiber composition in male and female track athletes. J. Appl. Physiol. 40:149–154.

Cuajunco, F. 1942. Development of the human motor end plate. Contrib. Embryol. (Nos. 187–197):129–152.

Davis, J. A., and J. Dobbing. 1974. Scientific Foundations of Paediatrics. London.

Dubowitz, V. 1963. Enzymatic maturation of skeletal muscle. Nature 197:1215.

Dubowitz, V. 1965. Enzyme histochemistry of skeletal muscle. Parts I and II. J. Neurol. Neurosurg. Psychiatry 28:516–524.

Dubowitz, V., and M. H. Brooke. 1973. Muscle Biopsy: A Modern Approach. Saunders, London.

Edström, L., and B. Ekblom. 1972. Differences in sizes of red and white muscle fibres in vastus lateralis of musculus quadriceps femoris of normal individuals and athletes. Relation to physical performance. Scand. J. Clin. Lab. Invest. 30:175–181.

Edström, L., and B. Nyström. 1969. Histochemical types and sizes of fibres in normal human muscles. A biopsy study. Acta Neurol. Scand. 45:257–269.

Engel, W. K. 1962. The essentiality of histo- and cytochemical studies of skeletal muscle in the investigation of neuromuscular disease. Neurology (Minneap.) 12:778–784.

Essén, B. 1978. Regulation of metabolism in human skeletal muscle: Intermittent exercise as an experimental model. Thesis, Karolinska Institutet, Stockholm.

Essén, B., and J. Henriksson. 1974. Glycogen content of individual muscle fibres in man. Acta Physiol. Scand. 90:645–647.

Essén, B., E. Jansson, J. Henriksson, A. W. Taylor, and B. Saltin. 1975. Metabolic characteristics of fiber types in human skeletal muscle. Acta Physiol. Scand. 95:153–165.

Fenichel, G. M. 1963. The B fiber of human fetal skeletal muscle. Neurology (Minneap.) 13:219–226.

Goldspink, G. 1969. Succinic dehydrogenase content of individual muscle fibers at different ages and stages of growth. Life Sci. 8 (Part II):791–808.

Gollnick, P. D., R. B. Armstrong, C. W. Saubert IV, K. Piehl, and B. Saltin. 1972. Enzyme activity and fiber composition in skeletal muscle of untrained and trained men. J. Appl. Physiol. 33:312–319.

Gordon, E. E., K. Kowalski, and M. Fritts. 1967. Adaptations of muscle to various exercises. Studies in cats. JAMA 199:103–108.

Guth, L. 1968. Trophic influences of nerve on muscle. Physiol. Rev. 48:645–687.

Gutmann, E. 1976. Neurotrophic relations. Annu. Rev. Physiol. 38:177–216.

Gutmann, E., J. Melichna, A. Herbrychowá, and J. Stichová. 1976. Different changes in contractile and histochemical properties of reinnervated slow soleus muscles of the guinea pig. Pfluegers Arch. 364:191–194.

Hedberg, G., and E. Jansson. 1976. Skeletal muscle fiber composition (in Swedish). Report 54, Pediatric Institute, Umeå, Sweden.

Karlsson, J. 1971. Lactate and phosphogen concentrations in working muscle of man. Acta Physiol. Scand. Suppl. 358.

Kamieniecka, Z. 1968. The studies of development of human fetal muscles with reference to some muscular diseases. J. Neurol. Sci. 7:319–329.

McArdle, J. J., and F. M. Sansone. 1977. Re-innervation of fast and slow twitch muscle following nerve crush at birth. J. Physiol. 271:567–586.

Nyström, B. 1967. Postnatal structural and functional development in the efferent neuromuscular system of the cat. Thesis, Karolinska Institutet, Stockholm.

Purves, D. 1976. Longterm regulation in the vertebrate peripheral nervous system. In R. Porter (ed.), International Review of Physiology. Vol. 10. Neurophysiology II. University Park Press, Baltimore.

Ringqvist, M., I. Ringqvist, and L.-E. Thornell. 1977. Differentiation of fibres in human masseter, temporal and biceps brachii muscles. A histochemical study. J. Neurol. Sci. 32:265–273.

Schmalbruch, H., and U. Hellhammer. 1976. The number of satellite cells in normal human muscles. Anat. Rec. 185:229–288.

Schmalbruch, H., and Z. Kamieniecka. 1974. Fiber types in the human brachial biceps muscle. Exp. Neurol. 44:313–328.

Sjögaard, G., E. Nygaard, M. Houston, and B. Saltin. 1978. Human skeletal muscle: Subgrouping of fast twitch fibres. Acta Physiol. Scand. 102:D10.

Sréter, F. A., J. Gergely, S. Salmons, and F. C. A. Romanul. 1973. Synthesis by fast muscle of myosin light chain characteristics of slow muscle in response to long-term stimulation. Nature (New Biol.) 241:17–19.

Tomanek, R. J., and A.-S. Colling-Saltin. 1977. Cytological differentiation of human skeletal muscle. Am. J. Anat. 149:227–246.

Wohlfart, G. 1937. Concerning the occurrence of various kinds of muscle fibers in the skeletal musculature of man and some mammals (in German). Acta Psychiatr. Neurol. Scand. (Suppl. 12).

Human Muscle Morphology with Emphasis on the Fine Structure of Different Fiber Types and Effects of Physical Training—A Review

M. Sjöström

This short morphological review attempts to summarize some recent advances in striated skeletal muscle ultrastructural research aimed at increasing our understanding about the functional specificity of human muscle fibers of different types. It deals only with the normal adult human muscle because detailed ultrastructural information of the kind here related are, unfortunately, not yet available concerning the growing child. Progress in the development of new methods is discussed. Certain structural features of importance for fiber type discrimination are described in detail and some relations between different ultrastructural variables are demonstrated. Effects of physical training are also considered since new light and electron microscopical data have been obtained that further enlighten the relation between structure and function of the different muscle fiber types.

More than 300 individual muscles can be distinguished in the human body. Each of these has a specific function and is therefore (?) characteristically composed of a mixture of fibers with different structural and functional properties (Figure 1). There are reasons to believe that each muscle adapts specifically to various functional demands and should thus be considered as an organ with its own characteristics. From this it follows that morphological, physiological, or biochemical results obtained in studies of a certain muscle are not necessarily representative for all the other muscles in the body, especially not when the data have been

The results and experiences presented in this review have been obtained in studies supported by grants from the Swedish Medical Research Council, the Research Council of the Swedish Sport Federation, and the Muscular Dystrophy Association of America.

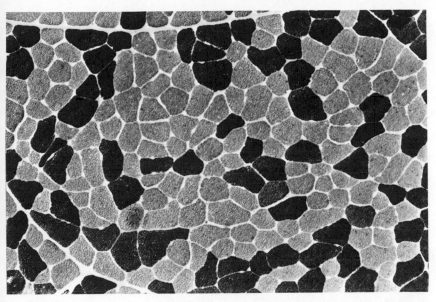

Figure 1.   Cross-sectioned human skeletal muscle (m. tibialis anterior). The section has been treated for visualization of myofibrillar ATPase at pH 9.4. Different fibers in the population of polygonally packed fibers show different staining properties. Two main categories (lightly stained type 1 fibers and heavily stained type 2 fibers) can be distinguished and can also be seen characteristically mixed. In this case, mATPase property is used, as a typical noncontinuous parameter, to discriminate the fibers of different types. Magnification × 125.

obtained from a homogenate or an otherwise poorly defined—with regard to fiber type composition—smaller or larger piece of muscle.

Different research groups are for many obvious reasons interested in and working with different muscles. The results are often generalized by the researchers themselves or by others and are too often compared with each other without any clear demonstration that this important fact has been considered. However, it is easy to understand why this unfortunate situation exists. Our knowledge about the detailed fiber composition of the muscles at light microscopical levels as well as about fiber characteristics at electron microscopical levels is insufficient. Actually, we do not have complete data about the fiber composition of any individual muscle in the human body and, so far, nobody has defined any ultrastructural feature that alone or in combination with other features can be used to distinguish the human fiber types, although some have tried.

How are the different fiber types distributed in the muscle? Homogeneously or heterogeneously? Which of the fiber properties are continuous and which are discontinuous? Are there differences in fiber properties (size, oxidative capacity, etc.) between superficial and deep portions or between proximal and distal parts of the muscle? For a meaningful detailed interpretation of metabolic and physiological results obtained from a certain muscle such information should be essential. Let us hope that systematically collected morphological data will be available in the future, e.g., in a computer in a reference bank, to be used by those who want to interpret sophisticated results from biochemical analyses, clinical examinations, and so on in structural terms.

For the electron microscopists, one of the most obvious aspects to start with for now is to enlighten the detailed ultrastructure of fibers of different types and the relation between structure and function of these fibers. Subcellular structures must be quantified and coupled to already well defined enzyme histochemical properties, contractile speed, etc. For this reason a number of methodological difficulties must be tackled and solved. Effects of changes in functional demands, extensively studied in parallel by the use of other methods, must then be clarified.

In this paper, examples are given that show how to approach these fundamental problems. The description is based mainly on results and experiences obtained by members of the Muscle Group, University of Umeå, and the Surgical Metabolical Laboratory, Sahlgren Hospital, Gothenburg, to whom I am indebted. I am also well aware of the fact that many readers of this review may be unfamiliar with ultrastructural terminology and methodology. Therefore certain basic structural features of the muscle fiber and some methodological comments are given initially to introduce the readers.

BASIC MORPHOLOGY OF THE STRIATED SKELETAL MUSCLE FIBER

The body of the typical cross-striated vertebrate skeletal muscle is made up of many parallel fibers of 50–100 μm diameter and these may extend the whole length of the muscle. Each fiber is a multinucleate cell and contains the common organelles of any animal cell, but the fiber is, of course, characterized by an abundance of cell filaments. These are organized into cylindrical myofibrils of 1–2 μm diameter (Figure 2). The bulk of each fiber is therefore composed of many parallel myofibrils and in between these myofibrils are located the nuclei, mitochondria, membranous systems, and other cell organelles and particles (Figure 2). The different fibers within one and the same muscle, especially in most animal muscles, are characterized by obvious differences in content of mitochondria and glycogen, among other things, and also by several more recently discovered differences in the myofibrillar architecture that are referred to later.

The cross-striations are due to the presence of repeating units (sarcomeres) in the myofibrils themselves (Figure 3). It was shown early by Huxley and Hanson (1954) and Huxley and Niedergerke (1954) that each sar-

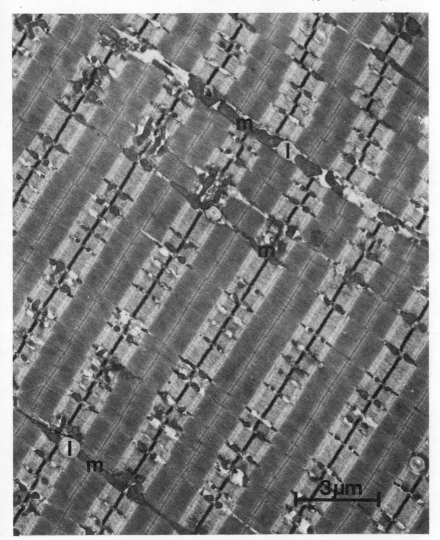

Figure 2.   Electron micrograph of plastic embedded and longitudinally sectioned human striated muscle fiber (m. tibialis anterior). The bulk of the fiber is composed of many parallel myofibrils and in between these myofibrils are located mitochondria (m) and other cell organelles and particles. Lipid droplets (l). The cross-striations are due to the presence of repeating units (sarcomeres) in the myofibrils themselves (see Figure 3). Magnification × 7000.

comere is composed of two main types of muscle filaments, that the arrangements of these filaments gives rise to the characteristic striation pattern, and that relative sliding of these filaments causes shortening of the muscle. The two types of filaments are referred to as the thick (or myosin) filaments and the thin (or actin) filaments.

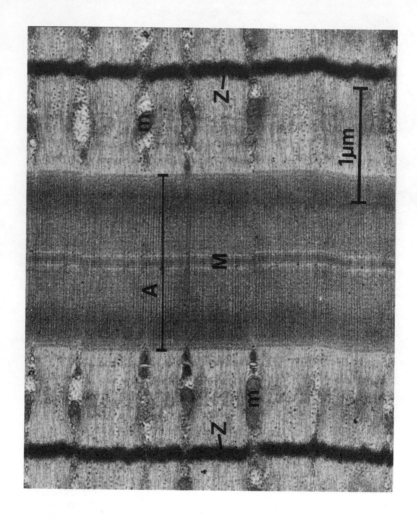

Figure 3.   Micrograph of the repeating unit, the sarcomere, of a few myofibrils from a conventionally prepared (see Table 1) human muscle fiber. The Z bands (Z), A band (A), and M band (M) are fully explained in the text to Figure 4. Magnification ×30,000.

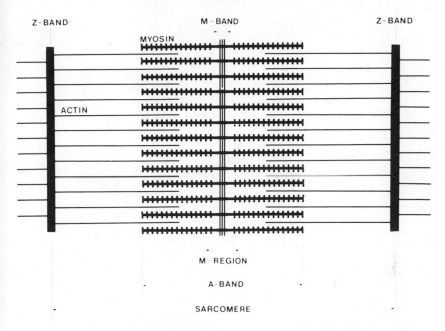

Figure 4.   The sarcomere schematically drawn. It is defined as the unit between one Z band and the next Z band along the myofibril. The sarcomere is composed of two main types of myofilaments that are referred to as the thick filaments (or myosin filaments) and the thin filaments (or actin filaments). Many thick filaments are grouped together to form the A band, in the middle of which the M region is located. In the M region the thick filaments are cross-linked together by an M band composed of, among other things, M bridges.

The A Band

The bipolar thick filaments are roughly cylindrical in shape, about 1.6 μm long and about 15 nm in diameter. Many such filaments are grouped together to form an array called the A band (Figures 3 and 4), in which they are arranged in axial register on a hexagonal lattice. The thick filaments are composed principally of myosin molecules. These consist of a rod-shaped region about 150 nm $\times$ 2 nm on one end of which are situated one (or more) globular regions. These latter form the "head" of the molecule, which has been shown to possess ATPase activity and to be capable of interacting with actin. The red part (or tail) is relatively inactive and is insoluble under normal physiological conditions. For these reasons it is thought that the myosin tails aggregate to form the cylindrical backbones of the myosin filaments and that the myosin heads are equivalent to the projections of cross-bridges that can be seen in micrographs to cover most of the surface of the filaments and that can interact with actin. In fact, projections on the thick filaments occur everywhere except in a region called the bare zone, about 160 nm long, that is situated in the center, or middle, of the filaments. This bare zone has also been termed the M region. The thick myofilaments are cross-linked to each other in the M region, by a structure called the M band (Figure 4).

The M Band

The M band consists primarily of M bridges that join any filament to its six neighbors in the hexagonal filament array. The M bridges occur on up to five lines each, separated by about 22 nm, thus giving the M band a maximum axial width of about 88 nm. The M bridges and other parts of the M band are composed of the so-called M proteins, which have not yet been identified or characterized unambiguously. Other proteins also occur in the thick filaments but are not considered further in this section.

The Z Band

Interdigitating with each end of the A band are two arrays of thin (actin) filaments. Such a thin filament array (about 1 μm long) is joined to a similar array in the next sarcomere by a cross-linking structure called the Z band (Figures 3 and 4). The sarcomere is therefore defined as the repeating unit between one Z band and the next Z band along the myofibril. The detailed architecture of the Z band has not yet been fully elucidated and the associated nonstructural proteins have only been characterized to a certain extent.

When a muscle contracts the two thin filament arrays are drawn into the two ends of the A band and the Z bands move closer together. Clearly this results in an overall shortening of the myofibrils and therefore of the whole muscle. It is thought that the relative movement of the thin and thick filaments is brought about by the action of projections (cross-bridges) that occur on the surfaces of the thick (myosin) filaments. It is thought that these cross-bridges attach to the actin filaments, change their angle of attachment, thereby causing a relative sliding movement between the filaments, and then detach again. Such a force-generating cross-bridge cycle (powered by ATP hydrolysis) is repeated frequently by a single cross-bridge when a muscle is stimulated. Different cross-bridges go through their cycles at different times so that a steady average sliding force is produced. Cross-bridge activity is controlled in the muscle by regulation of the concentration of Ca^{2+} ions in the sarcomere, and this in turn is controlled by the nervous input to the muscle.

Quantification of Ultrastructural Parameters

Different methods are available for quantification of subcellular structures of interest. Obviously, the easiest way of measuring the size of a component is to use a ruler or other more sophisticated, often optical, instrument giving two-dimensional information. However, since biological material never shows sharp edges, difficulties may emerge during the measurements. To take measurements of the Z band width as an example, the detailed architecture has not, at least concerning the human muscle fiber, been fully elucidated, primarily because of the existence of the associated nonstructural, fuzzy material mentioned above (see also Figure 3). Therefore, no criterion for definition of the edges of the Z band has been established. This introduces subjective estimates into the measurements, and results from different observers may thus be difficult to compare.

A more objective way of obtaining morphological data is by the use of the point-counting method of stereology. This method has been applied to vertebrate skeletal muscle tissue and extensively discussed by Eisenberg et al. (1974) and Eisenberg and Kuda (1975, 1976), as well as by others (Weibel, 1972; Hoppeler et al., 1973; Kiessling et al., 1973, 1974, 1975; Stonnington and Engel, 1973; Mobley and Eisenberg, 1975). Various theories and techniques have been used. However, our own experience with the stereological techniques is essentially in accordance with that of Eisenberg and co-workers (1974, 1975, 1976). The reader is referred to their papers for further details. Examples of results obtained using this method are given in the following sections.

FINE MORPHOLOGY OF DIFFERENT FIBER TYPES

Almost all vertebrate muscles, including human muscles, are composed of a mixture of fibers with different properties (see Figure 1). The human fibers are often classified into two, or (perhaps more often) three, main types: Type 1 and Type 2, or Type 1, Type 2A, and Type 2B. This classification was originally made on enzyme histochemical grounds (Padykula and Herman, 1955; Dubowitz and Pearse, 1960; Brooke and Kaiser, 1970). Traditionally, other terms (Type 1–red, slow-twitch, etc.) are also used, paradoxically, even by electron microscopists, although they obviously can not see color or contraction speed in their microscopes.

Human Muscle

Since the original histochemical classification was made, a number of workers have attempted to distinguish the main fiber types by their ultrastructure. In 1966 Shafig et al. reported that red fibers (Type 1) in m. vastus lateralis of relatively young subjects (ages 8–32 years) had a greater content of mitochondria than white fibers (Type 2). Details about the criteria used for classification were not given, however. Similarily, Ogata and Murata (1969) found that a clear difference between red and white muscle fibers existed in that the shape and size of the mitochondria varied between the different fiber types. In red fibers the mitochondria were plump and multiform; in white they were slender and elongated. These authors distinguished between the fibers on the basis of the extent of mitochondrial chains found among the myofibrillar spaces. This feature has more recently provided the basis for identification of fiber types of control muscle at the ultrastructural level (Payne et al., 1975). However, since this distinction between the fiber types at the ultrastructural level is based on mitochondrial content and distribution, any variation in the experimental situation or pathologic condition that alters the amount and distribution of these organelles would make fiber typing difficult and even impossible. Obviously, such a situation exists in studies of the effects of physical training or insufficient blood and oxygen supply to the muscles. The use of other criteria for fiber discrimination is therefore a prerequisite.

Shafig et al. (1966) were of the opinion that the amount of sarcoplasmic reticulum could not be used as an indication of fiber type, but Ogata and Murata (1969) found Type 2 fibers to contain more sarcoplasmic reticulum, even if it was poorly developed in all fibers. Garamvölgyi (1972) concluded that it was the size of the Z band that was the most reliable criterion. Saltis and Mendell (1974) described ultrastructural differences in the morphology of Type 1 and Type 2 fibers on the basis of staining properties with diaminobenzidine. They found that the average Z band width was clearly different for fibers of Type 1 (121 nm) and Type 2 (81 nm). However, sufficient overlap existed, making identification on the basis of Z band width alone inconclusive. Similarly, Cullen and Weightman (1975) were unable to confirm that fibers could be distinguished on the basis of the size of the Z line or of the amount of sarcoplasmic reticulum, and concluded that no single ultrastructural feature could be used to distinguish fiber types reliably. If two factors were measured and certain assumptions were made, it was found possible to classify about 50% of the fibers examined. In their study fibers from four different muscles, each from a different subject, were analyzed. However, there are, as is shown in a later section, fine structural differences between different fibers, not only in the same muscle, but also between different muscles in the same individual. Furthermore, the importance of other factors, such as age and sex, for the volume densities of subcellular structures has been pointed out elsewhere (Hoppeler et al., 1973; Kiessling et al., 1973).

Animal Fibers

For animal muscles the distinction between different fiber types is clearer than in human muscles. Convincing results have recently been reported in a series of stereological analyses of muscles from guinea pigs (Eisenberg and co-workers, 1975, 1976, 1977). Three different muscles (the soleus and the red and white vastus muscles), each composed predominantly of one histochemically defined type (Types 1, 2A, and 2B, respectively), were studied. Above all, it was shown by the use of statistical methods that the entire fiber population could be separated with about 90% success on the basis of the mitochondrial volume together with Z band width (Eisenberg and Kuda, 1976). It follows that if similar studies could be performed on fibers from the same muscle, separation should be possible with still better success.

ALTERNATIVE METHODS OF PRESERVING MUSCLE FOR ELECTRON MICROSCOPY

There are at least three principal types of procedure for preserving muscle for electron microscopy: 1) the muscle specimen is chemically fixed, dehydrated, embedded in plastic, and ultrathin sectioned (the conventional method); 2) it is frozen with or without any previous treatment and sectioned (cryo-ultramicrotomy); and 3) its components are separated either mechanically or chemically and then contrasted (negative staining). These alternative methods of specimen preservation are summarized below. Irrespective of the procedure used, the first step is clearly to obtain a biopsy from the muscle. It is of the utmost importance that great care be taken not to damage the muscle fibers mechanically during this step. Otherwise it is unlikely that any meaningful structural information will be obtained from them, no matter how much care is taken in the subsequent processing.

Muscle Preparation

It is our experience that the surgical method (open biopsy) is much to be preferred to the use of percutaneous needle biopsy or other related instruments, a point that cannot be overemphasized. In the latter cases the samples obtained are too small, are difficult to orient, and are impossible to stretch correctly. Open biopsy is done under local anaesthesia. An incision about 20–30 mm in length is made over the belly of the muscle in the direction of the fibers. The fascia is then cut to expose the muscle. When this has been done a segment of muscle can be removed by grasping one end with forceps and cutting a cylinder with a pair of scissors. Alternatively a strip of muscle can be isolated by tying sutures at each end, after which it is removed together with the sutures. The excised muscle is then stretched slightly under a dissection microscope before being mounted onto a sheet of cork or wood, using pins. Maintaining the muscle in a slightly stretched state throughout fixation is important for the preservation of the subcellular organization. A convenient alternative technique is to make use of a pair of clamps with a defined separation, each of which is put on to opposite ends of the muscle strip. The ends of the muscle are then cut.

The Conventional Method of Preservation

This method of preserving muscle for electron microscopy is summarized in Figure 5 and Table 1. Sections obtained in this way have yielded a considerable amount of information on muscle ultrastructure, but, at the

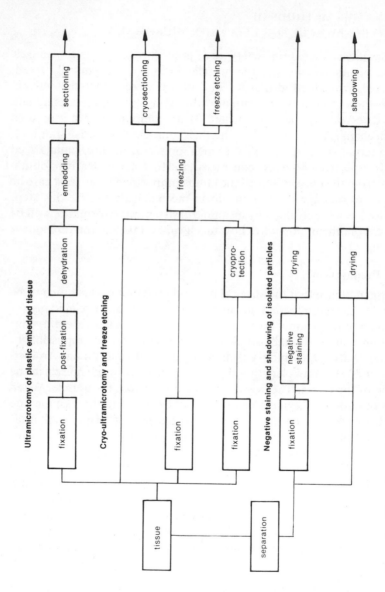

Ultramicrotomy of plastic embedded tissue

Cryo-ultramicrotomy and freeze etching

Negative staining and shadowing of isolated particles

Figure 5.   Alternative methods of specimen preservation for electron microscopy. For further explanations, see text.

Table 1.   The conventional method for preparing skeletal muscle for electron microscopy

---

Prefixation with glutaraldehyde, 1%–5% in a Ringer or a buffer solution, at 4°C
    for 40 min to 24 hr.
Rinsing for 5–15 min in the corresponding buffer.
Postfixation with osmium tetroxide, 1% for 2 hr.
(Uranyl acetate staining *en bloc*).
Dehydration 15 min in each of 45%, 70% , 95%, and 100% acetone or ethanol.
Plastic infiltration using Vestopal, Epon, etc.
Polymerization at 60°C.
Trimming, cutting of semithick (1 μ) survey sections, contrasting with toluidine
    blue, and examination in the light microscope.
Trimming and cutting of ultrathin (50–150 nm) sections of selected areas. Con-
    trasting and examination in the electron microscope.

---

same time, every electron microscopist must be aware of the fact that what he/she can see in the electron microscope, especially at higher resolution, is only a relic or ghost of what the muscle was like in vivo. Because of the harsh preparative procedures involved in obtaining plastic-embedded muscle, electron micrographs of muscle have tended to show a large amount of disorder. Because of this their resolution has been relatively poor and it has been difficult to obtain from them detailed information, for example, about the macromolecular arrangements of the myofibrils. Therefore, differences eventually occurring between fibers within the same muscle have not been demonstrated convincingly. The deterioration of macromolecular structures as the muscle is taken through the various preparative steps has been investigated by the use of X-ray diffraction (Sjöström and Squire, 1977b). It has been found that the main features of the X-ray diffraction pattern are reasonably well preserved after brief treatment with glutaraldehyde, but subsequent treatment in OsO_4 and/or dehydration cause many of the X-ray reflections to become weaker and some to disappear, indicating that the structure has been partly destroyed. The final preparative step of embedding the fixed tissue in epoxy resin (e.g., Araldite or Epon) destroys the true structure of the muscle still further. There has therefore been a great incentive to find less harmful procedures for preparing skeletal muscle for electron microscopy.

Negative Staining of Isolated Components

The structure of individual subcellular components can be seen more clearly by separating these components either mechanically or chemically, collecting them on a carbon-coated grid, and then contrasting them either by the negative staining procedure or by heavy metal shadowing (Figure 5). In the former method the stain tends to collect in depressions or to pile up against edges of the particles being studied. This tends to mask any

Table 2.   The method of cryo-ultramicrotomy in the study of muscle fine structure (according to Sjöström and Squire, 1977b)

Careful dissection of the muscle.
Stabilization with 1%–5% glutaraldehyde in a Ringers, Tryode's, or other buffer solution for 5–15 min (or more) at 4°C.
Glycerol treatment, 30% for 30 min to 1 hr at room temperature.
Rapid freezing by immersion in liquid nitrogen-chilled Freon 12.
Sectioning with a cryo-ultramicrotome at −70 to −110°C (specimen) and about −50°C (knife) using glass knives equipped with trough containing 50% DMSO or 60% glycerol in water.
(Enzyme histochemistry or immunocytochemistry.)
Negative staining of the sections using 0.5% uranyl acetate (pH 4.6) or 2% ammonium molybdate (pH 7.3). Removal of excess solution with the aid of a filter paper.
Air drying, storage in a dry atmosphere, and examination in the electron microscope.

positive staining that may occur so that the protein components in the particles are effectively unstained features embedded in an enveloping matrix of stain. Much valuable information on the myofibrillar material has been obtained in this way and the resolution has been relatively good (for references see Elliott et al., 1976), but inevitably the mechanical and chemical preparative procedures tend to destroy the very particles that are being isolated and even those particles that remain sufficiently intact to provide useful structural information are usually visibly disordered in some way. Furthermore, it must be remembered that homogenates of human muscle characteristically contain a mixture of components of fibers of different types. It may therefore, since a certain component may differ from one fiber type to another, be difficult to know, or to prove, from what type of fiber the particle originates.

Cryo-ultramicrotomy and Freeze Etching

The conventional embedding procedures for preparing tissue are used primarily to render the tissue sufficiently rigid to make it possible to cut ultrathin sections. An alternative method of rendering the tissue rigid is to freeze it. In a procedure that we have found effective for preservation of myofibrillar fine structure, the tissue is first fixed for a few minutes with glutaraldehyde. As mentioned above, brief fixation of this kind is known to alter relatively little the structure as seen by X-rays. It is then put into a glycerol solution, which acts as a cryoprotective agent, and frozen by rapid immersion in one of the fluorocarbons cooled by liquid nitrogen. In this way the formation of large, potentially disruptive, ice crystals can be avoided. The frozen tissue is then sectioned on a cryo-ultramicrotome using a cooled knife. The steps in this procedure are summarized in Figure 5 and Table 2. Alternatively the frozen tissue can be fractured, etched, and replicated using the normal freeze etching technique (Rayns, 1972).

Figure 5 shows that there are a number of important variations of the cryosectioning method in which either or both the steps of prefixation and cryoprotection are left out. Taking all of these possibilities together, the cryosectioning method has the following intrinsic advantages over conventional sectioning methods:

1. It avoids the steps of postfixation, dehydration, and plastic embedding.
2. Sections to be used for the study of myofibrillar fine structure can be contrasted by the negative staining method, which can give a good resolution. (In fact the stain also seems to support the structures of interest to some extent when the sections are dried before viewing in the electron microscope, and it therefore serves another useful purpose as a kind of embedding medium.)
3. Because of the rapidity of the freezing step a living fiber can be instantaneously frozen. The sections obtained from this, if appropriately handled, can be used for elemental analysis by X-ray microanalysis.
4. Because the cryo-sectioning method does not involve the use of an embedding medium, in situ enzyme or immunocytochemistry can be carried out directly on the cryosections in which the components of interest are exposed.

Further discussions of these and other potential advantages and uses of the technique have been given elsewhere (Sjöström and Squire, 1977a, 1977b). The usefulness of the method is demonstrated in the next section.

RECENT MORPHOLOGICAL FINDINGS AIMED AT CHARACTERIZING DIFFERENT MUSCLE FIBER TYPES

So far I have mainly described and discussed common morphological features of muscle fibers and alternative techniques that can be applied to the study of muscle fiber ultrastructure in general. In this section I describe the nature and relevance of some of my recently obtained data of particular interest for the study of myofibrillar fine structure of different fibers. A technique that has been very useful in this respect is that of cryo-ultramicrotomy (see previous section). All of the ultrastructure details, e.g., in the A band, that are visible in the plastic sections can also be seen in cryosections (Figure 6), but much additional information is present in the cryosections for which there is little or no evidence in plastic sections.

Cryosectioning Results on M Band Structure

One of the most striking improvements in the preservation of detail using the cryosectioning method occurs in the M region of the A band (see Figure 7). Figures 7a and 7b compare the M regions in a good plastic section and a typical cryosection from the same type of muscle fiber. It can

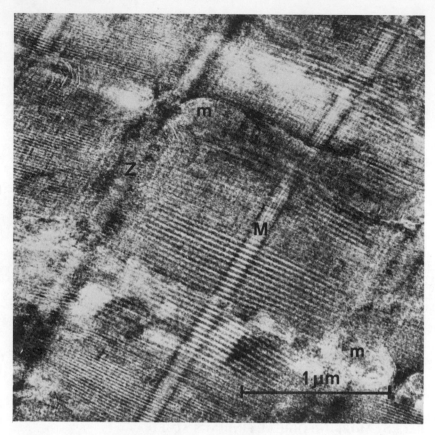

Figure 6.   Section of muscle obtained by the use of cryo-ultramicrotomy. The section has been stained using a technique similar to that used when isolated particles are negatively stained (ammonium molybdate). In the cryosection, protein appears clear against a dark (stained) background, whereas in positively stained sections of plastic embedded tissue the reverse is true. A certain amount of mental adjustment by those used to studying plastic sections is therefore necessary. All ultrastructural details in and around the myofibrils that are visible in the plastic sections can also be seen in the cryosections. Z band (Z), M band (M), and mitochondria (m). Magnification × 45,000.

be seen that the five strong lines of M bridges are apparent in both types of sections. In Figure 7c these lines have been numbered M1, M4, and M6 as in the scheme proposed by Sjöström and Squire (1977a). The line M3, which is usually weaker than the five strong M bridge lines, can also be seen in both types of sections. Lines M1, M3, M4, and M6 are, reasonably, all due to the presence of additional M proteins that interact with myosin to form the M band (see also Luther and Squire, 1978). In addition to these lines the cryosectioned M region shows an abundance of

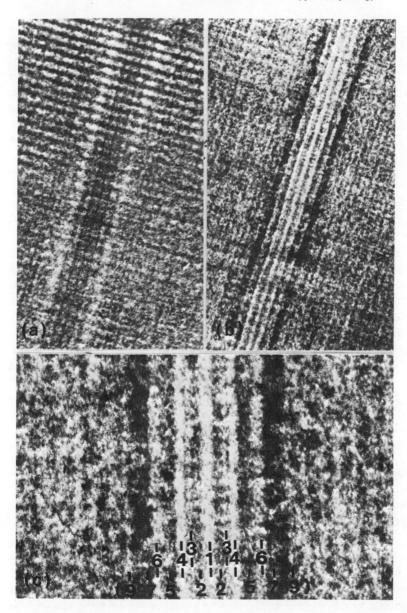

Figure 7.   M region in a plastic section (a) compared with an M region from the same type of human muscle fiber in a cryosection (b). A most striking improvement in the preservation of detail can be seen. The five strong lines of M bridges (M1, M4, M6) are apparent in both types of sections, but in addition to these lines the cryosectioned M region shows an abundance of other striations (M2, M3, M5, M7, M8, and M9) and these are not apparent (except for M3 and M9) even in the best plastic sections. (From Sjöström and Squire, 1977b.)

other striations (i.e., M2, M5, M7, M8, and M9 in Figure 7c, plus some weak striations superimposed on M1, M4, and M6), and these are not apparent even in the best plastic sections. These weak lines fit onto one of two periodic arrays of spacing of about 14.5 nm. The presence of two overlapping arrays is clearly consistent with Huxley's model (Huxley, 1963), in which antiparallel packing of myosin molecules occurs in the filament-bare zone (M region).

Since cryosections show such good structural preservation of the M region it has been possible to carry out a very detailed comparative M region study between different fiber types in the same muscle and between different muscles in the same subject (see also Sjöström and Squire, 1977b). We have found that characteristic differences occur in the appearances of the M region such that in fibers of different types and from different muscles the M bridge lines M1, M4, and M6 can have markedly different relative densities and widths. Within a given fiber the M region appearance in different myofibrils is always similar, but abrupt changes in pattern can occur between one fiber and the next in the same muscle. It has therefore been concluded that M region appearance is a characteristic of the muscle and fiber type from which the section has been taken.

On the other hand, despite these obvious characteristic differences in density of lines M1, M4, and M6 in different M bands, the weak lines in the M region generally occur in very similar positions in all of the M regions that have been studied. The important conclusion has therefore been reached that, despite differences that may occur in the M band structure (presumably as a consequence of variations in the number, distribution, and type of M proteins present), the underlying myosin packing arrangement in the bare zone of the thick filaments appears to be a constant feature. This is also in accordance with the model previously presented by Squire, 1973.

M Band Appearance in Different
Enzyme Histochemically Defined Fiber Types

From the cryosectioning results it was evident that the M band should be most useful as fiber type indicator. However, direct proofs for the usefulness of this criterion had to be found, i.e., a certain M band appearance had to be coupled to other structural or functional properties. The most immediate way of obtaining the desired evidence should be to analyze the same fiber both with enzyme histochemical and ultrastructural techniques. Different reports describing methods permitting combined histochemical and ultrastructural studies on the same fiber are available (Pierobon Bormioli and Schiaffino, 1975; Banks et al., 1977; Eisenberg and Kuda, 1977; Ingjer, 1977). Our methodological approach was as follows. Frozen biopsy specimens were serially cross-sectioned. The thawed sections were prepared either for enzyme histochemistry or for

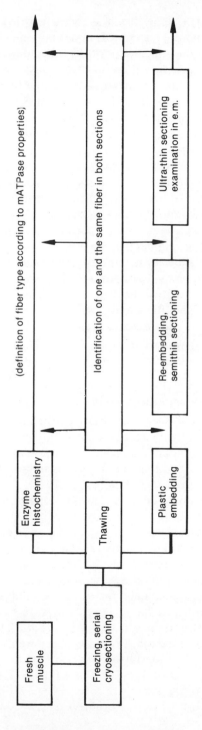

Figure 8.   Methodological approach for the study of the same muscle fiber with both enzyme histochemical and ultrastructural techniques.

electron microscopy. The same fiber was then identified in all serial sections and its ultrastructure examined under the electron microscope (Figure 8). Concerning the appearance of Z band and M band the following results were obtained (a detailed report from this study has been given elsewhere by Sjöström et al., in preparation): in the same fiber all myofibrils showed the same Z as well as M band structure. On the other hand, it was evident that these structures varied from fiber type to fiber type in the same muscle and that their appearance covariated to a great extent. Figure 9 summarizes these and the following findings. Low level resolution of Type 1 fiber usually showed broad Z and M bands with five strong M bridge lines. In Type 2A fibers intermediate Z bands were observed. In the middle portion of the M bands three strong M bridge lines were distinguished, whereas the two outer lines were relatively weak. Finally, Type 2B fibers usually appeared with narrow Z bands. The three M bridge lines in the middle were strong whereas the two outer were very weak, if seen at all. Statistical analyses showed that about 30% of the fibers should have been correctly classified on the basis of the Z band width alone. When two independent observers classified the fibers on the basis of M band appearance more than 95% of the fibers were correctly classified. Thus both the Z and M bands were found to be useful as fiber type discriminators. However, the M band structure proved to be more reliable than the Z band width, and should therefore be used as fiber type indicator.

The Relation between M Band Appearance, Z Band Width, and Mitochondrial Volume

If conventionally prepared fibers were then classified according to their M band appearance and other subcellular structures were quantified, a number of data were obtained of relevance for the discussion about fiber type characteristics. Some of them are briefly summarized and discussed here. The reader is referred to Bylund et al. (1977), Sjöström et al. (in preparation), and Ängquist and Sjöström (in preparation) for more detailed descriptions.

Z Band Width   Within each fiber type there was a characteristic distribution of Z band widths. This is illustrated in Figure 10, which shows a histogram, based on the results of the measurements of all fibers ($N = 234$) from six healthy middle-age male subjects. Two peaks clearly appeared. One of these was mainly due to the distribution of widths of Type 1 fibers, and the other to that of Type 2 fibers. In each individual the typical Type 1 fibers showed the broadest Z bands and Type 2B the most narrow, whereas the Z bands in Type 2A fibers were of intermediate widths. Thus, the mean Z band width of Type 1 fibers for the entire population was greater than that of Type 2A fibers (125 ± 11 and 101 ± 9 nm, respectively; $p < 0.001$). The mean width for Type 2A fibers was in turn greater than that of Type 2B fibers (86 ± 8 nm; $p < 0.001$). A certain

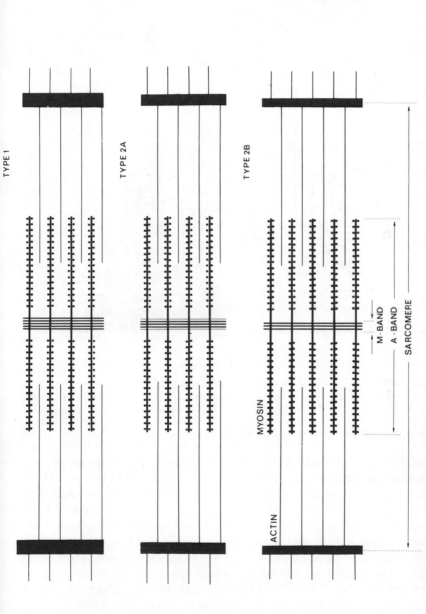

Figure 9.   Schematic drawing showing the Z and M band appearances in different types of human muscle fibers. For a complete description, see text.

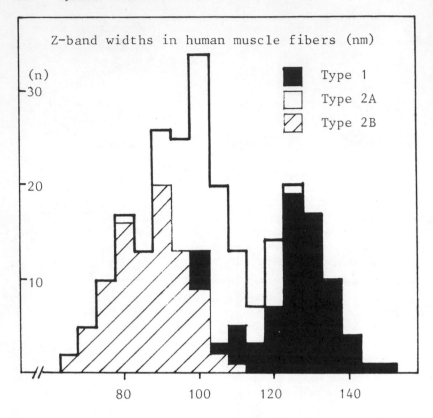

Figure 10.   Diagram showing results of measurements of the Z band width of 234 fibers from m. vastus lateralis of six clinically healthy middle-age men. Two peaks clearly appear. One of these was found to be mainly due to the distribution of widths of type 1 fibers (classified according to the appearance of the M band), and the other to that of type 2 fibers. An obvious overlapping occurs between type 2A and type 2B.

amount of overlapping occurred between the Type 1 and Type 2A populations and, more particularly, between 2A and 2B (see Figure 10). However, there was no overlapping in any individual between Type 1 and Type 2B. By the use of discriminant analysis it was found that, if the M band structure in each individual had been used to determine the three fiber types, 76% to 87% (mean 83%) of the fibers would have been correctly classified on the basis of the Z band width alone. The misclassification mainly concerned Type 2A fibers. Usually, these fibers were allocated to Type 2B, but sometimes also to Type 1. On the other hand, no Type 1 fibers were allocated to Type 2B and vice versa (see also Table 4).

The usefulness of the Z band as fiber type discriminator has previously been discussed by Payne et al. (1975). In their work the M and Z band appearances in fibers from diseased muscles was described; each showed a deficiency in at least one of the major histochemical fiber types.

Table 3.   Mitochondrial mean volumes with range (in parentheses) in percent of muscle fiber volume from m. vastus lateralis (VL) and from m. tibialis anterior (TA) of male untrained middle-age subjects

	VL (10 subjects; 389 fibers)	TA (20 subjects; 810 fibers)
Total	4.0 (3.4–5.0)	4.3 (6.0–3.4)
Type 1	5.6 (4.3–6.4)	4.7 (6.6–3.6)
Type 2	3.3 (2.6–4.8)	3.4 (5.9–2.6)
Type 2A	4.0 (2.7–5.7)	3.6 (6.0–2.5)
Type 2B	2.8 (2.3–4.3)	3.1 (5.5–1.6)

Very little is known about whether or not changes in enzyme properties develop in parallel with the fine structure of the myofibrils. However, in this context it should be mentioned that it was shown that Type 1 fibers had wide Z and M bands (95 and 89 nm, respectively). Type 2A had narrow Z bands (74 nm) and wide M bands (79 nm) and Type 2B had narrow Z and M bands (69 and 60 nm, respectively). It was concluded from this that Type 1 fibers could be distinguished from Type 2 fibers on the basis of Z band width. This should be compared with our result, obtained by the use of statistical methods, of about 94%. Furthermore, Type 2A fibers should, according to Payne et al. (1975), preferably be distinguished from Type 2B on the basis of M band width. This is also in agreement with our results described above, suggesting that the Z band is poorer (83%) as a discriminator when sorting Type 2A and Type 2B fibers than when sorting Type 1 and Type 2 fibers.

   Mitochondrial Volume   The mean values on relative mitochondrial volume (i.e., volume of mitochondria in percent of fiber volume, or more correctly, the mitochondrial volume density) obtained in studies from two different muscles of untrained middle-age male individuals are given in Table 3. As can be seen Type 1 fibers show the highest value and Type 2B the lowest value in both materials. The differences between Type 1 and Type 2A, and also between Type 2A and Type 2B, are significant ($p < 0.001$). However, there is a great deal of overlap with regard to mitochondrial volumes between the different fiber types. This is illustrated in Figure 11, which shows the results of measurements of 234 fibers from six of the individuals whose data are given in Table 3 and from which the specimens had been obtained from the m. vastus lateralis. These data have then been further analyzed by the use of statistical methods (Sjöström et al., in preparation). Discriminant analyses showed that, if the M band appearances had been used to determine the three fiber types, data on mitochondrial volume densities would have been, when compared with Z band widths, poor as fiber discriminators. Only 23% to 47% (mean 37%) of the fibers would have been correctly classified if sorted per individual according to the amount of mitochondria. However, if the

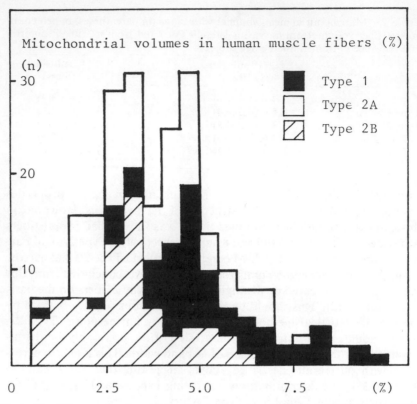

Figure 11.   Diagram showing results of measurements of mitochondrial volume of 234 fibers from m. vastus lateralis of six clinically healthy middle-age men. Type 1 fibers show the highest value and type 2B the lowest. A great deal of overlap between the different fiber types is demonstrated.

amount of mitochondria in each subject had been used to distinguish Type 1 fibers from Type 2 fibers (i.e., 2A plus 2B), 56% to 77% (mean 69%) of the fibers would have been correctly allocated. Type 2A could not be distinguished at all from Type 2B by the amount of mitochondria, since about only every second Type 2 fiber (19% to 67%, mean 47%) would have been correctly classified. If data on Z band widths and mitochondrial volumes per subject were combined, however, 79% to 92% (mean 86%) of the fibers would have been successfully categorized. Table 4 summarizes the results of discriminant analyses of data, which compared with those described previously have been extended in that they have been obtained twice from each of the individuals (i.e., both before and after a period of physical training).

Mitochondrial Volumes versus
Other Structural and Metabolic Variables

Mitochondrial volumes in different types of fibers seemed to be correlated with each other, at least in untrained individuals, i.e., if the individ-

Table 4. Summary of results of discriminant analysis of Z band width and mitochondrial volumes in muscle fibers classified according to M band appearance. The fibers (m. vastus lateralis; total number, 472) have been obtained twice from six healthy middle-age male subjects

Actual group		Predicted groups					
(M band pattern)		Z band width			Mitochondrial volume		
Type	N	Type 1	2A	2B	Type 1	2A	2B
1	149	123	26	0	124	15	10
2A	153	29	108	16	111	32	10
2B	170	0	23	147	107	33	30
Cases correctly classified		80%			39%		

ual had a high volume of mitochondria in Type 1 fibers, it is most likely that he had a high volume also in Type 2 fibers. Interestingly, however, the mitochondrial volumes did not correlate either with fiber type occurrences or with fiber diameters. The data on mitochondrial volumes were found to be correlated with a number of metabolic variables, e.g., in Type 2 fibers, in which they were significantly correlated to citrate synthase activity and to tissue concentration of phospholipids and carnitine. For further details on metabolic data, see Bylund et al. (1977). The relevance of some of the findings described in this section are discussed in the following section, in which some of the effects of physical training are considered.

EFFECTS OF PHYSICAL TRAINING ON THE ULTRASTRUCTURE AND METABOLISM OF DIFFERENT HUMAN FIBERS

"Physical training" is a broad expression that includes many qualitative and quantitative forms of activities aimed at increasing physical performance. The description that follows is limited to effects of endurance training not only for the sake of simplicity: the detailed ultrastructural reports so far available deal only with this type of physical training.

Endurance Training—A Methodological Consideration

It is well established that human skeletal muscles respond to endurance physical training by increasing their capacity for aerobic metabolism (e.g. Henriksson and Reitman, 1976; Holloszy and Booth, 1976; Saltin et al., 1976; Bylund et al., 1977; Jansson and Kaijser, 1977; Öhrlander et al., 1977). However, the events at the subcellular level with regard to fiber type are not fully elucidated. It is obvious that the different categories of fibers adapt selectively to various functional demands (Holloszy and Booth, 1976). This selectivity may be difficult to detect by applying conventional biochemical methods because the biopsy specimens consist of mixed muscles. Various approaches have been used to evaluate the adaptive responses of the various types of muscle fibers. One has been to determine the levels of enzymes histochemically by their staining intensity. However, this is basically a qualitative approach and is not useful when minor quantitative changes in metabolic activities are to be detected. Instead, for quantitative determinations of biochemical activities specimens that consist predominantly of a certain fiber type may be useful, but unfortunately in most human muscles the different types of fibers are too closely intermingled. A technique has recently been presented that permits biochemical studies on individual, histochemically defined fibers (Essén et al., 1975). Put briefly, this involves the dissection of portions of single muscle fibers from freeze-dried biopsy specimens, or sections of them, and analysis using microanalytical methods and enzyme histochemistry in parallel.

An advantage of the alternative method presented in a previous section in this paper, which combines enzyme histochemistry and electron microscopy (see also Sjöström et al., in preparation), is that the fine structure of the fibers can be inspected before the quantitative analyses are performed because the subcellular architecture is still intact and the fiber is located in its in situ position. This also means that pathologically changed fibers may either be included in the material or excluded as described. It is possible within the same fiber to measure different parameters, such as volumes of mitochondria and sarcoplasmic reticulum as well as the amount of contractile material. The volume contribution of an organelle of a certain fiber type to a unit volume of the muscle can be calculated by combining the stereologic data with the data obtained during the morphometric analyses of the histochemically treated sections. This also makes it possible to perform a meaningful comparison of biochemical data on enzyme activities conventionally obtained from a homogenate of muscle tissue. However, it also emphasizes the importance of the fact that the relative occurrences and the diameters of the different fiber types may vary from muscle to muscle and that metabolic data and morphometric results, obtained without regard to individual fiber types, on different muscles must therefore be compared with caution.

Effects on Fine Structure with Regard to Fiber Type

Six healthy sedentary middle-age men participated in a 6-month training program (Bylund et al., 1977; Sjöström et al., in preparation). The physical training consisted of warm-up calisthenics followed by leg exercise, jogging, running, and basketball for 60 min once a week. Twice a week the men did a 4-km cross-country run on a well defined course. The number of exercise repetitions and the intensity of exercise were increased progressively during the training period. The training was supervised by a physiotherapist and a physician taking part in the training program. Each training session was adjusted to correspond to 80%–90% of the maxi-

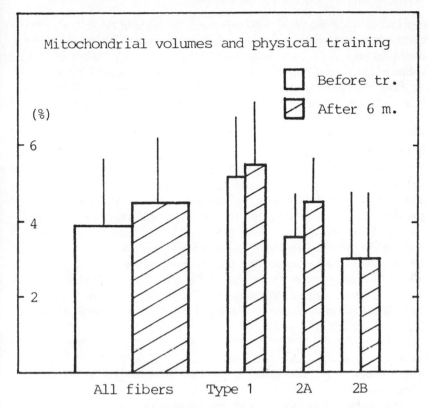

Figure 12.   Example showing changes in mitochondrial volumes ($\pm$ SD) after a period of 6 months of physical training (dynamic endurance training). The population of fibers ($N = 234$ and 238, respectively) have been obtained from six healthy male subjects (see Figures 10 and 11). The advantages of subdivision of fibers into different types is here clearly demonstrated. As can be seen, different fibers respond differently to this very type of training. For further comments, see text.

mum working capacity as judged from the heart rate during training. When the program started running time (4 km) was 31.4 ± 2 (SD) min for the whole group. This value was improved to 23.6 ± 3 min after the completed training period. Meanwhile, oxygen uptake increased from 2.93 ± 1.57 liters/min to 3.68 ± 0.97 liters/min and heart rate at a work load of 150 W decreased from 149 ± 21 to 129 ± 14 b.p.m.

When the period of physical training had been completed the fiber diameters had increased, especially those of Type 2 fibers, but the fiber type ratio remained unchanged. The Z band widths showed a distribution that was very similar to that obtained before training. Significant increases in the mitochondrial volumes were found in Type 1 and Type 2A but not in Type 2B fibers (Figure 12). Quantitatively, the most dramatic increase (about 25%) concerned Type 2A fibers. This differentiation of the adaptive response to physical training became more clear if the proportion of mitochondria was expressed as mitochondrial volume per tissue volume. Finally, a number of correlations were demonstrated between the morphometric and metabolic data. In brief, the mitochondrial volumes were correlated to the activities of mitochondrial enzymes and the fiber sizes and numbers were correlated to cytoplasmic variables. For further details, see Sjöström et al., in preparation.

The Relevance of Data on Mitochondrial Volumes

It has been frequently reported that oxidative enzyme activity, concerning the muscle fiber population as a whole, is related to relative volume of mitochondria (Morgan et al., 1971; Kiessling et al., 1974, 1975; Öhrlander et al., 1977). However, whether or not the mitochondrial volume and oxidative capacity develop perfectly in parallel has not been fully elucidated. It is obvious from many studies that different enzymes involved in oxidative metabolism do not change to the same degree, which has been interpreted as being due to a qualitative rearrangement rather than a quantitative adaptation (Holloszy and Booth, 1976). Such an optimizing may not be detectable as a change in mitochondrial volumes. However, there is sufficient evidence to suggest a covariation between mitochondrial volume densities and enzymes. Mitochondrial volumes may therefore be considered as reflecting the oxidative capacity of muscle tissue. In the work by Sjöström et al. (in preparation), a number of further correlations between morphometric and oxidative metabolic variables were found supporting this view.

However, it should be noted that the majority of these correlations appeared after the training, suggesting that the relationships between structural and functional variables are more obvious after adaptation to higher functional demand.

It has been suggested that endurance training mainly involves Type 1 fibers. A significant hypertrophy of these fibers has been found and a selective loss of glycogen from them has been demonstrated (Gollnick et al., 1972, 1973, 1974; Saltin et al. 1976). It was therefore somewhat surprising that the data obtained in this work concerning mitochondrial volumes indicated changes mainly of Type 2A fibers. However, the exercise program followed by the subjects was not a pure endurance training program. It was designed so as to correspond to a more popular type of physical training (dynamic endurance training). Furthermore, hypertrophy of muscle fibers and increases in mitochondrial volumes, both induced by the training, may reflect two quite distinct adaptive responses in the muscle. Increases in diameters with increasing functional demands were demonstrated in this work for both Type 1 and Type 2 fibers. This finding supports the hypothesis that the physical condition for muscle contraction. i.e., the tension over the muscle belly, is involved in the control of the synthesis and degradation of myofibrillar proteins (Tabary et al., 1972; Goldspink, 1977; Schiaffino, 1974; Munsat et al., 1976). The other type of adaptive response induced by the dynamic endurance training was signs of increased oxidative capacity, i.e., the increases of mitochondrial volumes, which mainly concerned Type 2A fibers and which seemed to be induced without any relation to increases in muscle fiber sizes. Little is known about why physical exercise enhances the oxidative enzyme capacity of the muscle tissue, and the role of this increase is not well understood. Similar conclusions about the ability of Type 2A fibers to adapt to high oxidative demands have been shown by others (Henriksson and Reitman, 1976; Jansson and Kaijser, 1977). It has been suggested that the enzymes are of importance for the utilization of oxygen by the tissues and may thus play a role in the extraction of oxygen. For example, femoral vein oxygen content has been found to be higher during exercise in untrained as compared to trained legs (Saltin et al., 1976). The stimulus that induces increases in mitochondrial oxidative enzymes may be the relative hypoxia, since patients with peripheral arterial insufficiency seem to increase their oxidative capacity (Holm et al., 1972).

SUMMARY AND CONCLUSION

This review initially described why there is a need for further light as well as electron microscopical information about human muscle fibers of different types. A main point was the intention of the ultrastructuralists to provide data detailed enough to make possible an adequate interpretation of the increasingly sophisticated functional data obtained by those working in the fields of muscle physiology and biochemistry. A possible approach has now been outlined. Techniques for the study of muscle fine structure have been briefly summarized and some new relevant information about the macromolecular structure of the myofibril has been described. The importance of objective quantification of subcellular structure has been emphasized. Type-specific structural characteristics, which make fiber typing possible at ultrastructural level with a reasonable degree of success, have been described. The relationships between some of these discriminating properties have been analyzed by the use of statistical methods both before and after physical training.

Much interesting information has already been obtained, to a certain extent, thanks to recently discovered new and very detailed data obtained by the use of cryo-ultramicrotomy. However, it must conclusively be pointed out that there is a great deal of further information to be found even in conventionally prepared muscle specimens, especially if quantitative morphometric techniques are applied and the data are appropriately tackled using statistics.

REFERENCES

Banks, R. W., D. W. Harker, and M. J. Stacey. 1977. A study of mammalian intrafusal muscle fibers using a combined histochemical and ultrastructural technique. J. Anat. 123:783–796.

Brooke, M. H., and K. K. Kaiser. 1970. Muscle fiber types: How many and what kind? Arch. Neurol. 23:369–379.

Bylund, A.-C., T. Bjurö, G. Cederblad, J. Holm, K. Lundholm, M. Sjöström, K. A. Ängqvist, and T. Scherstén. 1977. Physical training in man. Skeletal muscle metabolism in relation to muscle morphology and running ability. Eur. J. Appl. Phys. 36:151–169.

Cullen, M. J., and D. Weightman. 1975. The ultrastructure of normal human muscle in relation to fiber type. J. Neurol. Sci. 25:43–56.

Dubowitz, V., and A. G. E. Pearse. 1960. A comparative histochemical study of oxidative enzyme and phosphorylase activity in skeletal muscle. Histochemie 2:105–117.

Eisenberg, B. R., and A. M. Kuda. 1975. Stereological analysis of mammalian skeletal muscle. II. White vastus muscle of the adult guinea pig. J. Ultrastruct. Res. 51:176–187.

Eisenberg, B. R., and A. M. Kuda. 1976. Discrimination between fiber population in mammalian skeletal muscle by using ultrastructural parameters. J. Ultrastruct. Res. 54:76–88.

Eisenberg, B. R., and A. M. Kuda. 1977. Retrieval of cryostat sections for comparison of histochemistry and quantitative electron microscopy in a muscle fiber. J. Histochem. Cytochem. 25:1169–1177.

Eisenberg, B. R., and A. M. Kuda, and J. B. Peter. 1974. Stereological analysis of mammalian skeletal muscle. I: Soleus muscle of the adult guinea pig. J. Cell Biol. 60:732–754.

Elliot, A., G. Offer, and K. Burridge. 1976. Electron microscopy of myosin molecules from muscle and non-muscle sources. Proc. R. Soc. Lond. [Biol.] 193: 45–53.

Essén, B., E. Jansson, J. Henriksson, A. W. Taylor, and B. Saltin. 1975. Metabolic characteristics of fiber types in human skeletal muscle. Acta Physiol. Scand. 95:153–165.

Garamvölgyi, N. 1972. Slow and fast muscle cells in human striated muscle. Acta Biochim. Biophys. Acad. Sci. Hung. 7:165–172.

Goldspink, D. F. 1977. The influence of immobilization in stretch on protein turnover of rat skeletal muscle. J. Physiol. 264:267–282.

Gollnick, P. D., R. B. Armstrong, B. Saltin, C. W. Saubert, W. L. Sembrowich, and R. E. Shephard. 1973. Effect of training on enzyme activity and fiber composition of human skeletal muscle. J. Appl. Physiol. 34:107–111.

Gollnick, P. D., R. B. Armstrong, C. W. Saubert, K. Piehl, and B. Saltin. 1972. Enzyme activity and fiber composition in skeletal muscle of untrained and trained man. J. Appl. Physiol. 33:312–319.

Gollnick, P. D., K. Piehl, and B. Saltin. 1974. Selective depletion pattern in human muscle fibers after exercise of varying intensity and at varying pedaling rates. J. Physiol. (Lond.) 241:45–51.

Henriksson, J., and J. S. Reitman. 1976. Quantitative measures of enzyme activities in Type I and Type II muscle fibers of man after training. Acta Physiol. Scand. 97:392–397.

Holloszy, J. O., and F. W. Booth. 1976. Biochemical adaptions to endurance exercise in muscle. Annu. Rev. Physiol. 38:273–291.

Holm, J., P. Björntorp, and T. Scherstén. 1972. Metabolic activity in human skeletal muscle. Effect of peripheral arterial insufficiency. Eur. J. Clin. Invest. 2:321–325.

Hoppeler, H., P. Lüthi, H. Claassen, E. R. Weibel, and H. Howald. 1973. The ultrastructure of the normal human skeletal muscle. A morphometric analysis on untrained men, women and well-trained orienteers. Pfluegers Arch. 344: 217–232.

Huxley, H. E. 1963. Electron microscope studies on the structure of natural and synthetic protein filaments from striated muscle. J. Mol. Biol. 7:281–308.

Huxley, H. E., and J. Hanson. 1954. Changes in the cross-striations of muscle during contraction and stretch and their structural interpretation. Nature 173: 973–976.

Huxley, A. F., and R. Niedergerke. 1954. Structural changes in muscle during contraction. Interference microscopy of living muscle fibers. Nature 173:971–973.

Ingjer, F. 1977. A method for correlating ultrastructural and histochemical data from individual muscle fibers. Histochemistry 54:169–172.

Jansson, E., and L. Kaijser. 1977. Muscle adaptation to extreme endurance training in man. Acta Physiol. Scand. 100:315–324.

Kiessling, K.-H., L. Pilström, A.-C. Bylund, K. Piehl, and B. Saltin. 1975. Effects of chronic ethanol abuse on structure and enzyme activities of skeletal muscle in man. Scand. J. Clin. Lab. Invest. 35:601–607.

Kiessling, K.-H., L. Pilström, A.-C. Bylund, B. Saltin, and K. Piehl. 1974. Enzyme activities and morphometry in skeletal muscle of middle-aged men after training. Scand. J. Clin. Lab. Invest. 33:63–69.

Kiessling, K.-H, L. Pilström, J. Karlsson, and K. Piehl. 1973. Mitochondrial volume in skeletal muscle from young and old physically untrained and trained healthy men and from alcoholics. Clin. Sci. 44:547–554.

Luther, P., and J. Squire. 1978. Three-dimensional structure of vertebrate muscle M-region. J. Mol. Biol. 125:313–324.

Mobley, B. A., and B. R. Eisenberg. 1975. Sizes of components in frog skeletal muscle measured by methods of stereology. J. Gen. Physiol. 66:31–45.

Morgan, T. E., L. A. Cobb, F. A. Short, R. Ross, and D. R. Gunn. 1971. Effects of long-term exercise on human muscle mitochondria. In: B. Pernow and B. Saltin (eds.), Muscle Metabolism during Exercise, pp. 87–95. Plenum Publishing Corp., New York.

Munsat, T. L., D. McNeal, and R. Waters. 1976. Effects of nerve stimulation on human muscle. Arch. Neurol. 33:608–617.

Ogata, T., and F. Murata. 1969. Cytological features of three fiber types in human striated muscle. Tohoku J. Exp. Med. 99:225–245.

Öhrlander, J., K.-H. Kiessling, J. Karlsson, and B. Ekblom. 1977. Low intensity training, inactivity and resumed training in sedentary men. Acta Physiol. Scand. 101:351–363.

Padykula, H. A., and E. Herman. 1955. Factors affecting the activity of adenosine triphosphatase and other phosphatases as measured by histochemical techniques. J. Histochem. Cytochem. 3:161–167.

Payne, C. M., L. Z. Stern, R. G. Curless, and L. K. Hannapel. 1975. Ultrastructural fiber typing and diseased human muscle. J. Neurol. Sci. 25:99–108.

Pierobon Bormioli, S., and S. Schiaffino. 1975. A procedure for correlated histological, histochemical and ultrastructural study of skeletal muscle tissue. J. Submicrosc. Cytol. 7:361–371.

Rayns, D. G. 1972. Myofilaments and cross-bridges as demonstrated by freeze-fracturing and -etching. J. Ultrastruct. Res. 40:103–121.

Saltin, B., K. Nazar, D. L. Costill, E. Stein, E. Jansson, B. Essén, and P. O. Gollnick. 1976. The nature of the training response: Peripheral and central adaptations to one-legged exercise. Acta Physiol. Scand. 96:289–305.

Saltis, L. M., and J. R. Mendell. 1974. The fine structural differences in human muscle fiber types based on peroxidatic activity. J. Neuropathol. Exp. Neurol. 5:632–640.

Schiaffino, S. 1974. Hypertrophy of skeletal muscle induced by tendon shortening. Experientia 30:1163–1164.

Shafig, S. A., M. Gorycki, L. Goldstone, and A. T. Milhorat. 1966. Fine structure of fiber types in normal human muscle. Anat. Res. 156:283–302.

Sjöström, M., and J. Squire, 1977a. Fine structure of the A band in cryo-sections. The structure of the A-band in ultra-thin cryo-sections negatively stained. J. Mol. Biol. 109:49–68.

Sjöström, M., and J. Squire. 1977b. Cryo-ultramicrotomy and myofibrillar fine structure. A review. J. Microsc. 111:239–279.

Squire, J. M. 1973. General model of myosin filament structure. III. Molecular packing arrangements in myosin filaments. J. Molec. Biol. 77:291–323.

Stonnington, H. H., and A. G. Engel. 1973. Normal and denervated muscle. A morphometric study of fine structure. Neurology 23:714–724.

Tabary, J. C., C. Tabary, C. Tardieu, G. Tardieu, and G. Goldspink. 1972. Physiological and structural changes in the cat's soleus muscle due to immobilization at different lengths by plaster casts. J. Physiol. (Lond.). 224:231–244.

Weibel, E. R. 1972. A stereological method for estimating volume and surface of sarcoplasmic reticulum. J. Microsc. 95:229–242.

Muscle Substrates, Muscle Enzyme Activities, and Muscle Structure in Infants with Symptomatic Ventricular Septal Defects

B. O. Eriksson, L.-G. Friberg, and G. Mellgren

An infant with a ventricular septal defect (VSD) and a large left-to-right shunt will incur heart failure at the age of 4 to 6 weeks (Talner, 1977; Rowe and Izukawa, 1978). This heart failure can be long lasting and pronounced in some patients and is one of the reasons for early surgical correction. The symptomatology of this heart failure includes, among many other things, muscular weakness, delayed gross motor development, and impaired growth (for references, see Talner, 1977; Keith, 1978). The latter is most marked in regard to weight gain. In many respects these infants resemble children with celiac disease and other types of malnutrition (Naeye, 1965). They also exhibit gross motor disturbances similar to those found in children with neuromuscular disorders—the "floppy infant syndrome." Because these latter diseases are accompanied by muscle metabolic disturbances, it was considered of interest to study these infants with heart failure caused by a large VSD and with muscular symptoms to determine if they also had any disturbances in their skeletal muscle metabolism.

SUBJECTS

Fourteen children, eight boys and six girls, ages 2–13 months were studied. Twelve of these infants had an isolated VSD, and the other two had a VSD with infundibular pulmonary stenosis and left-to-right shunt (acyanotic tetralogy of Fallot) and a cerebral AV fistula with a large left-to-right shunt, respectively. (These two infants had the same problem with heart failure due to their large left-to-right shunts.) All 14 infants were studied in relation to diagnostic heart catheterization. Twelve of them had been on digitalis from 1 week to 11 months prior to the study. All showed major or minor signs and symptoms of heart failure. A weight deviation greater then -1 SD was present in 11 infants, and a height deviation of more than -1 SD was found in six (Table 1). Some hemodynamic variables are also included in Table 1. A control group consisting of 25 children ages 1 month to 11 years was also studied. These children were hospitalized for minor surgical problems such as inguinal hernia or undescended testicle. A further description of this group is given elsewhere (Lundberg et al., 1979a).

PROCEDURES

Muscle biopsies were taken from the gracilis muscle simultaneously with the diagnostic heart catheterization. This muscle is very close to the saphenous vein that was used for the catheterization. Thus, the biopsy was made in the same cut-down as for the heart procedure. The muscle sample taken weighed around 25 mg. In the control subjects, a needle biopsy was performed from the vastus lateralis muscle using the method described by Bergström (1962). One muscle sample was immediately frozen in liquid nitrogen for later analyses of muscle substrate concentrations and muscle enzyme activities. Another sample was frozen in isopenthan, cooled by liquid nitrogen. This sample was used for the histochemical stainings.

METHODS

The frozen biopsies were stored at $-80°C$ until analyzed. They were weighed at $-20°C$ and then analyzed for adenosine triphosphate (ATP), creatine phosphate (CP), glycogen, glucose, glucose 6-phosphate, and lactate according to the modified Lowry methods as described by Karlsson (1971). The activities of the muscle enzymes, succinate dehydrogenase (SDH), lactate dehydrogenase (LDH), and phosphorylase were determined according to the methods of Cooperstein et al. (1950), Karlsson et al. (1968), and Lowry and Passonneau (1964), respectively. All values obtained were expressed as wet weight (w.w.) values.

The muscle samples for histochemical analysis were cut in a cryostat at $-20°C$ after careful orientation of the muscle fiber direction. Serial sections were cut and mounted on cover glasses. Staining for myosine ATPase at pH 10.3 was done according to the method of Padykula and Herman (1955). A photomicroscopy technique was used for getting photoprints of the sections for classifying type I and type II fibers. Fiber size was determined by "lesser diameter" as described by Brooke and Engel (1969).

Table 1. Some variables in infants with VSD (cases 1–12), cerebral AV fistula (case 13), and a VSD with infundibular pulmonary stenosis and left-to-right shunt (case 14)

Case	Age (years)	Pulmonary artery pressure (mm Hg)	$\dot{Q}_p:\dot{Q}_s$	Height deviation (in SD units)	Weight deviation (in SD units)	Digitalis treatment before biopsy (months)
1	0.48	55/20 m = 35	2.3:1	−0.5	+0.5	2.0
2	0.43	80/40 m = 55	3.6:1	−0.2	−2.7	3.0
3	0.17	84/32 m = 50	4.1:1	0	−1.5	2.0
4	0.44	28/8 m = 14	2.0:1	−1.7	−2.8	—
5	1.15	86/39 m = 62	2.4:1	−1.3	−2.8	11.0
6	0.38	55/15 m = 32	2.7:1	−0.6	−1.2	1.5
7	0.25	56/16 m = 32	2.7:1	−1.5	−2.3	0.5
8	1.01	45/16 m = 24	3.2:1	−1.0	−3.5	0.5
9	0.76	22/12 m = 16	1.7:1	−1.0	−1.0	6.0
10	0.51	40/10	2.6:1	+1.5	0	—
11	0.29	79/20 m = 42	5.5:1	0	−3.0	0.3
12	0.13	65/25 m = 35	8.0:1	−0.5	−1.5	0.3
13	0.24	32/21 m = 22		+1.1	−0.8	1.0
14	0.33	not entered	1.5:1	−2.0	−5.0	1.5

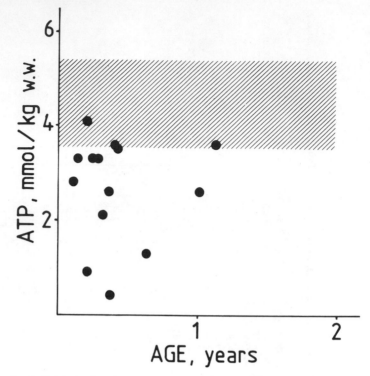

Figure 1.   Individual values for muscle ATP concentrations in infants with VSD. Included are also ± 1 SD for the control group (Lundberg et al., 1979b).

RESULTS

The concentration of ATP was found to be low in 11 of the 14 infants (Figure 1); the mean value was 2.65 mmol/kg w.w. The mean CP concentration was also lower when compared to the control group; a mean value of 11.0 mmol/kg w.w. was found. In eight of the 14 infants with VSD, values for CP concentration were within ±2 SD, while the other six had values below −2 SD (Figure 2). The glycogen concentration was somewhat less influenced. However, in eight of the 14 infants, values below −2 SD were obtained (Figure 3). No significant deviation from the control group was found for the glucose, glucose 6-phosphate, and lactate.

Regarding the muscle enzyme activities, very low values were obtained in most cases for the SDH activity (Figure 4). The lowest value was found in a 4-month-old girl in whom the diagnosis of heart failure and VSD was not suspected initially. She had been diagnosed as having a metabolic disease with liver and spleen enlargement and extreme muscular weakness. Phosphorylase activity was moderately decreased (Figure 5), whereas only a minor decrease was found for the LDH activity (Figure 6). A normal proportion of type I and type II fibers was found—50.0% of

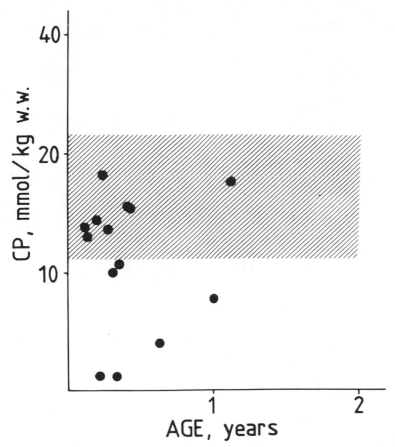

Figure 2.   Individual values for CP concentration in skeletal muscle in infants with VSD. Also included, in the shadowed area, are values ± 1 SD for a control group. (Lundberg et al., 1979b).

each as a mean. The fiber sizes were also normal when compared to the control subjects (Figure 7). The mean values for type I and type II fibers were found to be 18.8 μ and 16.5 μ, respectively. No obvious pathological changes were found in the specimens.

DISCUSSIONS

Heart failure in an infant has an influence on the entire organism. Under-nourishment due to an inadequate food intake, in combination with an in-testinal malabsorption caused by lymphedema in the intestines, can often be found (Jones, 1961; Talner, 1977). Another finding is a metabolic dis-turbance characterized by a lower insulin response to glucose administra-tion and a higher sympathomimetic activity with higher catecholamine levels in serum (Hait et al., 1972; Downing et al., 1977). Clinically, these

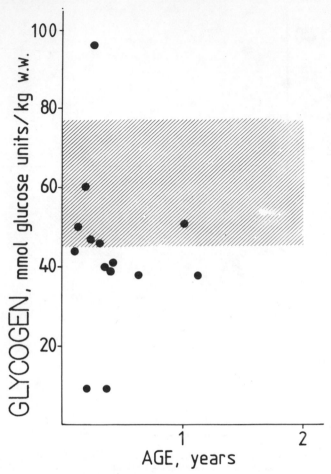

Figure 3.   Individual values for muscle glycogen concentration in infants with VSD. Also included, in the shadowed area, are values ± 1 SD for a control group (Lundberg et al., 1979b).

infants often resemble malnourished infants from underdeveloped countries, with their tiny arms and legs, reduced subcutaneous fat layer, and poor weight gain (Lees et al., 1965). Their muscles are usually more flaccid, and their gross motor development is delayed.

In this study, these metabolic disturbances were shown to be accompanied by a rather marked decrease in the substrate energy levels in the skeletal muscle. It is possible that these obtained values are only attributable to the malabsorption present. Similar but not so marked results have also been found in children with celiac disease (Lundberg et al., 1979a; Lundberg, this volume). Another possible explanation could be that the decreased muscle blood flow, which is caused by the heart failure, provides too poor a supply of nutrients to the muscle, so that the formation

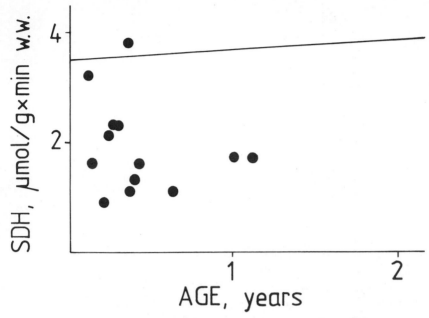

Figure 4. Individual values for SDH activity in infants with VSD. The regression line ($y = 3.52 + 0.16\ x$) for the control subjects is also given.

of these energy-rich compounds is reduced. Since there were no data on the muscle blood flow in these infants, this question cannot be answered. However, it is reasonable to assume that a combination of these two factors could at least partly explain the obtained results.

With a decreased blood flow to an extremity, a limitation in muscular activity exists. This was the case in the clinical finding in these infants. A reduced muscular activity may lead to a reduction in substrate energy levels. Therefore, it is very difficult to determine which of these factors were the most important in these infants. Children with a late walking debut, and thus reduced muscular activity in the legs, show similar but less marked results regarding the muscle subtrate energy levels in the leg muscles (Lundberg et al., 1979b). On the other hand, the less active conditions found in the VSD infants were not so marked as in the late walking children. Thus, this theory does not fully explain the result obtained in the VSD infants. A combination of the effect of a reduced muscular blood supply and the effect of inactivity seems more probable. Whether or not these two factors fully explain the deviation found is uncertain.

In infants with the "floppy infant syndrome," an underlying neuro-muscular or metabolic disease is usually found (Dubowitz and Brooke, 1973). When a neuromuscular disease is present, hypotrophy or atrophy of either type I or type II fibers or both occurs. The proportion of the fibers is also changed (Dubowitz and Brooke, 1973). It is quite obvious

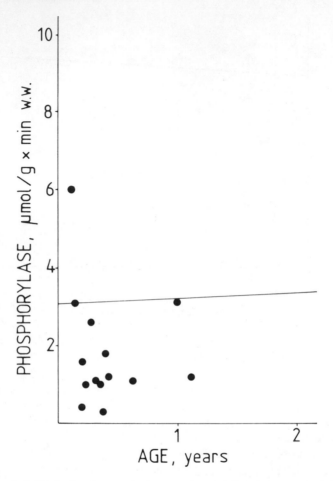

Figure 5.   Individual values for muscle phosphorylase activity in infants with VSD. The regression line ($y = 3.04 + 0.16 \, x$) for the control subjects is also given.

that none of these alterations were present in these VSD infants (Figure 7). If any deviation from the normal size of the muscle fibers was present, larger muscle fibers were found. However, it is dangerous to draw too many conclusions from these findings. The fiber size of the normal group that the VSD infants were compared with belonged to a group of children admitted for a suspected neuromuscular disorder who had some symptoms, but in whom no definitive diagnosis of abnormality had been made. Also included were results from biopsies of brothers and sisters of affected children in whom muscle biopsies were performed in order to determine whether or not they also had a disease. Thus, the biopsy material of Brooke and Engel (1969) cannot be looked on as normal material. [Further support for this view can be found in the reports by Colling-

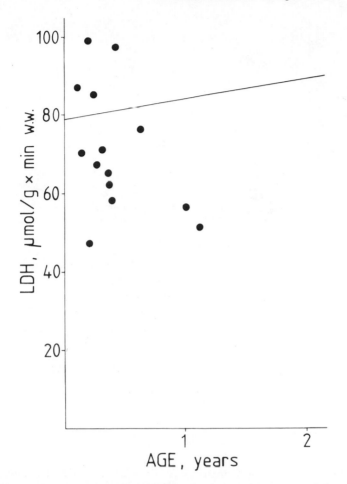

Figure 6.   Individual values for LDH activity in the muscles of infants with VSD. The regression line ($y = 78.7 + 5.20\,x$) for the control subjects is also given.

Saltin (1978), Lundberg et al. (1979a), and Lundberg et al. (1979b).] It can thus be stated that, with regard to muscle morphology, a normal situation existed in the VSD infants.

The marked decrease in SDH activity (Figure 4) that was found in these infants was not accompanied by the same degree of decrease regarding LDH and phosphorylase. These two latter enzymes are involved in anaerobic glycolysis. In a situation involving a decreased supply of oxygen, a stronger demand for anaerobic energy delivery will exist. This explains why these enzymes deviated much less than SDH. One can also ask why SDH activity was decreased to such an extent. With a reduced blood supply, as in slight to moderate claudicatio intermittens patients, an increased SDH activity is found (Holm et al., 1973). Only with a severe re-

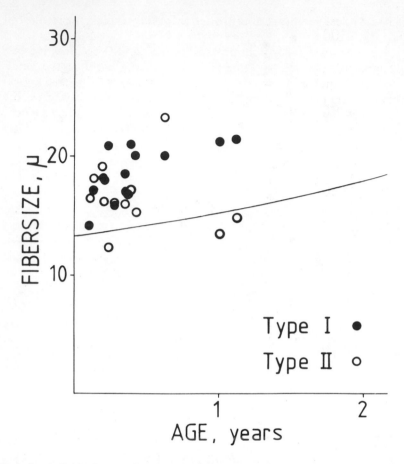

Figure 7.   Individual mean values for muscle fiber sizes, expressed as "lesser diameter" according to the method of Brooke and Engel (1969) in infants with VSD. Solid circles denote type I fibers and open circles type II fibers. The curved line denotes "normal muscle fiber size" according to Brooke and Engel (1969).

duction of muscle blood flow—as in severe claudicatio intermittens—has a reduction of the SDH activity been found. This reduction is not so marked as the one present in these VSD infants. Therefore, it is reasonable to assume that other factors may play an important role in these VSD infants. One such factor could be inactivity. Henriksson (1977) has shown that inactivity leads to a marked reduction of the SDH activity, whereas physical training has the opposite effect. In the studies of Häggmark (1978), a reduction in SDH activity was also found after immobilization of an extremity with plaster. Thus, inactivity may contribute to a reduction of SDH activity. Perhaps reduced muscle blood supply in combination with inactivity produces these results. Other factors, such as the effect of malabsorption or the lack of nutritive substances, may also play important roles. Further studies are needed to fully explain the results obtained.

It is obvious that early surgical correction of VSD becomes increasingly important. A successful operation dramatically improves the condition of the infant with heart failure (Talner, 1977). It has also been known for many years that a VSD infant will improve spontaneously between 1 and 2 years of age. Almost all muscular symptoms disappear and a catch-up in weight gain takes place. It is not known whether surgical repair and spontaneous improvement accomplish catch-up to the same degree regarding muscle substrate levels and muscle enzyme activities. A follow-up study is needed to answer these questions. However, three of these children were re-examined at the ages of 8, 12, and 22 months. All of their pathological values had normalized, and they did not show any gross motor disturbances. Thus, the abnormal findings in symptomatic infants seem to be reversible, and a surgical closure of the VSD will probably also lead to normalization. This could be a further reason for recommending early surgical closure of VSD in infants with heart failure.

REFERENCES

Bergström, J. 1962. Muscle electrolytes in man. Scand. J. Clin. Lab. Invest. 14, Suppl. 68.

Brooke, M. H., and W. Engel. 1969. The histograph analysis of human muscle biopsies with regard to fiber types. Neurology (Minneap.) 19:591–605.

Colling-Saltin, A.-S. 1978. Skeletal muscle differentiation during fetal life in man (in Swedish). Thesis, Karolinska Institutet, Stockholm.

Cooperstein, S. J., A. Lazarow, and N. J. Kurfess. 1950. A microspectrophotometric method for the determination of succinic dehydrogenase. J. Biol. Chem. 186:129–139.

Downing, S. E., J. C. Lee, and R. P. Ricker. 1977. Mechanical and metabolic effects of insulin on newborn lamb myocardium. Am. J. Obstet. Gynecol. 127: 649–656.

Dubowitz, V., and M. H. Brooke. 1973. Muscle Biopsy: A Modern Approach. W. B. Saunders, Ltd., London.

Häggmark, T. 1978. A study of morphological and enzymatic properties of the skeletal muscles after injuries and immobilization in man. Thesis, Karolinska Institutet, Stockholm.

Hait, G., M. Corpus, F. R. Lamarre, Y. Shang-Hsien, J. Kypson, and G. Cheng. 1972. Alteration of glucose and insulin metabolism in congenital heart disease. Circulation 46:333–346.

Henriksson, J. 1977. Human skeletal muscle adaptation to physical activity. Thesis, Karolinska Institutet, Stockholm.

Holm, J., A. G. Dahlöf, P. Björntorp, and T. Scherstén. 1973. Enzyme studies in muscles of patients with intermittent claudicatio. Effect of training. Scand. J. Clin. Lab. Invest. 31(Suppl. 128):201–205.

Karlsson, J. 1971. Lactate and phosphagen concentrations in working muscle of man. Acta Physiol. Scand., Suppl. 358.

Karlsson, J., B. Diamant, and B. Saltin. 1968. Lactate dehydrogenase activity in muscle after prolonged severe exercise in man. J. Appl. Physiol. 25:88–91.

Keith, J. D. 1978. Physical growth in infants and children with congenital heart disease. In: J. D. Keith, R. D. Rowe, and P. Vlad (eds.), Heart Disease in Infancy and Childhood. 3 Ed., pp. 185–199. Macmillan Publishing Co., Inc., New York.

Lees, M. H., J. D. Bristow, H. E. Griswold, and R. W. Olmsted. 1965. Relative hypermetabolism in infants with congenital heart disease and undernutrition. Pediatrics 36:183–191.

Lowry, O. H., and J. V. Passonneau. 1964. The relationship between substrates and enzymes of glycolysis in brain. J. Biol. Chem. 239:31–42.

Lundberg, A., B. O. Eriksson, and G. Jansson. 1979. Muscle abnormalities in coeliac disease: Studies on gross motor development and muscle fiber composition, size and metabolic substrates. Eur. J. Pediatr. 130:93–103.

Lundberg, A., B. O. Eriksson, and G. Mellgren. 1979. Metabolic substrates, muscle fiber composition and fiber size in late walking and normal children. Eur. J. Pediatr. 130:79–92.

Naeye, R. L. 1965. Organ and cellular development in congenital heart disease and in alimentary malnutrition. J. Pediatr. 67:447–458.

Padykula, H. A., and E. Herman. 1955. The specificity of the histochemical method of adenosine triphosphatase. J. Histochem. Cytochem. 3:170–195.

Rowe, R. D., and T. Izukawa. 1978. The distressed newborn. In: J. D. Keith, R. D. Rowe, and P. Vlad (eds.), Heart Disease in Infancy and Childhood. 3rd Ed., pp. 185–199. Macmillan Publishing Co., Inc., New York.

Talner, N. S. 1977. Heart failure. In: A. J. Moss, F. H. Adams, and G. C. Emmanouilides (eds.), Heart Disease in Infants, Children and Adolescents. 2nd Ed., pp. 660–675. Williams & Wilkins Co., Baltimore.

Muscle Metabolism during Exercise in Men Operated on for Coarctation of the Aorta in Childhood

B. O. Eriksson and E. Hansson

The abnormal hemodynamic situation resulting from coarctation of the aorta is not completely normalized with surgery. Thus, one often finds a remaining hypertension in the upper part of the body (Nanton and Olley, 1976), and this is frequently the case in spite of a good anatomical result (Hansson and Eriksson, in preparation). Furthermore, a remaining blood pressure difference between the arms and legs is often found, which is pronounced on exercise (Hansson and Eriksson, in preparation). Thus, an impaired blood flow to the legs, i.e., a situation resembling a mild claudicatio intermittens, could be suspected. In looking for differences between the muscles in the arms and legs in a group of operated coarctation patients an increased activity of the oxidative enzyme succinate dehydrogenase (SDH) was found in the legs (Eriksson et al., in preparation). Such an increased SDH activity has also been found in patients with mild claudicatio intermittens (Holm et al., 1973), and in physically well trained subjects (Varnauskas et al., 1970). It was therefore felt to be of interest to study muscle metabolism in the legs in patients operated on for coarctation of the aorta.

SUBJECTS

Sixteen young men operated on for an isolated coarctation of the aorta during childhood were the subjects for this investigation. Their mean age

This study was supported by the Tielman Foundation for Pediatric Research and Svenska Läkarsällskapet.

at the time of the study was 21 years (range, 16–28 years). Their mean age at the time of surgery was 10 years (range, 6–14 years); an average of 11 years (range, 6–14 years) had elapsed since surgery.

PROCEDURES

Exercise tests were performed on an electrically braked bicycle ergometer (Elema) at a pedaling rate of 60 r.p.m. Heart rates were recorded from ECG recordings. Expired air was collected in Douglas bags and the volumes were measured with a gas clock. Analyses of the expired air were made using the micro-Scholander technique (Scholander, 1947). Blood lactate concentrations were determined with an enzymatic method (Scholtz et al., 1959) on samples obtained from a prewarmed fingertip. Muscle samples from the vastus lateralis portion of the quadriceps muscle were obtained by needle biopsy (Bergström, 1962) and immediately frozen in liquid nitrogen. Analyses for glycogen, glucose, glucose 6-phosphate (G-6-P), adenosine triphosphate (ATP), creatine phosphate (CP) and lactate were made according to the modified Lowry methods as described by Karlsson (1971). All concentrations were expressed as wet weight values.

An exercise test was performed prior to the biopsy study. The men performed a graded leg exercise at three or more submaximal loads (50, 100, and 150 W) before the maximal load, which was defined as the highest work load the subjects could perform for at least 3–4 min and until exhaustion. At the maximal load, two bags of expired air were collected during the last 1–2 min of exercise. The values for maximal oxygen uptake in each subject were the mean values obtained from those two bags, each analyzed twice. As further criteria of having obtained maximal values for oxygen uptake, a respiratory quotient exceeding 1.0, a ventilatory quotient ($\dot{V}_E / \dot{V}_{O_2}$) exceeding 30, and a blood lactate concentration exceeding 8.0 mmol/liter were required (Åstrand and Rodahl, 1970).

The biopsy studies were made on another day. Biopsies were taken at rest, after 6 min of work at the submaximal loads, and at the end of the maximal exercise, which was performed at an average of 226 W (175–300 W). Exercise time at maximal exercise was on the average 5 min (range = 3–8). The biopsies taken at rest were done with the patients lying down, and those taken during work were done while they were seated on the bicycle. Blood for lactate analyses was taken from a prewarmed fingertip at the same time that the biopsies were done. Expired air for determination of oxygen uptake was collected during the last 1 or 2 min of work.

In order to make all values for the muscle metabolites comparable to values obtained in the same situation in normal subjects, all submaximal work levels were expressed in terms of percentage of the maximal oxygen uptake (see Karlsson, 1971).

Table 1. Mean values with SD and SEM for muscle substrates and metabolites at rest and during exercise in 16 young men operated on for coarctation of the aorta during childhood (also included are values for oxygen uptake and blood lactate concentrations)

		$\dot{V}O_2$ (l/min)	ATP (mmol/ kg w.w.)	CP (mmol/ kg w.w.)	Glycogen glucose units (mmol/ kg w.w.)	Glucose (mmol/ kg w.w.)	G-6-P (mmol/kg w.w.)	Muscle lactate (mmol/kg w.w.)	Blood lactate (mmol/l)
At rest	$\bar{x}$	0.28	5.26	19.30	85.4	0.66	0.44	1.69	1.76
	SD	0.05	1.35	4.65	25.7	0.42	0.23	0.54	0.80
	SEM	0.01	0.34	1.16	6.4	0.11	0.06	0.14	0.20
50 W	$\bar{x}$	0.99	4.88	15.97	74.7	1.12	0.69	2.64	2.11
	SD	0.14	0.99	4.59	24.3	0.63	0.35	0.90	0.87
	SEM	0.03	0.25	1.15	6.1	0.17	0.09	0.22	0.22
100 W	$\bar{x}$	1.48	4.81	13.38	66.9	1.21	0.82	5.01	3.02
	SD	0.16	1.03	3.92	22.0	0.34	0.29	2.56	0.93
	SEM	0.04	0.27	0.98	5.5	0.08	0.07	0.64	0.23
150 W	$\bar{x}$	2.12	4.41	8.97	54.8	1.66	0.96	11.12	5.83
	SD	0.13	1.29	4.86	18.1	0.70	0.45	6.29	2.35
	SEM	0.03	0.32	1.21	4.5	0.18	0.11	1.57	0.59
Maximum exercise, at 225 W (range = 175–300)	$\bar{x}$	2.87	3.25	4.95	35.4	2.59	0.94	18.25	11.66
	SD	0.34	0.89	1.73	19.7	0.66	0.70	3.90	2.17
	SEM	0.09	0.22	0.43	4.9	0.16	0.17	0.98	0.54

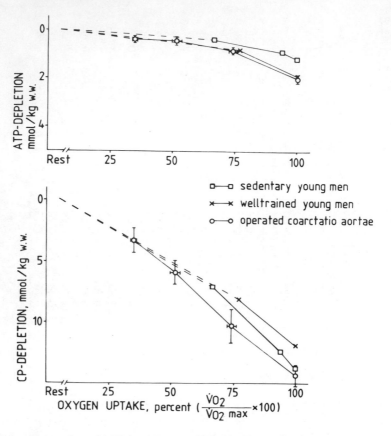

Figure 1.   Mean values with SE for ATP and CP depletion in relation to relative work load in 16 young men operated on for coarctation of the aorta in childhood. Also included are values for healthy well trained young men (data from Karlsson, 1971).

RESULTS

Mean values with SD and SEM are given in Table 1. The mean ATP concentration at rest was 5.26 mmol/kg w.w. A small decrease was found during exercise (Figure 1), down to 3.25 mmol/kg w.w. at maximal exercise (Table 1). The mean value for CP concentration at rest was 19.30 mmol/kg w.w., and it decreased gradually down to an average of 5.0 mmol/kg w.w. (Figure 1). The pattern of depletion of these energy-rich phosphagens was similar to that seen in normal subjects (Karlsson, 1971). The glycogen concentration decreased with increasing work load, from 85.4 down to 35.4 mmol glucose units per kg w.w. (Figure 2). The glycogen depletion was as expected based on conclusions from data obtained in healthy men (Karlsson, 1971). The values for glucose and G-6-P fell within normal limits both at rest and during exercise.

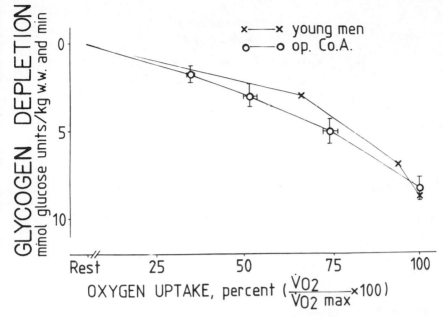

Figure 2.   Mean values with SE for glycogen depletion in relation to relative work load in 16 young men operated on for coarctation of the aorta in childhood. Also included are values for healthy young men (data from Karlsson, 1971).

The muscle lactate concentration at rest was 1.69 mmol/kg w.w. During light exercise it increased slowly, but with work loads exceeding 50% a greater accumulation was found (Figure 3). The mean value at maximal exercise was 18.25 mmol/kg w.w. The blood lactate increased in a similar manner, from a mean value of 1.76 mmol/liter at rest up to 11.66 mmol/liter at maximal exercise (Figure 4).

DISCUSSION

The maximal oxygen uptake in the 16 patients operated on for coarctation of the aorta was, on the average, 2.87 liters/min or 43 ml/kg•min, which is normal or somewhat low compared to Swedish standards (Ekblom et al., 1968; Nordesjö, 1974). Comparing the metabolic data of these 16 young men with the data reported for healthy subjects by other authors, some differences were found. The resting mean value for ATP (but not for CP) was high ($p < 0.001$) compared to that for sedentary young men reported by Karlsson et al. (1970) and Karlsson et al. (1972); it was comparable to the high values found by these authors in well trained subjects. The depletion of ATP at maximal exercise was high (2.0 mmol/kg w.w.). The significance of this is uncertain. Karlsson et al. (1970) reported such a high ATP depletion in one group of well trained young men, but, on the other hand, they found a lower depletion and no difference in the deple-

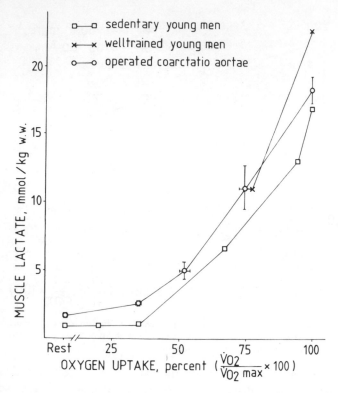

Figure 3.   Mean values with SE for muscle lactate concentration in relation to relative work load in 16 young men operated on for coarctation of the aorta in childhood. Also included are values for healthy sedentary young men and well trained young men (data from Karlsson, 1971).

tion after training in another group of young men (Karlsson et al., 1972). These different magnitudes of depletion are probably due to different degrees of exhaustion. The muscle lactate concentration at maximal exercise was on the average somewhat higher than in the sedentary group, but not as high as in the well trained group studied by Karlsson (1971). These differences are probably due to differences in the ability to sustain lactate in the muscle. Blood lactate increases were similar in the coarctation group and the two groups studied by Karlsson (1971).

On relating the blood lactate to the muscle lactate taken simultaneously, one finds that the operated coarctation patients, like the well trained group, had a somewhat lower blood lactate at a given muscle lactate than the sedentary group (Figure 5). Similar but more marked findings have been reported in patients with uncorrected tetralogy of Fallot (Bjarke et al., 1974) and in patients with claudicatio intermittens (Pernow et al., 1975). The reason for this lowered blood:muscle lactate ratio is not known, but an impaired blood flow to the legs and an increased metabo-

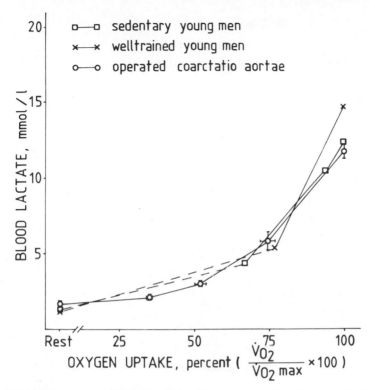

Figure 4.   Mean values with SE for blood lactate concentration in relation to relative work load in 16 young men operated on for coarctation of the aorta in childhood. Also included are values for healthy sedentary young men and well trained young men (data from Karlsson, 1971).

lism of lactate have been discussed (Pernow et al., 1975: Karlsson et al., 1972).

Hemodynamic studies in these patients (Hansson and Eriksson, in preparation) have revealed that the femoral arterial mean blood pressure hardly increases at all during exercise in patients operated on for coarctation of the aorta. However, this seems not to create any obvious problems for the exercising muscles, judged by the metabolic responses to exercise. The only differences found, compared to normal individuals, were changes of the metabolism toward that of well trained subjects. However, this is not accompanied by corresponding high maximal oxygen uptake. It could be hypothesized that the operated coarctation patients have a somewhat impaired blood flow to the legs, that is only partially compensated for by a well trained condition in their legs. This would mean that they would have reached a higher maximal oxygen uptake if they had not been forced to stop leg work prematurely because of this impaired blood flow. However, full knowledge of the blood flow distribution to the legs during

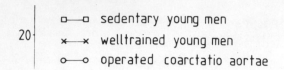

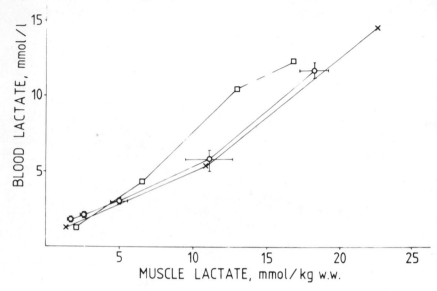

Figure 5. Mean values with SE for blood lactate concentration during exercise in relation to muscle lactate concentration in 16 young men operated on for coarctation of the aorta in childhood. Also included are values for healthy sedentary young men and well trained young men (data from Karlsson, 1971).

exercise demands direct flow measurements in the legs combined with determination of the cardiac output.

REFERENCES

Åstrand, P.-O., and K. Rodahl. 1970. Textbook of Work Physiology. McGraw-Hill Book Co., New York.

Bergström, J. 1962. Muscle electrolytes in man. Scand. J. Clin. Lab. Invest. 14, Suppl. 68.

Bjarke, B., B. O. Eriksson, and B. Saltin. 1974. ATP, CP and lactate concentrations in muscle tissue during exercise in male patients with tetralogy of Fallot. Scand. J. Clin. Lab. Invest. 33:255–260.

Ekblom, B., P.-O. Åstrand, B. Saltin, J. Stenberg, and B. Wallström. 1968. Effect of training on circulatory response to exercise. J. Appl. Physiol. 24: 518–528.

Holm, J., A.-G. Dahlöf, P. Björntorp, and T. Scherstén. 1973. Enzyme studies in muscles of patients with intermittent claudication: Effect of training. Scand. J. Clin. Lab. Invest 31(Suppl. 128):201–205.

Karlsson, J. 1971. Lactate and phosphagen concentration in working muscle of man with special reference to oxygen deficit at the onset of work. Acta Physiol. Scand., Suppl. 358.

Karlsson, J., B. Diamant, and B. Saltin. 1970. Muscle metabolites during submaximal and maximal exercise in man. Scand. J. Clin. Lab. Invest. 26:385–394.

Karlsson, J., L.-O. Nordesjö, L. Jorfelt, and B. Saltin. 1972. Muscle lactate, ATP and CP levels during exercise after physical training in man. J. Appl. Physiol. 33:199–203.

Nanton, M. A., and P. Olley. 1976. Residual hypertension after coarctectomy in children. Am. J. Cardiol. 37:769–772.

Nordesjö, L.-O. 1974. A comparison between the Thornwall maximal ergometer test, submaximal ergometer tests and maximal oxygen uptake. Försvarsmedicin 10:3–10.

Pernow, B., B. Saltin, J. Wahren, R. Cronestrand, and S. Ekeström. 1975. Leg blood flow and muscle metabolism in occlusive arterial disease of the leg before and after reconstructive surgery. Clin. Sci. Mol. Med. 49:265–275.

Scholander, P. F. 1947. Analyses for accurate estimation of respiratory gases in one-half cubic centimeter samples. J. Biol. Chem. 167:235–250.

Scholtz, R., H. Schmitz, T. Bücher, and J. O. Lampen. 1959. Uber die Wirkung von Nystatin auf Bäckerhefe. Biochem. Z. 331:71–86.

Varnauskas, E., P. Björntorp, M. Fahlen, I. Prerorsky, and J. Stenberg. 1970. Effects of physical training on exercise blood flow and succinic oxidase activity in skeletal muscle. Cardiovasc. Res. 4:418–422.

Exercise Studies of Handicapped Children

Exercise Studies of Children with Chronic Diseases

C. A. R. Thorén

The modern conception of the care of children with chronic diseases emphasizes their maximal participation in a normal way of life. Overprotective care of these children may be reflected in deviations in their emotional development as well as in an improper approach to society, which then becomes an additional handicap. The degree of physical fitness often proves to be a limiting factor—or even a hindrance—keeping a handicapped child from being an equal member of the community of children. Physical education must be adaptable to the needs of individual handicapped pupils who often are exempted from physical training. Schoolchildren with asthma, diabetes, obesity, and neurocirculatory dysfunctions are still often excluded from regular school gymnastics, although physical training is in fact an important element in the treatment of these complaints. Pupils with constitutional weaknesses, with motor handicaps due to congenital or acquired defects, and with chronic diseases generally have difficulties participating in the ordinary class gymnastics. Lack of individualization is also one of the main reasons for certain pupils being excluded from meaningful physical training in school.

It is of importance to know how a chronic disease or a handicap may have an influence on a child's physical fitness. From a physiological point of view, it is also necessary to understand and to take into consideration the different factors that may influence exercise tests and determination of working capacity. Problems in exercise testing of children with different chronic diseases are discussed in this article.

This paper is dedicated to Prof. Rolf Zetterström, a great pediatric scientist, on his 60th birthday.

This research was supported by grants from the Solstickan Foundation and the H. & G. Jeanson Foundation.

ASTHMATIC CHILDREN

There is general agreement that asthmatic children can sustain physical exertion relatively well (Thorén et al., 1973). There are no changes due to exercise in the mechanism of breathing in asthmatics. However, asthmatics are predisposed to react with bronchospasm on exercise, causing so-called exercise-induced asthma (EIA), which has been studied thoroughly during the last decade (Fitch and Godfrey, 1976). Reduced $FEV_{1.0}$, metabolic acidosis, and higher blood lactate have been reported in asthmatics during exercise. The studies of ventilation during exercise revealed that ventilation was greater in asthmatics than in healthy subjects at the same work load. Ventilation studies have shown that the $\dot{V}E:\dot{V}O_2$ ratio is higher in asthmatics, and the alveolar ventilation is adequate for the increased gas exchange, and the alveolar PCO_2 remained within the standard range of healthy children (Vávra et al., 1971).

In several asthmatic children in the asymptomatic period, maximal oxygen uptake was reported to be 20% to 30% lower than in healthy children. However, this reduction did not come from the disease itself, but was due to insufficient physical training of asthmatics (Vávra et al., 1971). On the contrary, Bevegård et al. (1971), when examining seriously asthmatic children, failed to find any significant difference in working capacity compared with healthy children. The Australian Olympic Swimming Team of 1976 had no less than eight out of 28 members who were asthmatic, and Olympic champion Dawn Fraser won gold medals in three successive games despite her asthma (Fitch, 1978). These facts exemplify that aerobic capacity is not a limiting factor for fitness in asthmatic persons.

A basic condition for attaining comparable values is to perform the exercise tests only in asymptomatic periods. Even then the great variability of asthma, influenced by environmental factors (e.g., season or emotional situation in family, school, and laboratory), may affect the results and make evaluation more difficult. The subjective improvement by regular physical training reported by patients is often the consequence of their improved emotional state.

The following factors have an influence on the exercise performance and the risk for EIA in asthmatic children:
Type and degree of asthma and bronchospasms
Lung functions: FEV %, $FEV_{1.0}$, VC, FRC
Pharmacological therapy and/or prophylaxis
Type of exercise; leg and/or arm, bicycle, running, swimming
Work intensity, humidity, temperature
Warm-up to reduce the risk of EIA
Parental overprotection

OVERWEIGHT CHILDREN

Obesity is the most common nutritional disturbance in childhood in industrialized countries. The incidence is about 2.6% to 3.3% among urban schoolchildren in Sweden and is lower in rural areas (Thorén, 1971; Lindgren, 1976).

In 1962, Börjeson showed that obese schoolboys in Stockholm had lower physical working capacity in relation to body weight and smaller heart volume and total hemoglobin than boys with normal weight. He also pointed out that this subnormal capacity may account for a low habitual physical activity and that overweight children cannot be expected to match the performance of normal children.

Mocellin and Rutenfranz (1971) have shown that physical working capacity decreased linearly with increasing overweight without any sexual differentiation. They also found that almost all overweight children had a PWC_{170} value below -2 SD when the degree of overweight reached more than 40%. Secondary inactivity may cause this deterioration. However, up to a certain degree of overweight in schoolboys (about 30% to 40%), there seems to be a normal relationship between working capacity and circulatory dimensions. Figure 1 shows the relation between heart volume and work capacity for 26 obese boys with a mean age of 11.4 years (range, 10.8–12.5 years) and a mean overweight of $+2.18\pm0.81$ SD (range, 2.5–5.7), i.e., 21.8%. The correlation coefficient between PWC_{170} and heart volume was 0.69. Calculated on the 19 boys with an overweight between $+2.5$ and $+4$ SD (i.e., 25%–40% overweight), the correlation coefficient increased to 0.71. The heart volume showed a stronger correlation to lean body mass, with $r=0.83$ for the total group (Figure 2). However, the same strong correlation ($r=0.85$) was found between heart volume and body surface area. In another series of 43 obese boys with a mean age of 9.23 years (range, 8.3–10.8 years) and a mean overweight of $+3.21\pm0.72$ SD (range, 2.1–5.4) (Blomquist et al., 1965), the correlation coefficient was found to be 0.86 (Figure 3). That even the fat-free weight often is increased in obese children has been confirmed by others (Pařízková, 1977). From these observations it seems that slight overweight at the beginning of the development of obesity might act as a constant load and cause a sort of training as long as the child displays sufficient physical activity. From our studies of moderately obese prepubertal boys, no significant metabolic changes were found (Sterky, 1971), except a significantly lower blood lactate level during maximal exercise (Figure 4).

Heavy body weight must be considered in discussions of working capacity and the type of tests. However, we could not show any difference in maximal heart rate or blood lactate when comparing bicycle with tread-

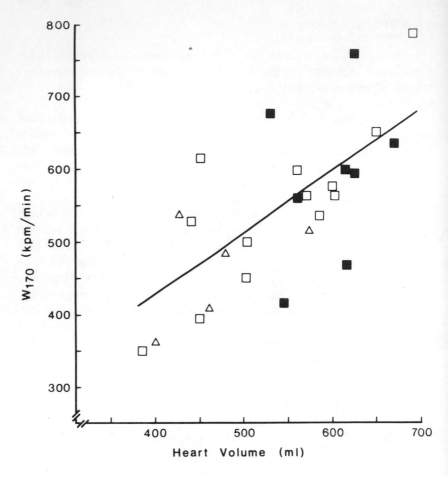

Figure 1.   Working capacity (W_{170}) related to heart volume (from supine position) in 26 obese boys, 11–12 years old. Individual values are given. Regression line ($y = 0.863x + 80.91$; $SD = 104.9$; $r = 0.71$) for boys with a body weight less than $+4$ SD is drawn. Symbols denote degree of overweight: $\triangle = +2.5$ to <3.0 SD; $\square = +3$ to <4 SD; $\blacksquare = 4$ to <5.7 SD.

mill exercise. On the latter, the mean oxygen uptake was still 12% higher (significant at $p < 0.05$) (Table 1).

Pařízková (1977) has studied the relationship between nutrition, body composition, and physical activity and has summarized the knowledge in a monograph. In considering data from human studies and animal experiments, she felt that nutritional status and fatness are mutually related to physical fitness and suggested that the degree of physical activity could have an important relationship to some pathological conditions involving fat metabolism.

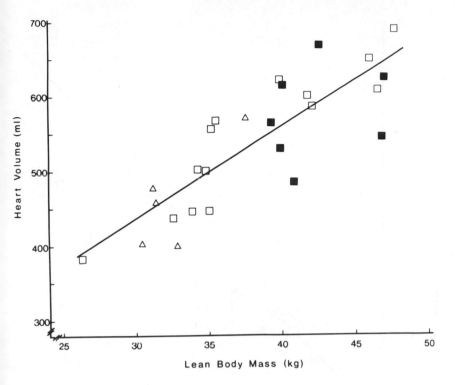

Figure 2.   Heart volume related to lean body mass calculated from body weight and skin-fold thickness. Individual values of 26 obese boys are given with regression line ($y = 79.1 - 12.2x$; SD $= 1.16$; $r = 0.83$). Symbols as in Figure 1.

From training studies, it can be stated that increased physical activity is an important means of preventing obesity from increasing and becoming entrenched (Thorén et al., 1973). Training should serve to improve fitness and combat the primary inactivity that often characterizes obesity. When the child's overweight increases, the mobility decreases, and the functional adaptation of circulatory dimensions to body weight will be ineffective. This secondary inactivity increases the progress of the deterioration in physical condition—a kind of snowballing process very difficult to reverse. There are many observations to date showing that the obese child's low working capacity is secondary.

In summary, the following factors are of importance for the working capacity and exercise performance in obese children:

Degree of overweight and lean body weight
Duration and biochemical alterations
Type of exercise: short, prolonged, bicycle, treadmill, swimming

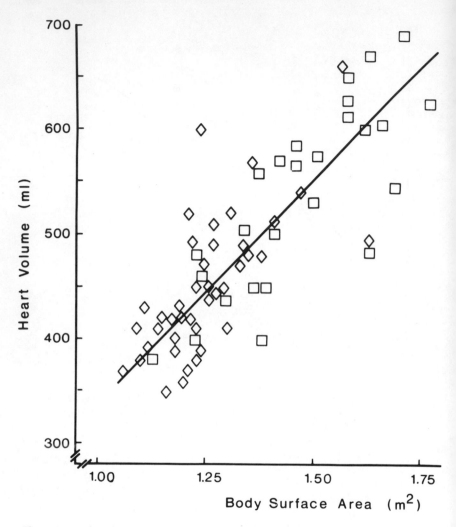

Figure 3.   Heart volume related to body surface area in 69 obese boys, 9–12 years old. Individual values and regression line ($y = 429x - 91.3$; SD = 88; $r = 0.86$) are given. Symbols: □ 11–12 years; ◇ 8–10 years.

Mechanical efficiency and body temperature
Psychological motivation

CHILDREN WITH DIABETES

In an investigation of adolescent girls with diabetes, Larsson et al. (1962) reported that they had a lower working capacity compared with a control

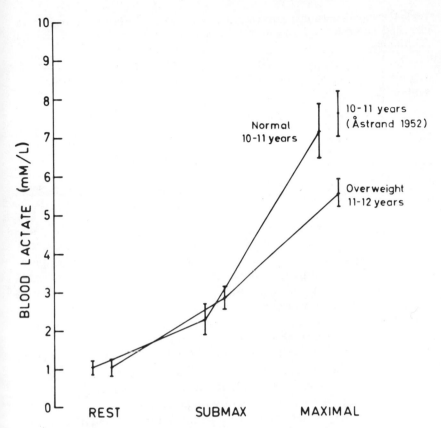

Figure 4.   Blood lactate during exercise to exhaustion on bicycle ergometer in 14 obese boys, 11–12 years old. Mean maximal value was 5.97 ± 1.62 mM for the obese and 7.14 ± 0.74 for boys with normal body weight and of the same age.

group of the same age and body size. The difference was most evident in the older girls. Sterky (1963) enlarged the study to include all diabetic schoolchildren in Stockholm and compared them with matched controls. After puberty, the diabetic children of both sexes had higher heart rates than the controls at the same work loads. Children with a brief history of diabetes and a higher age at onset of the disease displayed better physical fitness. Inadequate physical training was suggested to be the main reason for the inferior physical working capacity in diabetic children in adolescence.

During prolonged physical training of diabetic teenagers, a marked improvement in diabetes control was evident, with a striking increase in the occurrence of aglycosuria, despite a 50% increase in caloric intake and unchanged insulin supply (Larsson et al., 1964a). After rigorous cross-

Table 1.   Individual and mean values in five obese boys for heart rate, oxygen uptake, and blood lactate during maximal bicycle (B) exercise and maximal treadmill (T) running

Subject	Degree of overweight (SD)	Heart rate (b.p.m.)		Oxygen uptake (l/min)		Blood lactate (mM)	
		B	T	B	T	B	T
MK	4.1	207	207	2.67	2.67	4.61	5.35
PN	2.5	200	202	2.49	2.78	6.16	6.02
LN	3.5	202	199	2.11	2.57	5.03	5.52
FA	3.5	212	219	2.38	2.78	5.38	5.85
TK	2.4	203	200	2.85	3.22	8.02	7.66
$\bar{x}$	3.2	204.8	205.8	2.50	2.80	5.84	6.08

country skiing for more than 3 hr at a mean intensity level of 66% of maximal capacity, no significant differences were shown between diabetic adolescents and controls in heart rate, blood pressure, and body temperature. The FFA utilization was similar in both groups during maximal exercise of short duration, but the postexercise rise was somewhat greater in the diabetics. During prolonged skiing, the diabetics derived more energy from the oxidation of carbohydrates and seemed to be more dependent than nondiabetics on an abundant carbohydrate intake during prolonged strenuous exercise. The ability to mobilize fat, however, might be less well developed in diabetics (Larsson et al., 1964b). An insufficient energy supply therefore entails the risk of hypoglycemia, conceivably the most important limiting factor for diabetics in performing prolonged, high-intensity work. Experimental studies on adult males who had juvenile diabetes have also revealed that glucose tolerance is more normal after severe exercise (Maehlum and Pruett, 1973). On the basis of the studies reviewed and from many years of experience in the physical training, children with diabetes can be said to display responses and improvements in functional capacity similar to nondiabetics. The metabolic liability that often characterizes juvenile diabetes in adolescents is counteracted by exercise. Physical training also increases the child's self-confidence and dispels the feeling of being handicapped—an important psychological prerequisite for a normal and relatively asymptomatic life with normal physical development.

The following factors are of importance when exercising a diabetic child:

Duration of diabetes and degree of physical activity
Blood-glucose level and ketonemia
Intensity of exercise
Psychological motivation

CHILDREN WITH CEREBRAL PALSY

Children handicapped by cerebral palsy are prone to physical inactivity and poor working capacity and are easily fatigued by the exertion of daily life activity. In a recent study of 11–12-year-old children with spastic diplegia, Lundberg (1978) found 50% lower values in physical working capacity (determined as PWC_{170}) for handicapped children than for healthy controls. Maximal oxygen uptake in relation to body weight was 11% and 18% lower for the handicapped boys and girls, respectively.

There are both *quantitative* and *qualitative* differences between children with motor handicaps and nonhandicapped children. The relatively small total muscle mass in relation to body dimensions plays a quantitative role. From a qualitative point of view, the ineffectiveness of neuromuscular function is of importance. Extra energy is required for the constant increase in muscle tonus, involuntary muscle activity, and postural stabilizing maneuvers. All these factors explain the low mechanical efficiency reported by Lundberg (1975). For submaximal work the mechanical efficiency in the spastic group was as low as 50% of normal values on the bicycle ergometer.

Recently, Landin et al. (1977) observed that patients with moderate hemiparesis had pronounced qualitative changes of muscle metabolism and substrate utilization in the paretic muscle during exercise. The rates of uptake of oxygen, glucose, and free fatty acid (oleic acid) were 40%–50% lower for the paretic leg. They also found that during one-legged exercise the difference was only significant for lactate release. The metabolic derangements found in paretic muscles may partly be explained by the increased activity and the number of type II muscle fibers, and by changes of muscle mitochondria, which were also found. The decrease of peripheral blood flow in the paretic leg may also have consequences for the working muscle.

The working capacity in children with cerebral palsy is more likely to be related to qualitative circumstances, as was found in the studies mentioned, than to quantitative properties. However, physical training may increase performance capacity in spite of even more severe motor handicaps, as was shown in the study by Berg (1970).

Exercise performance of children with cerebral palsy depends on:

Type and severity of CP
Type of exercise
Coordination disturbances: ataxia, athetosis, dystonia
Mechanical efficiency
Metabolic rate
Body composition

CHILDREN WITH CONGENITAL HEART DISEASE

Children with congenital heart disease are usually asymptomatic during their school age years. Despite this, they are often considered to have "decreased" exercise tolerance and are restricted in their everyday activities, including physical education. The deprivation during these years and parental anxiety undoubtedly have negative effects, both physical and psychological. Ergometry has become very useful as a noninvasive method for functional examination of children with congenital heart disease free from parental influence and the tendency of these children to dissimulate. Many children with congenital heart disease do have a reduced endurance and functional capacity. Limiting factors for exercise performance are:

Type and severity of malformation
Effort intolerance
Arterial oxygen saturation and acidosis
Maximal heart rate
Rhythm disturbances
Cardiac output; stroke volume
Blood pressure, systemic and pulmonary
Parental overprotection

Not the least important is a lower HR_{max}, with mean values in the range of 175 b.p.m. (Goldberg et al., 1966; Bjarke, 1974; Mocellin and Bastanie, 1976). However, on treadmill endurance tests, Cumming found a normal HR_{max} in children with congenital heart disease, except in the cyanotics (1978, personal communication). There is surely considerable individual variation of maximal heart rate, and for clinical purposes it is not necessary to perform maximal exercise or endurance tests. A normal exercise tolerance is often observed even in cases of severe *valvular stenosis* created by a compensatory mechanism, with accompanying abnormal ventricular pressure or volume load. The rise of systolic pressure in the right ventricle for the patient with pulmonary stenosis can be very marked during exercise but is related to the resting pressure (Ikkos et al., 1966). If the valve anomaly is known, the response to exercise can be predicted from resting catheterization data. In spite of increased pressure, the stroke volume is small, and the systolic ejection time is prolonged. The peripheral circulation is adapted to an efficient distribution and high oxygen utilization, which are all compensatory factors typical for hypokinetic circulation (Jonsson, 1973). In congenital valvular aortic stenosis, the working capacity during exercise is often normal. In cases with moderate to severe stenosis, the exercise ECG may show ST-T changes reflecting left ventricular hypertrophy with myocardial ischemia during or after exercise, which is indeed of importance in following the clinical course and helping to identify those who need surgery (James et al., 1976). The low systolic blood pressure during exercise is a constant and may be the only sign of an abnormal dynamic in aortic valvular stenosis.

In patients with large *atrial septal defects,* the respiratory frequency may increase abnormally during exercise and the working capacity may be decreased because of a reduced left ventricular stroke volume.

In patients with *tetralogy of Fallot,* right ventricular pressure is equal to aortic pressure and the right-to-left shunt is determined by the degree of pulmonary stenosis. The maximal aerobic power is usually severely reduced. The compensatory mechanisms of a decreased mixed venous saturation and increase of hemoglobin concentration cannot overcome the effect of the reduced arterial oxygen saturation. During heavy exercise, the arterial oxygen saturation does not decrease further and is not the absolute limiting factor. Another limiting factor is the acidosis due to carbon dioxide accumulation secondary to low pulmonary blood flow, as shown by Bjarke (1974). Thus, the criteria of maximal work are different in cyanotic patients compared with noncyanotic patients. In a follow-up study of successfully—but late in adolescence—corrected Fallot patients, Bjarke also found that the $\dot{V}o_{2\,max}$ was reduced up to 60% compared to normal values, with a mean value of 28 ml/kg of body weight. During exercise, the patients had normal cardiac output at a given $\dot{V}o_2$, but the stroke volume was small. Mocellin et al. (1975) confirmed this finding in children operated on during school age. They noted that only half of the children took part in physical training at school and the parents showed an overprotective attitude against exercise even many years after heart surgery. In a study of the response to exercise in corrected cases of Fallot, an inverse relationship was found between maximal working capacity and age at surgery (James et al., 1976). The cardiovascular function after corrective heart surgery may, during the years of growth, more or less normalize, which also speaks in favor of early correction. This circumstance is illustrated by a monozygotic twin with tetralogy of Fallot totally corrected at the age of 5 years, who showed a successive catch-up of his working capacity following repair. He reached the fitness of his healthy twin brother after 4 years (Thorén, 1978).

Any complete assessment of the results of heart surgery must consider the response to exercise, which has several different objectives (Thorén, 1976). After successful coarctectomy, for instance, the normalized blood pressure may rise abnormally during exercise and a residual hypertension may be revealed. In Mustard-corrected children with transposition of the great arteries, it is certainly important to use exercise tests, as a hidden arrhythmia may be revealed.

Children with congenital *complete heart block* without concomitant heart disease show a linear increase of both the ventricular and the atrial rates. The maximal ventricular rate may reach up to 135 b.p.m. as the

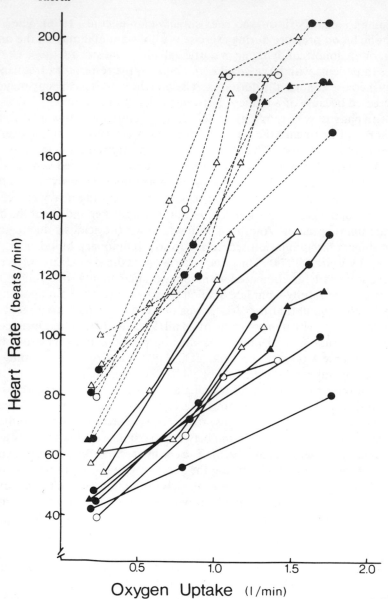

Figure 5. Ventricular rate (solid lines) and atrial rate (dashed lines) during exercise in eight patients with congenital complete heart block. Mean age 12.4 years (range, 9.4–15). Open symbols denote girls, triangles from Mocellin et al. (1975), and circles from author's unpublished data.

atrial rate increases to a normal level of 190–200 b.p.m. (Figure 5). However, there is wide individual variation in the atrial:ventricular rate index (Thorén et al., 1974). Exercise testing of these children provides important information concerning their functional capacity and the adaptation of their circulatory systems to their disease.

These examples of different chronic diseases in children show that exercise testing yields a good deal of valuable information and is of importance for therapy and rehabilitation.

REFERENCES

Berg, K. 1970. Effect of physical training of school children with cerebral palsy. Acta Paediatr. Scand., Suppl. 204.

Bevegård, S., B. O. Eriksson, V. Graff-Lonnevig, S. Kraepelien, and B. Saltin. 1971. Circulatory and respiratory dimension and functional capacity in boys aged 8–13 years with bronchial asthma. Acta Paediatr. Scand., Suppl. 217, pp. 86–89.

Bjarke, B. 1974. Functional studies in palliated and totally corrected adult patients with tetralogy of Fallot. Scand. J. Thorac. Cardiovasc. Surg., Suppl. 16.

Blomquist, B., M. Börjeson, Y. Larsson, B. Persson, and G. Sterky. 1965. The effect of physical activity on the body measurements and work capacity in overweight boys. Acta Paediatr. Scand. 54:566–572.

Börjeson, M. 1962. Overweight children. Acta Paediatr. Scand., Suppl. 132.

Fitch, K. D. 1978. Swimming medicine and asthma. In: B. Eriksson and B. Furberg (eds.), Swimming Medicine IV, pp. 16–31. International Series on Sport Sciences. Vol. 6. University Park Press, Baltimore.

Fitch, K. D., and S. Godfrey. 1976. Asthma and athletic performance. JAMA 236:152–157.

Goldberg, S. J., R. Weiss, and F. H. Adams. 1966. A comparison of the maximal endurance of normal children and patients with congenital cardiac disease. J. Pediatr. 69:46–55.

Ikkos, D., B. Jonsson, and H. Linderholm. 1966. Effect of exercise in pulmonary stenosis with intact ventricular septum. Br. Heart J. 28:316–330.

James, F. W., S. Kaplan, D. C. Schwartz, T.-C. Chou, M. J. Sandker, and V. Naylor. 1976. Response to exercise in patients after total surgical correction of tetralogy of Fallot. Circulation 54:671–679.

Jonsson, B. 1973. Circulatory adaptation to exercise in congenital heart disease. Proc. Assoc. Eur. Paediatr. Cardiol. 9:2–8.

Låndin, S., L. Hagenfeldt, B. Saltin, and J. Wahren. 1977. Muscle metabolism during exercise in hemiparetic patients. Clin. Sci. Mol. Med. 53:257–269.

Larsson, Y., G. Sterky, K. Ekengren, and T. Möller. 1962. Physical fitness and the influence of training in diabetic adolescent girls. Diabetes 11:109.

Larsson, Y., B. Persson, G. Sterky, and C. Thorén. 1964a. Functional adaptation to rigorous training and exercise in diabetic and nondiabetic adolescents. J. Appl. Physiol. 19:629–635.

Larsson, Y., B. Persson, G. Sterky, and C. Thorén. 1964b. Effect of exercise on blood lipids in juvenile diabetes. Lancet 1:350.

Lindgren, G. 1976. Height, weight and menarche in Swedish urban school children in relation to socio-economic and regional factors. Ann. Hum. Biol. 3:501–528.

Lundberg, A. 1975. Mechanical efficiency of bicycle ergometer work of young adults with cerebral palsy. Dev. Med. Child. Neurol. 17:434–439.

Lundberg, A. 1978. Maximal aerobic capacity of young people with spastic cerebral palsy. Dev. Med. Child. Neurol. 20:205–210.

Maehlum, S., and E. D. R. Pruett. 1973. Muscular exercise in male juvenile diabetics. II. Glucose tolerance after exercise. Scand. J. Clin. Lab. Invest. 32: 149–153.

Mocellin, R., and C. Bastanier. 1976. The reliability of W_{170} in calculating the working capacity of children with cogenital heart diseases (in German). Eur. J. Pediatr. 122:223–239.

Mocellin, R., C. Bastanier, H. Hofacker, and K. Bühlmeyer. 1975. Clinical and functional findings in children with totally corrected Fallot's tetralogy (in German). Monatsschr. Kinderheilkd. 123:363–365.

Mocellin, R., and J. Rutenfranz. 1971. Investigations of the physical working capacity of obese children. Acta Paediatr. Scand., Suppl. 217:77–79.

Pařízková, J. 1977. Body Fat and Physical Fitness. Martinus Nijhoff, B. V. Medical Division, The Hague.

Sterky, G. 1963. Physical work capacity in diabetic school children. Acta Paediatr. Scand. 52:1–10.

Sterky, G. 1971. Clinical and metabolic aspects on obesity in childhood. In: B. Pernow and B. Saltin (eds.), Muscle Metabolism during Exercise, pp. 521–527. Plenum Publishing Corp., New York.

Thorén, C. 1971. Physical training of handicapped school children. Scand. J. Rehabil. Med. 3:26–30.

Thorén, C. 1976. The role of exercise testing in children with congenital heart disease after surgery. In: Kidd and Rowe (eds.), The Child with Congenital Heart Disease after Surgery, pp. 344–351. Futura Publ. Comp., Mount Kisco.

Thorén, C. 1978. Exercise testing in children. Paediatrician 7:100–115.

Thorén, C., P. Herin, and J. Vávra. 1974. Studies of submaximal and maximal exercise in congenital complete heart block. Acta Paediatr. Belg. Suppl. 28: 132–143.

Thorén, C., V. Seliger, M. Mácek, J. Vávra, and J. Rutenfranz. 1973. The influence of training on physical fitness in healthy children with chronic diseases. In: Linnewaeh (ed.), Current Aspects of Perinatology and Physiology of Children, pp. 83–112. Springer, Berlin.

Vávra, J., M. Mácek, B. Mrzena, and V. Spičák. 1971. Intensive physical training in children with bronchial asthma. Acta Paediatr. Scand., Suppl. 217, pp. 90–93.

Exercise-induced Asthma:
A Review

S. Oseid

The basic defect in bronchial asthma appears to be an altered state of the bronchial tissues with resulting hyper-reactivity to a number of different trigger stimuli. Particularly in young individuals, immunological hypersensitivity is an important etiological factor, but infection, emotion, cold air, wind and temperature variations, air pollution, tobacco smoke, hyperventilation and hormonal factors may also trigger obstruction. Several of these factors may interact through biochemical or physiological mechanisms (Aas, 1978).

Bronchial obstruction triggered by physical exercise represents a major clinical problem and a severe handicap to young asthmatic children, restricting their normal physical and psychological development (Oseid and Haaland, 1978).

Exercise-induced asthma (EIA) or, rather, postexercise bronchial obstruction, can be prevented by prophylactic medication with selective β_2-sympathomimetic agents, methylated xanthines, or cromolyn sodium, but it can also be prevented by regular specific physical training or a combination of training and medication (Oseid et al., 1978).

This article reviews the established facts and recent new ideas about EIA, and discusses rational treatment of this condition, both prophylactically and therapeutically.

PREVALENCE AND DEFINITION

EIA is not a separate disorder, but rather one method of provoking an attack in an asthmatic subject. The reports of incidences of EIA vary considerably, mainly because so many factors influence the degree of EIA

277

(Godfrey et al., 1973), but also because different studies have used different techniques. The severity of asthma in the subjects may also influence the degree of EIA.

Using a 20% reduction in both peak expiratory flow rate (PEFR) and in forced expiratory volume in 1 sec ($FEV_{1.0}$) as an index of response, nearly 80% of asthmatic children are reported to develop EIA (Oseid and Haaland, 1978). On the other hand, Godfrey (1977) found a greater than 10% fall in PEFR in some 90% of his asthmatic children. Using a 15%-20% fall in $FEV_{1.0}$ as an index of response, other authors have found EIA in 60%-70% of the children tested (Eggleston and Guerrant, 1976; Fitch, 1975; Kawabori et al., 1976). These studies are not quite comparable, but reflect a high incidence of EIA, even if a 20% fall is used as a criterion.

Using a 10% fall in PEFR as the criterion of EIA, some false-positive cases might be diagnosed because there may be individual variations of more than 10% related to technique, motivation, and individual effort in repetitive testing of lung function (Aas, 1975). It therefore might not be justified to regard Godfrey's higher estimate of incidence as correct.

Thus, EIA may be defined as at least a 15% fall in pulmonary function during the postexercise period in individuals with an asthmatic predisposition.

PATTERNS OF RESPONSE

The response to exercise is very similar in most sensitive subjects provided that the lung function is near normal before the exercise stimulus, and that no drugs are administered. Initially there is a moderate bronchodilation followed by a mild bronchoconstriction after 3–4 min of exercise. However, a major increase in airway obstruction occurs after exercise stops due to a postexercise bronchoconstriction of increasing severity during the first few minutes after stopping. According to Godfrey et al. (1973), this is caused by a pronounced bronchial lability, which can be calculated by an index taking into account both the early bronchodilation and any subsequent increase of airway resistance in asthmatic subjects. The fall usually reaches its maximum some 2 to 5 min after exercise stops (Godfrey, 1978), but the maximum may occur later (Jones et al., 1962; Perison et al., 1975; Oseid and Haaland, 1978). Normal lung function is generally achieved spontaneously within 40 to 60 min. However, great individual variations are found.

THE EXERCISE STIMULUS

Several studies indicate that the severity of EIA depends on the type of exercise, its intensity, and its duration.

The clinical experience that free running is the exercise stimulus most likely to provoke EIA was first described by Jones et al. (1962), who found that 90% of asthmatic children developed EIA even when they set a 25% loss in lung function as a criterion. This was later confirmed by Anderson et al. (1971), who compared bronchoconstriction induced by cycling and running. Clinical experience has also shown that most asthmatics can swim without trouble; this has been confirmed in a series of controlled studies (Anderson et al., 1971; Fitch and Morton, 1971; Fitch and Godfrey, 1976). The low asthmogenicity—not only of swimming, but also of walking and kayak paddling—shown in these studies is of special interest, and these sports have later been applied in physical activity programs for asthmatic children with great success (Oseid et al., 1978). It is important to stress that the low asthmogenicity was obtained even though the metabolic rates were as high as those for running.

Another important observation is that 6 to 8 min of continuous, moderately hard running is the most provocative stimulus for EIA. This effect is less pronounced in intermittent, progressive, or alternating forms of exercise raising the heart rate to approximately 170 b.p.m., corresponding to about 70% of maximal aerobic power in nonathletic subjects. This explains why some sports that are episodic, for example, relay races and ball games, cause relatively little problem. This has also been confirmed in our training studies (Oseid et al., 1978).

So far no convincing explanation for the different asthmogenicity of various types of exercise has been given, but several hypotheses have been proposed (Anderson et al., 1975).

The effect on pulmonary function depends largely on the duration of exercise (Jones et al., 1962; Silverman and Anderson, 1972); but it is also affected by the intensity of effort (Katz et al., 1971). Silverman and Anderson (1972) showed increasing amounts of EIA with increasing duration of exercise up to 6 min, but not longer, and with increasing severity of work load up to about 60%–80% of their predicted maximal oxygen consumption. This corresponded to a heart rate of about 180 b.p.m. Eggleston and Guerrant (1976) reached a similar conclusion. This evidence has led to standardized testing procedures in the laboratory. Using either a treadmill or a bicycle ergometer as the exercise stimulus, a 6-min work load giving steady state exercise at about 70% of maximal aerobic power is now a widely accepted test procedure giving fairly reproducible responses of the individual to repeated testing. In some cases, however, the coefficient of variation appears to be about 20%–30%, and may rise to 50%–60% for repeated testing at intervals of 1 to 4 months or longer (Silverman and Anderson, 1972; Eggleston and Guerrant, 1976).

Another important finding in Silverman and Anderson's studies (1972) was that brief exercise provoked only mild EIA, and that there was no increase in EIA with tests lasting more than 6 min. Actually, there was a tendency for less EIA the longer the tests lasted, with some individuals having no EIA after a 12- to 16-min run, even though they became very wheezy after a 6- to 8-min run. These results confirm not only the clinical experience of children "running through their asthma" during prolonged exercise, but also the beneficial effect of brief intermittent exercises as applied in our activity programs.

Earlier studies have suggested that repeating exercise tests at short intervals diminishes the EIA response (McNeil et al., 1966; Chan-Yeung et al., 1971; James et al., 1976), and recently a very interesting study of this refractory period following EIA in asthmatic children has been published (Edmunds et al., 1978). These investigators found that the severity of EIA in the second of a pair of exercise tests of equal severity depended on the interval between the tests, with a reduction in EIA in the second test with shorter intervals. When the severity of the first exercise period was varied to produce different amounts of EIA, the response in the second constant severity test of the pair was inversely related to the EIA produced by the first test. This means that the amount of EIA in the first test was proportional to the work rate, whereas the EIA produced in the second (fixed work) test was lesser if the first test produced a great fall in lung function, and greater if the first work test was less asthmogenic, provided these tests were carried out 30 min apart.

These results are not only of theoretical interest, but also of great practical value in clinical work and in planning training periods and exercise programs for asthmatic children. They also support the hypothesis that EIA is the result of the release of a stored mediator whose resynthesis takes an appreciable amount of time (Godfrey, 1978). This is discussed later in this article.

THE MECHANISMS OF EIA

One of the earliest reports that physical exertion could alter pulmonary mechanics in asthmatic subjects was made by Herxheimer (1946), who postulated that the cause was related to arterial hypocapnia. The roles of hyperventilation, hypocapnia, and acidosis—believed to be possible triggers—were reviewed by Anderson et al. (1975), and none were thought to be clearly implicated. Of all the hypotheses put forth until recently, two are most amenable to investigation: reflex bronchoconstriction secondary to activation of airway vagal receptors, and direct narrowing as a result of the release of mediators as the type I immunological reaction.

McFadden et al. (1977) concluded that the airway response to exercise in asthmatics was heterogenous in terms of having a predominant site of flow limitation and that this factor appeared to relate to mechanisms. Five of the 12 subjects tested in his study had a predominant site of flow limitation in the large airways. This group had their EIA abolished by pretreatment with an anticholinergic agent. The remaining seven subjects had decreased flow ratios, indicating predominant small airway obstruction. Anticholinergic agents, although producing bronchodilation, did not alter their bronchospastic response to exercise. However, pretreatment with disodium cromoglycate did significantly diminish the response of this group.

The theory of bronchospasm being the result of release of a stored chemical mediator was suggested by Silverman and Andrea (1972), who showed that sodium cromoglycate, which inhibits mediator release from mast cells, could inhibit EIA if given immediately before exercise, but not if given immediately at the end of exercise. The mediator theory received further strong support from Edmunds et al. (1978), who showed that repeated exercise tests at short intervals diminished the EIA response, and that this response depended on the intensity of the previous test and the interval between the tests. They believed that these results were compatible with the hypothesis that EIA is the result of the release of a stored mediator whose resynthesis took an appreciable amount of time.

Based on this theory of mediator release, Godfrey (1977) constructed a hypothetical model of the pathways involved in EIA. This model suggests that during exercise there is both stimulation of mast cells to liberate stored mediators of bronchoconstriction and an increased sympathetic drive, which inhibits this constriction. In most cases, the sympathetic effect predominates in the earlier part of exercise, and there is net bronchodilation. Once the patient stops exercising, the sympathetic drive falls off and the full constrictor effect takes over, which could account for the peak of EIA occurring some 2 to 3 min after stopping. Once the mast cells have been discharged, it takes an hour or two to resynthesize the transmitter, and this accounts for the refractory period described above. It is likely that the transmitter is itself actively destroyed at a relatively rapid rate, so that, if exercise is prolonged, virtually all the transmitter is inactivated while the symphathetic drive is still present, and then on stopping there is little or no EIA—i.e., the patient has "run through" his asthma.

As pointed out by Oseid and Aas (1978), it is important to distinguish between obstruction following exercise in patients starting exercise with some clinical or subclinical bronchial obstruction, and the "true" EIA described by Godfrey. The former is a result of abnormal ventilation dynamics, whereas the latter appears to be caused by the release or activation of biochemically active agents, and occurs even when exercise is started with completely normal lung function. In many patients, however, both mechanisms may be at work in producing obstruction following physical exertion. It is important to make such a distinction, since pharmacological management of the two forms and the approaches to prophylaxis and treatment are different.

Recently, another interesting observation has been reported by Bar-Or et al. (1977), who studied asthmatic children exercising on a treadmill in a climatic chamber at a temperature of 25°–26°C and relative humidities of 25% and 90%. The mean fall in postexercise maximum midexpiratory flow rate was 26% in the drier climate and only 5% in the humid climate.

A similar conclusion was reached by Chen and Horton (1977), who studied asthmatics exercising on a treadmill breathing air supplied at various combinations of temperature up to 37°C and humidity up to 100%. They showed a convincing relationship between the severity of EIA and the calculated amount of heat loss from the respiratory tract.

The influences of temperature variations and humidity have been further studied by Strauss et al. (1977), who showed that when asthmatics breathe subfreezing air during exercise, the bronchospastic response that develops is greatly accentuated when compared with that resulting from breathing air at standard room conditions. This potentiating effect of cold air was not reflexly mediated, but appeared to be due to the penetration of incompletely conditioned air into intrathoracic airways (Deal et al., 1978). Under these circumstances, the temperature of the mucosa is likely to be lowered far below its normal value during inspiration because considerable quantities of both heat and water must be transferred from the surface of the airways to bring the inspired air to body conditions before it reaches the alveoli. These observations suggested that airway cooling was an important initial local stimulus to the development of obstruction.

In a subsequent study, Strauss et al. (1978) demonstrated that the magnitude of the airway obstruction was inversely proportional to the water content of the inspirate through temperature ranges of 25°-37°C. Thus, the chief factor that related to the development of EIA, and the principal cause of mucosal cooling, was the vaporization of water. Strong additional support for this reasoning came from the reports of Bar-Or et al. (1977), Chen and Horton (1977), and Weinstein et al. (1976) showing that, if asthmatics inhale air at high humidity while exercising, the degree of airway obstruction that develops is markedly attenuated.

Analyses of these observations lead Deal et al. (1979a) to hypothesize that it was the total heat flux in the tracheobronchial tree during exercise that determined the degree of postexertional obstruction in asthma. Their studies showed that the magnitude of EIA was directly proportional to the thermal load placed on the airways, and that this reaction was quantifiable in terms of respiratory heat exchange.

Because the level of ventilation is an important determinant of the quantity of heat transferred from the mucosa, studies on hyperpnea and heat flux were performed (Deal et al., 1979b). They showed that the major stimulus for EIA was the heat loss from the mucosa, with subsequent cooling precipitated by the hyperpnea of exercise, but not exercise per se.

The studies referred to above are of great interest and explain the clinical experience of swimming as an almost ideal activity for those who develop EIA by running or cycling, provided that the air temperature is high enough and the pool or sea surroundings are reasonably free of irritants or allergens. The findings are in contrast to the general view that dry climates are good for asthmatics, but this assumption might have been raised because of the detrimental effect of the existing air pollution in humid outdoor climates.

THE SITE OF CONSTRICTION IN EIA

Studies to elucidate the site of airway obstruction in EIA in children and in some adults have suggested that the predominant site of airway obstruction is in the larger, central airways (Benatar and Koenig, 1974; McFadden et al., 1977). Other studies, however, have suggested the small airways as the primary site of obstruction. Furthermore, McFadden et al. (1977) noted that the subjects with predominately small airway response were helped by pretreatment with sodium cromoglycate, but not by the anticholinergic drug SCH 1000, whereas those with the large airway response were more likely to be helped by SCH 1000. They suggested that chemical mediators might be affecting small airways in EIA, whereas the effect on large airways was reflexly mediated through the vagus. In summary, it seems likely that both large and small airways are involved in EIA to a varying degree in different subjects; this might account for some of the differences in response to drugs such as atropine that have been observed (Godfrey, 1978).

DRUGS AND EIA

EIA can be prevented, totally or partially, by a number of different drugs. The general pattern of response to four agents (salbutamol, theophylline, sodium cromoglycate, and atropine) was reported by Anderson et al. (1975). The most widely used drugs are selective β_2-adrenoreceptor stimulants and sodium cromoglycate, which when administered as a pre-exercise prophylactic medication will reduce or abolish EIA in the majority of asthmatics (Fitch and Godfrey, 1976; Oseid and Haaland, 1978). According to Morton and Fitch (1974), approximately 45% of asthmatics will achieve complete protection from EIA, and on the average the drug will reduce EIA by about 70%. The effect, however, declines progressively over 4–6 hr. In my experience, the effect is very good for the first hour, but little useful protection remains after 2 hr. This means that regular, four times a day medication employed to manage clinical asthma must be supplemented by an additional pre-exercise dose to obtain suppression of EIA.

Godfrey (1978) states in his review article that the exact role of anticholinergic agents in provoked asthma remains uncertain despite continuing work in this field. Thus, the study by Borut et al. (1977) showed that both atropine and SCH 1000 were powerful bronchodilators when the subject was at rest, but that some constriction from the elevated baseline occurred after exercise. Chan-Yeung (1977) found that SCH 1000 inhibited EIA without showing much initial bronchodilator effect, which is rather difficult to understand. In relation to antigen-induced asthma, most recent work suggests that, after allowing for their initial bronchodilator effect, neither atropine nor SCH 1000 cause significant inhibition (Krell et al., 1976; Fish et al., 1977). In view of the results of McFadden et al. (1977), it is possible that the observed differences are due to intersubject differences in the site of airway obstruction.

Corticosteroids, whether given by mouth, intravenously, or by inhalation, have little effect on EIA (Koenig et al., 1974).

Methylated xanthines have some effect in suppressing EIA (Jones et al., 1963). Recent studies have demonstrated that high-dose theophylline therapy could inhibit EIA (Pollock et al., 1977), and that the effect was related to the blood level achieved. However, high doses may give undesirable gastric symptoms and are therefore not advisable in this context.

EIA AND TRAINING PROGRAMS

From a clinical point of view, bronchial obstruction induced by physical exercise represents a major handicap, particularly in children and young adults. In these age groups, physical activity is essential for balanced physical, psychological, and social development. EIA may largely contribute to the negative impact of the disease on social adaptation and psychological development. Assessment of EIA should be one of the routine diagnostic procedures for physicians specializing in the care of asthmatic individuals. Today, the ergometer bicycle, and possibly also the treadmill, have become as important as equipment for the etiological diagnosis of asthma as are bronchial inhalation and lung function testing equipment.

In pure EIA in young individuals, emphasis should be put on physical rehabilitation programs, thus enabling the individual to tolerate higher physical loads without developing asthma. This can be achieved by different training programs of the interval type, which increase the aerobic capacity and the exercise tolerance limit. (Oseid et al., 1978). Such programs give these children the opportunity to take part in play, sport, and other recreational activities that are natural for their age group. The training must be enjoyable, and not competitive blood, sweat, and tears. By accepting play as a form of training, one can give asthmatic children the opportunity for a more enjoyable form of training, which is part of their natural development. This is especially important for asthmatic children, who are reluctant to take part in physical activities because of EIA and poor general fitness. They need to be motivated by stimulating and enjoyable training programs they can master, and that motivate for further training, not only in the institution, but also at home and at school. This does not mean that play reduces the demands put on the child. Learning correct swimming techniques, for example, makes pool activities more effective and more fun.

Three basic principles must be followed in all training sessions (Oseid et al., 1978):

1. Premedication must be given prior to all physical activity (this applies to most, not all, children).
2. There should be a long warm-up period of mild intensity (10–15 min) to prevent rapid development of bronchial obstruction.
3. Training should be in intervals with submaximal work loads to attain a heart rate of from 160–170 b.p.m. in prepubertal children up to 180 b.p.m. in younger children.

A training session should last 45–60 min. Circuit training, relay races, ball games, movement-free dance, swimming, kayaking or canoeing, and skiing are examples of activities that are beneficial for children with asthma. Such programs cause an increase in endurance and muscle strength, and less bronchial obstruction following exercise, provided that the children are tested on identical work loads before and after the training period (Oseid et al., 1978).

Beneficial psychological and social effects are even more impressive and convincing, as is reported by Graff-Lonnevig et al. (1979). The fact that asthmatic children can participate in physical training programs in institutions and at school reduces the overprotective attitude of parents and teachers, and the children become more self-confident and social, and integrate more easily with children without a handicap.

A more detailed description of EIA and training principles is given in the film, "Exercise-induced Asthma: Rehabilitation of the Asthmatic Child" (Oseid, 1977). This film is available through Fisons Ltd. in most countries.

CONCLUSION

The basic mechanisms of EIA are yet not fully understood.

The prominent prophylactic effect of cromoglycate has led to speculation that mast cells are involved in inducing asthma during and after exercise, as is discussed in detail by Godfrey (1978). However, one cannot exclude the possibility that cromoglycate acts on some undefined enzyme important both for mast-cell degranulation and for the activation, inactivation, or metabolism of some important chemical agent in the bronchii. Thus, unknown biochemical events leading to EIA may not necessarily be related to mast-cell degranulation. The response to EIA is easily reversible and not inflammatory, whereas mast-cell degranulation seems to release agents also taking part in inflammation (Austen et al., 1976). EIA may also be caused by some mechanisms involving altered lung metabolism of known or unknown bronchodilators or bronchoconstrictors.

The pathophysiology and pharmacochemistry of EIA are probably not fully representative of that of bronchial asthma. This adds to the complexity of asthma as far as our understanding extends today. Future compilation of data of this kind, combined with data from other experimental models, may finally lead to a simple explanation, as, for example, one single error of metabolism.

REFERENCES

Aas, K. 1975. In: The Bronchial Provocation Test, pp. 61, 64. Charles C Thomas, Springfield, Illinois.

Aas, K. 1978. Biochemical and immunological basis of bronchial asthma. Triangle 17:103–107.

Anderson, S. D., N. M. Connolly, and S. Godfrey. 1971. Comparison of bronchoconstriction induced by cycling and running. Thorax 26:396–401.

Anderson, S. D., M. Silverman, P. Koenig, and S. Godfrey. 1975. Exercise induced asthma. Br. J. Dis. Chest 69:1–39.

Austen, K. F., S. I. Wasserman, and E. J. Goetz. 1976. Mast cell derived mediators: Structural and functional diversity and regulation of expression. In: S. G. O. Johansson, K. Strandberg, and B. Uvnaes (eds.), Molecular and Biological Aspects of the Acute Allergic Reaction. Plenum Publishing Corp., New York.

Bar-Or, O., I. Neuman, and R. Dotan. 1977. Effects of dry and humid climates on exercise induced asthma in children and adolescents. J. Allergy Clin. Immunol. 60:163–168.

Benatar, S. H., and P. Koenig. 1974. Maximal expiratory flow and lung volume changes associated with exercise induced asthma in children and the effect of breathing a low-density gas mixture. Clin. Sci. Mol. Med. 46:317–329.

Borut, T. C., D. P. Tashkin, T. J. Fischer, R. Katz, G. Rachelefsky, S. C. Siegel, E. Lee, and C. Harper. 1977. Comparison of aerosolized atropine sulphate and SCH 1000 on exercise induced broncospasm in children. J. Allergy Clin. Immunol. 60:127–133.

Chan-Yeung, M. 1977. The effect of SCH 1000 and disodium cromoglycate on exercise induced asthma. Chest 71:320–323.

Chan-Yeung, M. M. W., M. N. Vyas, and S. Grzybowski. 1971. Exercise induced asthma. Am. Rev. Respir. Dis. 104:915–923.

Chen, W. Y., and D. J. Horton. 1977. Heat and water loss from the airways and exercise induced asthma. Respiration 34:305–313.

Deal, E. C., E. R. McFadden, R. H. Ingram, and J. J. Jaeger. 1978. Effects of atropine on potentiation of exercise-induced bronchospasm by cold air. J. Appl. Physiol: Respirat. Environ. Exercise Physiol. 45(2):238–243.

Deal, E. C., E. R. McFadden, R. H. Ingram, R. H. Strauss, and J. J. Jaeger. 1979a. Role of respiratory and heat exchange in production of exercise-induced asthma. J. Appl. Physiol.: Respirat. Environ. Exercise Physiol. 46(3):467–475.

Deal, E. C., E. R. McFadden, R. H. Ingram, and J. J. Jaeger. 1979b. Hyperpnea and heat flux: Initial reaction sequence in exercise-induced asthma. J. Appl. Physiol: Respirat. Environ. Exercise Physiol. 46(3):476–483.

Edmunds, A. T., M. Tooley, and S. Godfrey. 1978. The refractory period following exercise induced asthma. Am. Rev. Respir. Dis. 117:247–254.

Eggleston, P. A., and J. L. Guerrant. 1976. A standardized method of evaluating exercise induced asthma. J. Allergy Clin. Immunol. 58:414–425.

Fish, J. E., R. R. Rosenthal, W. R. Summer, H. Menkes, P. S. Norman, and S. Permutt. 1977. The effect of atropine on acute antigen-mediated airway constriction in subjects with allergic asthma. Am. Rev. Respir. Dis. 115:371–379.

Fitch, K. D. 1975. Comparative aspects of available exercise systems. Pediatrics 56(Suppl.):904–907.

Fitch, K. D., and S. Godfrey. 1976. Asthma and athletic performance. JAMA 236:152–157.

Fitch, K. D., and A. R. Morton. 1971. Specificity of exercise in exercise-induced asthma. Br. Med. J. 4:577–581.

Godfrey, S. 1977. Exercise induced asthma. In: T. J. H. Clark and S. Godfrey (eds.), Asthma. Chapman & Hall, London.

Godfrey, S. 1978. Exercise-induced asthma. Review article. Allergy 33:229–237.

Godfrey, S., M. Silverman, and S. Anderson. 1973. Problems of interpreting exercise induced asthma. J. Allergy Clin. Immunol. 52:199–209.

Graff-Lonnevig, V., S. Bevegård, B. O. Eriksson, S. Kraepelin, and B. Saltin. 1979. Two years' follow-up of asthmatic boys participating in a physical activity program. Acta Paediatr. Scand. In press.

Herxheimer, H. 1946. Hyperventilation asthma. Lancet 1:83–87.

James, L., J. Faciane, and R. M. Sly. 1976. Effect of treadmill exercise on asthmatic children. J. Allergy Clin. Immunol. 57:408–416.

Jones, R. S. 1966. Assessment of respiratory function in the asthmatic child. Br. Med. J. 2:972–975.

Jones, R. S., M. H. Buston, and M. J. Wharton. 1962. The effect of exercise on ventilatory function in children with asthma. Br. J. Dis. Chest. 56:78–86.

Jones, R. S., M. J. Wharton, and M. H. Buston. 1963. The place of physical exercise and bronchodilator drugs in the assessment of the asthmatic child. Arch. Dis. Child. 38:539–545.

Katz, R. M., B. J. Whipp, E. M. Heimlich, and K. Wasserman. 1971. Exercise-induced bronchospasm, ventilation and blood gases in asthmatic children. J. Allergy 47:148–158.

Kawabori, I., W. E. Pierson, L. L. Conquest, and C. W. Bierman. 1976. Incidence of exercise induced asthma in children. J. Allergy Clin. Immunol. 58:447–455.

Koenig, P., P. Jaffe, and S. Godfrey. 1974. The effect of corticosteroids on exercise induced asthma. J. Allergy Clin. Immunol. 54:14–19.

Krell, R. D., L. W. Charrin, J. R. Wardell, J. McCoy, and E. Giannone. 1976. The effect of cholinergic agents on a canine model of allergic asthma. J. Allergy Clin. Immunol. 58:19–30.

McFadden, E. R., R. H. Ingram, R. L. Haynes, and J. J. Wellman. 1977. Predominant site of flow limitation and mechanisms of post-exertional asthma. J. Appl. Physiol. 42:746–752.

McNeil, R. S., J. R. Nairn, J. S. Millar, and C. G. Ingram. 1966. Exercise-induced asthma. Q. J. Med. 35:55–67.

Morton, A. R., and K. D. Fitch. 1974. Sodium cromoglycate in the prevention of exercise induced asthma. Med. J. Aust. 2:158–162.

Oseid, S. 1977. Exercise-induced asthma. Rehabilitation of the asthmatic child (motion picture). 20 min, 16 mm, optical sound. Fisons Ltd. Pharmaceutical Division.

Oseid, S., and K. Aas. 1978. Exercise-induced asthma. Allergy 33:227–228.

Oseid, S., and K. Haaland, 1978. Exercise studies on asthmatic children before and after regular physical training. In: B. O. Eriksson and B. Furberg (eds.), International Series on Sport Sciences. Vol. 6: Swimming Medicine IV, pp. 32–41. University Park Press, Baltimore.

Oseid, S., M. Kendall, R. B. Larsen, and R. Selbekk. 1978. Physical activity programs for children with exercise-induced asthma. In: B. O. Eriksson and B. Furberg (eds.), International Series on Sport Sciences. Vol. 6: Swimming Medicine IV, pp. 42–51. University Park Press, Baltimore.

Perison, W. E., G. G. Shapiro, and C. W. Bierman. 1975. Modification of cyclo-ergometer-induced bronchospasm with cromolyn sodium. Pediatrics 56 (Suppl.):927–929.

Pollock, J., F. Kiechel, D. Cooper, and M. Weinberger. 1977. Relationship of serum theophylline concentration to inhibition of exercise induced bronchospasm and comparison with cromolyn. Pediatrics 60:840–844.

Silverman, M., and S. D. Anderson. 1972. Standardization of exercise tests in asthmatic children. Arch. Dis. Child. 47:882–889.

Silverman, M., and T. Andrea. 1972. Time course of effect of disodium cromoglycate on exercise induced asthma. Arch. Dis. Child. 47:419–422.

Strauss, R. H., E. R. McFadden, R. H. Ingram, E. C. Deal, and J. J. Jaeger. 1978. Influence of heat and humidity on the airway obstruction induced by exercise in asthma. J. Clin. Invest. 61:433–440.

Strauss, R. H., E. R. McFadden, R. H. Ingram, and J. J. Jaeger. 1977. Enhancement of exercise-induced asthma by cold air. New Engl. J. Med. 297:743–747.

Weinstein, P. E., J. A. Anderson, P. K. Kuale, and L. C. Sweet. 1976. Effects of humidification on exercise-induced asthma. J. Allergy Clin. Immunol. 57: 250–251.

Pulmonary Gas Exchange in Asthmatic Boys During and After Exercise

V. Graff-Lonnevig, S. Bevegård, and B. O. Eriksson

The respiratory function at rest in children with bronchial asthma is well documented (Kraepelien et al., 1958; Engström, 1964; von der Hardt et al., 1976). Obstructive impairments of varying degrees are often present, as well as increased functional residual capacity and residual volume. When obstructive impairment is present there may also be disturbances in the pulmonary gas exchange, as reflected in blood gas tension.

Surprisingly little is reported about pulmonary gas exchange during exercise in children with bronchial asthma (Katz et al., 1971). The aim of the present investigation was to analyze the pulmonary gas exchange during submaximal and maximal physical work in boys with bronchial asthma.

SUBJECTS AND METHODS

Fourteen boys with bronchial asthma were studied. Their mean age was 11.7 years (range, 9.8–13.8 years). Based on clinical observations, nine boys were considered to have severe bronchial asthma, three to have moderately severe bronchial asthma, and two to have mild bronchial asthma.

Leg exercise in a sitting position was performed on an electrically braked bicycle ergometer at one to three submaximal loads of 6-min duration prior to the maximal work load. Expired air was collected in Douglas bags and the volume measured in a balanced spirometer. Analyses of expired gases were made according to the micro-Scholander technique. Heart rates were obtained from ECG tracings, and the respiratory rates were determined by auscultation for at least 30 sec while collecting expired

289

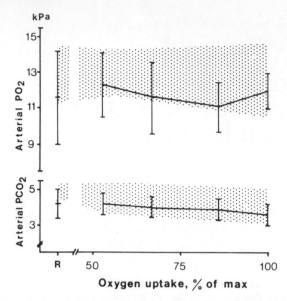

Figure 1.   Mean values (±2 SD) for arterial blood gases at rest (R) ($N = 14$) and during submaximal ($N = 12$, 14, and 7) and maximal ($N = 13$) exercise in asthmatic boys. The shaded area denotes ±2 SD for healthy boys. Adapted from Koch and Eriksson (1973).

air for gas analysis. Arterial blood gases were determined with a blood gas analyzer (Instrumentation Laboratory, Model 113) on samples drawn through a Teflon catheter placed in the brachial artery, before, during, and after exercise.

The physiological dead space was calculated using the Bohr equation and the alveolar oxygen tension from the alveolar gas equation, assuming the arterial P_{CO_2} was equal to the mean alveolar P_{CO_2}.

RESULTS

At rest, the asthmatic boys had a higher respiratory rate, lower arterial P_{O_2} and P_{CO_2}, and greater alveolar-arterial oxygen tension difference than healthy boys. The arterial P_{O_2} showed a large interindividual variation (Figure 1).

During submaximal and maximal exercise the arterial P_{O_2} and P_{CO_2} for the asthmatic boys remained somewhat low when compared with those of healthy boys (Koch and Eriksson, 1973) (Figure 1). The pH and standard bicarbonate were within normal limits during submaximal and maximal work. The total ventilation increased linearly during exercise and reached a maximal value of 69.6 liters/min (Figure 2), almost identical to values found for trained healthy boys, but somewhat larger than the values found for healthy untrained boys (Koch and Eriksson, 1973).

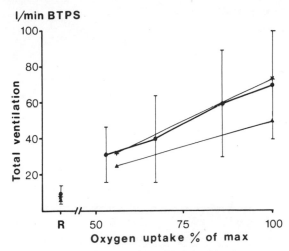

Figure 2.   Mean values (±2 SD) for the total ventilation at rest (R) (*N*= 6) and during sub-maximal (*N*= 12, 14, and 7) and maximal (*N*= 13) exercise in asthmatic boys. Mean values for healthy untrained (triangles) and trained (stars) boys are given. Adapted from Koch and Eriksson (1973).

The alveolar ventilation in the asthmatic boys also increased in the same way as in healthy children and reached a maximal value of 61.2 liters/min (Figure 3). The alveolar-arterial oxygen tension gradient decreased from a high resting value of 4.3 kPa to 2.7 and 3.7 kPa during submaximal work (Figure 4). During maximal work there was an increase to 4.2 kPa with a tendency to normalization at this level. Thus the alveolar-arterial oxygen tension difference was higher than in normal children both at rest and during exercise, but the difference decreased at maximal exercise levels.

Thus, in general, physical exercise did not have much influence on the arterial Po_2 in boys with bronchial asthma. In one boy, however, there was a dramatic fall in arterial Po_2 at a submaximal working level. The arterial Po_2 fell to its lowest value of 4.8 kPa after exercise.

DISCUSSION

Clinical evaluation of the present group of subjects, mainly comprised of boys with clinically severe bronchial asthma, showed that, in spite of this affliction, most of the boys had lung volumes within normal limits.

At rest total ventilation and alveolar ventilation were also within normal limits, but the respiratory rate was somewhat higher than in healthy boys (Koch and Eriksson, 1973). All of the asthmatic boys had an increased alveolar-arterial oxygen tension difference at rest, indicating an impaired gas exchange. The increased alveolar-arterial oxygen tension

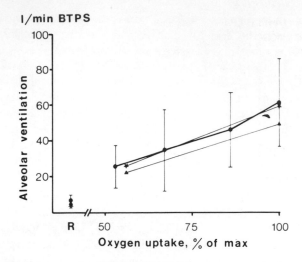

Figure 3.   Mean values (±2 SD) for alveolar ventilation at rest (R) ($N=6$) and during sub-maximal ($N=12$, 14, and 4) and maximal ($N=12$) exercise in asthmatic boys. Mean values for healthy untrained (triangles) and trained (stars) boys are given. Adapted from Koch and Eriksson (1973).

difference was due to the somewhat lower arterial oxygen tension at rest. The arterial P_{CO_2} was also somewhat low at rest, indicating a slight hyper-ventilation. Thus, there may be signs of impaired gas exchange at rest in asymptomatic asthmatic boys. This condition in asthmatics is also supported by the findings of Solymar et al. (1976), who found increased values for closing volume and pathological slopes of the alveolar plateau in asymptomatic asthmatic boys.

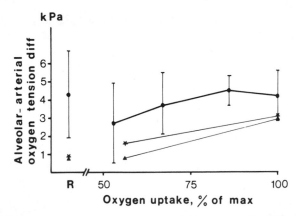

Figure 4.   Mean values (±2 SD) for alveolar-arterial oxygen tension difference at rest (R) ($N=6$) and during submaximal ($N=12$, 14, and 4) and maximal ($N=12$) exercise in asth-matic boys. Mean values for healthy untrained (triangles) and trained (stars) boys are given. Adapted from Koch and Eriksson (1973).

During submaximal and maximal work, the asthmatic boys increased their total ventilation and alveolar ventilation more than healthy untrained boys, mainly by increasing their tidal volume. They were more comparable to trained than to untrained healthy boys in this respect (Koch and Eriksson, 1973). The arterial P_{O_2} and P_{CO_2}, as well as the alveolar-arterial oxygen tension difference, tended to normalize during heavy work, indicating an improvement in the pulmonary gas exchange and ventilation:perfusion ratio. This may have been due to a better distribution of the pulmonary perfusion and a more even ventilation in the lungs by the opening of previously closed small airways. It can be concluded that, in boys with bronchial asthma, the pulmonary ventilation and alveolar gas exchange are well adapted to heavy physical work. The possibility of a sudden drop in arterial P_{O_2} should be kept in mind, however, when asthmatic children perform heavy physical work. They should, therefore, be closely supervised when participating in sports.

REFERENCES

Engström, I. 1964. Respiratory studies in children. XI. Mechanics of breathing, lung volumes and ventilatory capacity in asthmatic children from attack to symptom-free status. Acta Paediatr. Scand., Suppl. 155.

Katz, R. M., B. J. Whipp, E. M. Heimlich, and K. Wasserman. 1971. Exercise-induced bronchospasm, ventilation and blood gases in asthmatic children. J. Allergy 47:148–158.

Koch, G., and B. O. Eriksson. 1973. Effect of physical training on pulmonary ventilation and gas exchange during submaximal and maximal work in boys aged 11 to 13 years. Scand. J. Clin. Lab. Invest. 31:87–94.

Kraepelien, S., I. Engström, and P. Karlberg. 1958. Respiratory studies in children. II. Lung volumes in symptom-free asthmatic children 6–14 years of age. Acta Paediatr. Scand. 47:399–411.

Solymar, L., B. Bake, and J. Bjure. 1976. Closing volume and slope of alveolar plateau in asthmatic children. Scand. J. Respir. Dis. 95(Suppl.):31–38.

von der Hardt, H., F. Geubelle, and H. Hellweg. 1976. Static and dynamic lung compliance in asthmatic symptom-free children. Respiration 33:349–358.

Effect of a Physical Education Program on the Cardiopulmonary Function and Exercise Capacity of Boys with Bronchial Asthma

V. Graff-Lonnevig, S. Bevegård,
B. O. Eriksson, S. Kreapelien, and B. Saltin

Physical activity is considered to be essential for the development of the dimensions and function of the circulatory and respiratory systems in growing individuals. The physical activity of children with bronchial asthma may be limited because they are routinely exempted from physical education in schools and from sports in their leisure time. Parents and teachers are often overprotective and the children may become afraid of developing exercise-induced asthma (EIA). Physical inactivity in adolescence can lead to a low physical working capacity (Oseid and Haaland, 1978). Therefore, it seems important to encourage children with asthma to participate in regular physical activity in order to overcome their fear of developing EIA, and to allow them to develop as normally as possible.

Various conditioning programs for asthmatic children have been described; Strick (1969), Fitch (1974), and Oseid and Haaland (1978) have reviewed the literature in this field. In addition to psychological benefits, improvement in muscular strength and general fitness have been reported, but the effects on pulmonary function and maximal oxygen uptake are less evident.

The purpose of the present investigation was to design a physical conditioning program that could be used to adapt asthmatic children to regular physical education classes at school and to give further information on the influence of long-term physical training on asthma and on the cardiorespiratory system.

SUBJECTS AND METHODS

Eleven boys with bronchial asthma (mean age, 11.2 years) participated in a 20-month conditioning program. Seven boys were classified as having severe asthma and four of them were on long-term corticosteroid treatment. Only three of the boys participated regularly in physical education at school; two were occasional participants and six did not participate at all. Six boys performed some sort of sport activities during their leisure time, and five did not. Three were physically inactive both at school and during their leisure time.

Before, during, and after the training period, the 11 boys in the training group (TG) were investigated with respect to pulmonary dimensions and function; circulatory dimensions such as heart volume, blood volume, and total amount of hemoglobin; maximal oxygen uptake; and blood lactate concentration in the arterial blood. Exercise tests were performed in the sitting position on an electrically braked bicycle ergometer. The same investigations were made on nine untrained asthmatic boys, here referred to as the nontraining group (NTG).

The physical training was performed in an ordinary indoor gymnasium for 1 hr twice a week under the supervision of an experienced gymnastics teacher. During the first training sessions, the children's physician was present. No drugs were given before the physical training. The training program was designed to avoid triggering of EIA. Thus, during the warm-up period, no running was allowed. After 5 min of respiratory exercises, 20 min of "circuit-training," with increasing intensity, was performed at five different stations. The training session ended with a 20-min period of team games. After 5 months of conditioning training, the boys participated in a training camp during the winter in the mountains of northern Sweden (altitude, 600 m). During this training camp, the boys performed strenuous cross-country skiing at low temperatures.

RESULTS

All boys participated in the entire training program. A mean of nine of the 11 boys were present at each lesson. Two boys developed exercise-induced asthma (EIA) more often than the others, but they also trained more intensively than the others. EIA, when present, usually subsided within 5 to 10 min without medical treatment. Team games, such as basketball and soccer, were the commonest causes of EIA.

During the period of study, all values for respiratory and circulatory dimensions increased both in the training group and the nontraining group. During maximal exercise, cardiorespiratory function also increased and both groups showed good adaptation to heavy physical work.

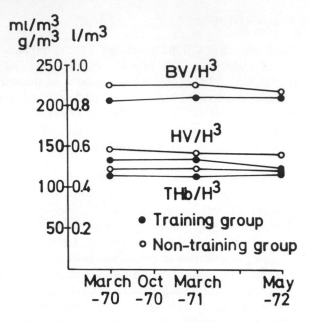

Figure 1.   Blood volume (BV), total amount of hemoglobin (THB), and heart volume (HV) corrected for body growth by dividing by the third power of body height (H^3) during the observation period. Training group (●); nontraining group (○).

In the TG, total ventilation rose from 59.6 to 79.6 liters/min; and in the NTG it rose from 64.4 to 70.5 liters/min. The maximal oxygen uptake was initially somewhat lower in the TG (1.59 liters/min) than in the NTG (1.74 liters/min), but it increased during the observation period by 29% and 22%, respectively. The maximal work load rose by 39% in the TG and by 29% in the NTG. However, since the boys were still growing, all values had to be corrected for height (von Döbeln and Eriksson, 1972). After this correction total amount of hemoglobin (THB), blood volume (BV), and heart volume (HV) were unchanged during the observation period (Figure 1). Also, lung function values such as total lung capacity (TLC), vital capacity (VC), functional residual capacity (FRC), residual volume (RV), and forced expiratory volume during 1 sec ($FEV_{1.0}$) were unchanged when corrected for body growth (Figure 2). Concerning maximal oxygen uptake, there were no significant changes during the period of study when the values were corrected for body growth (Figure 3).

During the 1-week winter training camp there was a small increase in the total ventilation ($\dot{V}_{E_{max}}$) ($p < 0.01$) and in the maximal work load ($p < 0.01$), but the maximal oxygen uptake was unchanged. Dynamic spirometry, using a Vitalograf, was performed before and 4 to 6 min after the daily ski race. All boys showed a reduction of the $FEV_{1.0}$ after the ski race. Thus, EIA was present in all cases. On the average, the $FEV_{1.0}$ was reduced by 19% after a 2000-m ski race.

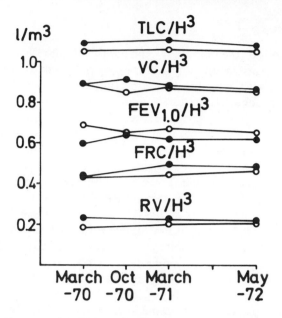

Figure 2.   Total lung capacity (TLC), vital capacity (VC), forced expiratory volume during the first second ($FEV_{1.0}$), functional residual capacity (FRC), and residual volume (RV) corrected for body growth (see Figure 1) during the observation period. Training group (●); nontraining group (○).

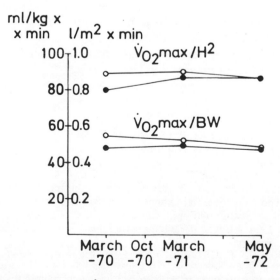

Figure 3.   Maximal oxygen uptake ($\dot{V}_{O_2 \, max}$) corrected for body growth by dividing by body height squared (H^2) and in relation to body weight (BW) during the observation period. Training group (●); nontraining group (○).

DISCUSSION

The dimensions of the pulmonary and cardiovascular systems were unaffected by the experimental physical training program. These findings are in accordance with more recent studies that have shown that, at around 12-13 years of age, increases in circulatory dimensions parallel body growth and working capacity are less affected by training than at other ages (Klissouras, 1976; Weber et al., 1976). On the other hand, the present findings are contrary to the opinion that physical training before and during puberty is essential for enhancement of maximal aerobic power (Åstrand et al., 1963; Ekblom, 1969). An increase in lung volumes has only been demonstrated after intensive training in swimming over a long period of time (Engström et al., 1971).

During winter training at low temperatures, all boys developed EIA after the 2000-m ski race. In spite of a high training intensity, there was no increase in $\dot{V}_{O_2\,max}$ after the training camp. However, the total ventilation at maximal work rose significantly and the maximal work performed increased. This suggests that it is possible to influence ventilatory function and working capacity if the training intensity is sufficiently high.

Fitch (1974) and Oseid and Haaland (1978) have reported that a high exercise intensity may improve pulmonary function and working capacity, but their children inhaled disodium cromoglycate (DSCG) before the training session. This made it possible to obtain a higher training intensity.

The present study shows that asthmatic boys can participate in a physical training program similar to the physical education given at school—without premedication—if minor modifications are made. If the aim of the physical training is to increase physical working capacity and aerobic power, it seems necessary to use drugs such as DSCG or β_2-receptor stimulators before the training sessions.

REFERENCES

Åstrand, P.-O., L. Engström, B. O. Eriksson, P. Karlberg, I. Nylander, B. Saltin, and C. Thorén. 1963. Girl swimmers. Acta Paediatr., Suppl. 147.
Ekblom, B. 1969. Effect of physical training on oxygen transport in man. Acta Physiol. Scand., Suppl. 328.
Engström, I., B. O. Eriksson, P. Karlberg, B. Saltin, and C. Thorén. 1971. Preliminary report on the development of lung volumes in young girl swimmers. Acta Paediatr. Scand. 60(Suppl. 217):73.
Fitch, K. D. 1974. Effects of exercise in asthma. Thesis, University of Western Australia, Nedlands.
Klissouras, V. 1976. Prediction of athletic performance: Genetic considerations. Can. J. Appl. Sport Sci. 1:195.
Oseid, S., and K. Haaland. 1978. Exercise studies on asthmatic children before and after regular physical training. In: B. O. Eriksson, and B. Furberg (eds.),

International Series on Sport Sciences. Vol. 6: Swimming Medicine IV, pp. 32–41. University Park Press, Baltimore.

Strick, L. 1969. Breathing and physical fitness exercises for asthmatic children. Pediatr. Clin. North Am. 16:31–42.

von Döbeln, and B. O. Eriksson. 1972. Physical training, maximal oxygen uptake and dimensions of the oxygen transporting and metabolizing organs in boys 11–13 years of age. Acta Pediatr. Scand. 61:653–660.

Weber, G., Kartodiharjie, and V. Klissouras. 1976. Growth and physical training with reference to heredity. J. Appl. Physiol. 40:211.

Physical Fitness and Trainability of Young Male Patients with Down Syndrome

J. Skrobak-Kaczynski and T. Vavik

This study was prompted by a number of recent investigations that have taken a stand against the old "helplessness-hopelessness" attitude toward patients with Down syndrome. The old and strong belief that these patients will remain permanently retarded—and preferably institutionalized—is slowly giving way. It has been shown that patients with Down syndrome have a large potential for trainability of their functional IQs (Aronson and Fällström, 1977). This evidence is stimulating to those who work for the integration of mentally retarded patients into schools and society.

However, total integration is impossible. There is no cure for organic mental retardation. We do not know any way to regenerate or replace brain tissue. The fact remains, therefore, that there is a limitation to the possible employment of integrated patients. For this group, choice of jobs is limited to simple manual tasks. Such tasks do not necessarily demand large muscular strength, but, rather, require static, monotonous and rhythmic exercises. Even at energy expenditure levels only a little above normal resting values, these tasks can be too tiring for persons with a low working capacity. This fact and reports of low physical capacity in mentally retarded persons (Nordgren, 1970; Bjørke et al., 1978) indicate the need for improvement of the physical status in such patients.

Unfortunately, we do not know much about the potential to increase physical working capacity in patients with Down syndrome. This aspect of care has not been given any attention: in the approximately 800 scientific papers on this syndrome published during the last 4 years, none is devoted to the problem of physical fitness.

The present study was limited to patients with Down syndrome for the following reasons:

1. Down syndrome is the most easily identifiable cause of mental retardation, and has a well-known etiology.
2. Patients with Down syndrome are the largest single group of mental retardates. They represent 10% of the patients in institutions, and about 6% of all individuals who are mentally retarded—about 3600 persons in Norway.
3. As the mortality associated with this syndrome dramatically decreases, this group will further increase in number.
4. The majority of patients with Down syndrome are only moderately retarded and hence respond well to developmental training.

The aim was to investigate the possibility of elevating the physical capacities of these patients by increased physical activity. The improvement in physical status of this group was considered equally important in the process of integration as developmental training aiming at an increase in functional IQ. If this program improved the physical status of the participating patients, it might be considered beneficial also for those with pronounced mental retardation who must remain in institutions.

METHODS

Subjects

Two groups of young male patients with Down syndrome were studied. The older group, Group 1, (mean age, 25 years; range, 16–31 years) consisted of 10 patients from the Ragna Ringdal Institution in Oslo. The younger group, Group 2, also 10 patients (mean age, 14 years; range, 11–17 years), stayed at the Radarveien Institution in Oslo. The older group was the better organized, and followed the leaders' instructions much better than the younger group, probably because of participation in regular organized physical training during the last 3–4 years. The two groups were, except for the difference in age, clinically and functionally fairly homogeneous. All the patients had spent most of their lives in institutions. The physical characteristics of the individuals in both groups are summarized in Table 1.

Training Program

The training program included two periods of 6 weeks each (1 hr 3 times per week). The aim of the training program was to increase aerobic capacity and muscular strength. A circuit-training program consisting of five stations was developed. The length of each working period was 2 min, ex-

Table 1.   Some physical characteristics of the subjects

Group	Subject	Age (years)	Height (cm)	Weight (kg)	Sum of skinfold thicknesses at 3 sites[a] (mm)
1	1	29	156	61	68
	2	28	157	60	48
	3	23	168	80	55
	4	28	164	62	60
	5	16	163	69	67
	6	31	157	57	43
	7	26	170	65	44
	8	19	155	57	60
	9	24	175	72	58
	10	24	156	69	90
2	1	13	152	48	44
	2	15	149	45	54
	3	15	151	51	37
	4	13	138	43	58
	5	17	167	91	122
	6	14	149	43	39
	7	15	162	60	46
	8	11	134	37	48
	9	13	145	39	31
	10	15	152	54	31

[a]Subscapula, triceps, and iliocrista.

cept for the bicycle ergometer station, which was programmed for 10 min (Figure 1).

The instructions were to keep the intensity of the exercise on the highest possible level that could be tolerated by the participants. The older group completed both training periods with a mean training time of 16 and 14 hr in the first and second training periods. Only six of the younger group completed both training periods. This was due to lack of interest among the personnel at the institution. Thus only the data for six persons are presented for this group.

Tests

Tests were performed at the beginning and at the end of both training periods. The tests included determinations of maximal oxygen uptake using the indirect submaximal method on a bicycle ergometer (Åstrand, 1960) and measurements of maximal isometric muscle strength, determined from trunk flexion and extension (Skrobak-Kaczynski et al., 1973). The test apparatus was the same as the one used for establishing norms for the general population of Norway. The same person performed measurements on both groups and on the control subjects.

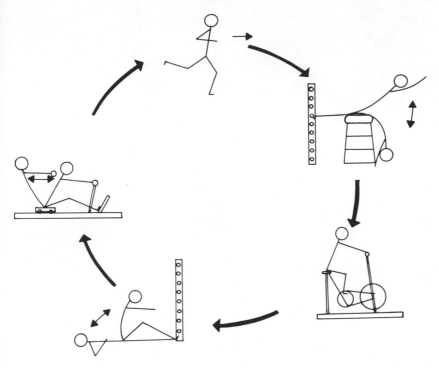

Figure 1.   The five stations of the circuit-training program.

In addition, height, weight, and skinfold thicknesses (sum of three sites—subscapula, triceps, and iliocrista) were collected.

RESULTS

Body Weight and Subcutaneous Fat

In Figure 2, the heights and weights of the two groups are plotted on a graph in relation to a distribution of Norwegian schoolchildren published by Brundtland et al. (1975). All the subjects were obese, but body weight decreased during the first training period. During the "normal" activity period (NA), Group 1 remained on this lower level, whereas Group 2 increased their body weight. During the second training period, Group 1 showed a further decrease, whereas Group 2 again increased in body weight. Total weight loss in Group 1 was 1.3 kg (Figure 3); in Group 2 the increase in weight was 1.6 kg (Figure 4).

The subcutaneous fat (Figures 3 and 4) decreased during the first training period in both groups. After the second training period, Group 1 had a further decrease; unfortunately we had no data for Group 2. The total decrease in Group 1 was significant ($p < 0.05$). During the NA

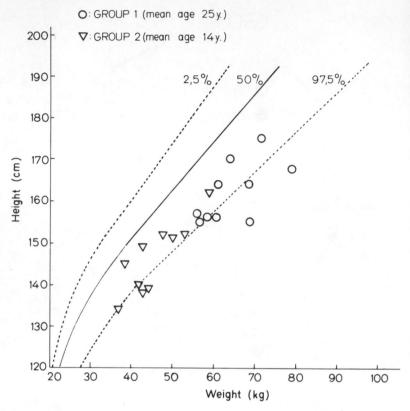

Figure 2.   Height:weight relationship in 20 young male patients with Down syndrome compared to data from normal Norwegian schoolchildren.

period the skinfold thicknesses remained unchanged in Group 1. They increased in Group 2, but this increase did not compensate for the decrease in the first period. However, the increase in body weight by 1.6 kg was followed by an increase in height of 3 cm. These height and weight changes indicated that this group also became slimmer.

Stature

Group 1 consisted of young men, 16–31 years of age; consequently, the growth process for most of them was completed. Only one boy, 16 years old, increased 0.7 cm in height during the period of study. Mean height in this group was 162 cm, which was 5 cm above the mean for a group of 22-year-old patients with Down syndrome studied by Rarick and Seefeldt (1974), and about 8 cm above the mean in older studies (Brousseau, 1928; Dutton, 1959).

The mean increase in height for Group 2 was 3 cm, and it did not seem to be influenced by the level of activity because the measure was

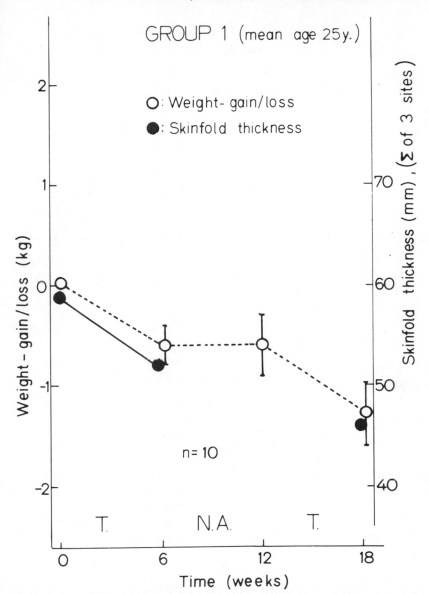

Figure 3.   Mean values of weight gain/loss and skinfold thicknesses of 10 older male patients (Group 1) during training (T) and normal activities at the institution (NA). Vertical bars indicate the range of 1 SE.

almost identical during training periods and at rest. Comparison with the boys in Rarick and Seefeldt's study (1974) revealed that our subjects were 10 cm taller than their American peers. Comparison with older data (Thelander and Pryor, 1966) reveals still larger differences.

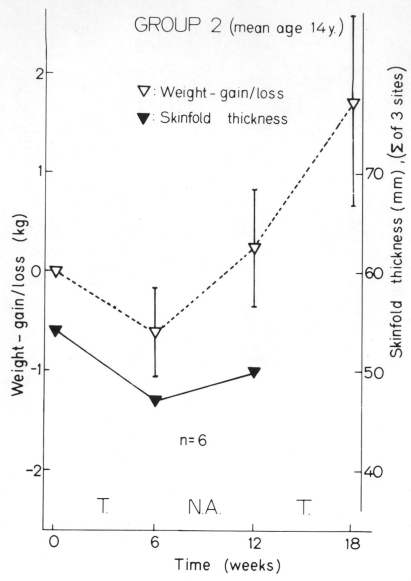

Figure 4.   Mean values of weight gain/loss and skinfold thicknesses of 10 younger male patients (Group 2) during training (T) and normal activities (NA). Vertical bars indicate the
range of 1 SE.

Strength: Trunk Extension

Group 1 had a 26% increase in muscle strength as measured by trunk extension during the first training period, the NA period showed no change,
and the second training period showed a further increase of 8%. The total
improvement was 38% ($p < 0.01$) (Figure 5).

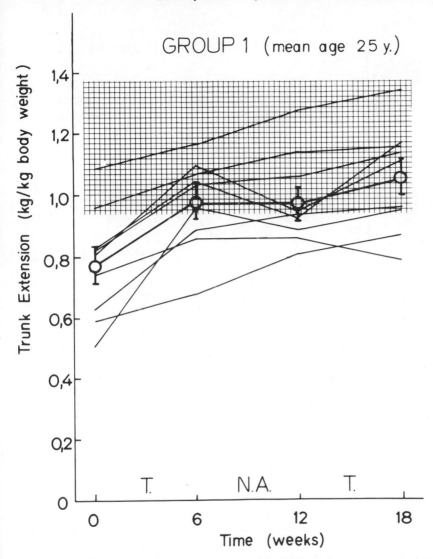

Figure 5.   Individual and mean values of strength of trunk extensors in Group 1. Shaded area indicates the average of Norwegian children, ± 2 SD. Vertical bars indicate the range of 1 SE. T = training, NA = normal activity.

Comparing Group 1 with published data for Norwegian young men (Lange-Anderson and Nesse, 1979), the relative muscle strength (kg/kg of body weight) in this group was only 66% of the normal value before the training program started. The final test showed an increase to 90% of normal. Analyses of individual data (Figure 5) reveal that at the start of our program only two individuals were within normal limits for Norwegian men of the same age group, whereas at the end of the study eight were within this limit. One of the boys was treated with sedatives during the last

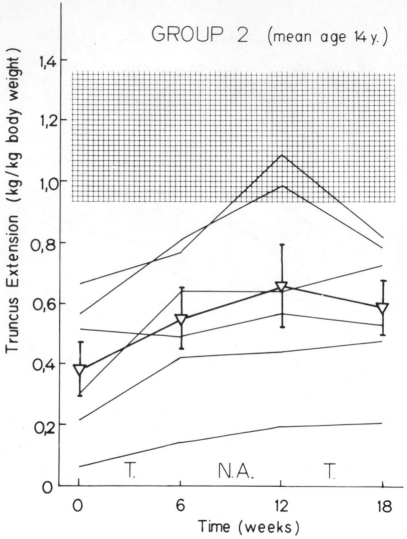

Figure 6.   Individual and mean values of strength of trunk extensors in Group 2. Shaded area indicates the average of Norwegian children ± 2 SD. Vertical bars indicate the range of 1 SE. T = training, NA = normal activity.

training period. He lost interest in training, became apathetic, and his muscle strength decreased.

Group 2 exhibited a marked increase in muscle strength during the first training period (44%) (Figure 6). Six weeks of normal activity brought about a further increase (10%). The strength of the trunk extensors increased by a total of 55% in this group. At the beginning of the study, the average muscle strength of Group 2 was 34% and at the end 53% when compared with healthy children. Because the data for healthy

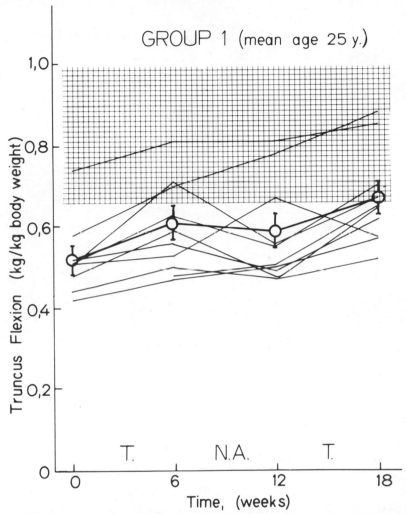

Figure 7.   Individual and mean values of strength of trunk flexors in Group 1. Shaded area indicates the average of Norwegian children, ± 2 SD. Vertical bars indicate the range of 1 SE. T = training, NA = normal activity.

children in the control subjects showed only a slight increase in this parameter in the age span 11–15 years (Skrobak-Kaczynski ct al., 1973), it is believed that the observed increase is an effect of training and not merely the result of growth. In spite of the described improvement at the end of the study, no individual was within two standard deviations of the average for healthy children (Figure 6).

Strength: Trunk Flexion

Development of strength of the trunk flexors (Figures 7 and 8) parallels the changes in strength of trunk extensors described above. Group 1 in-

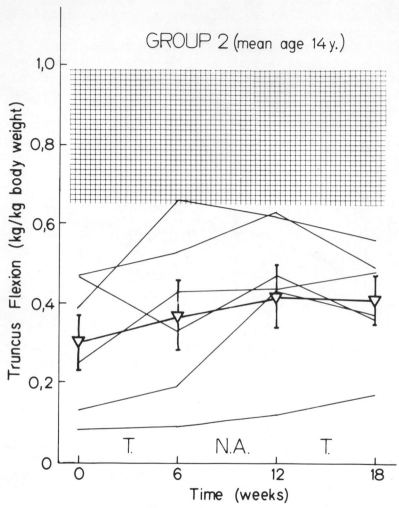

Figure 8.   Individual and mean values of strength of trunk flexors in Group 2. Shaded area indicates the average of Norwegian children ± 2 SD. Vertical bars indicate the range of 1 SE. T = training, NA = normal activity.

creased 28% ($p<0.02$); and the mean for Group 2 increased 37%. Expressing the means for both groups as a percentage of the expected value for Norwegian young men and schoolchildren in the control group, Group 1 increased from 62% to 80%, and Group 2 from 36% to 51%, respectively.

Maximal Oxygen Uptake

The first test of oxygen capacity showed no significant difference between the groups. The mean value was 36 ml/min·kg for Group 1 and 35 ml/

min•kg for Group 2. All the subjects were more than two standard deviations below the mean for normal persons.

Tests after the first 6 weeks of training revealed similar improvements in both groups. The mean was 39.8 ml/min•kg for Group 1 and 40 ml/min•kg for Group 2. The period of normal activity caused a slight decrease of $\dot{V}_{O_2\ max}$ in both groups (-1.6 and -3.7 ml/min•kg for Group 1 and Group 2, respectively).

The second period of training was distinctly more intensive for Group 1, which resulted in a significant increase of $\dot{V}_{O_2\ max}$ in this group ($p < 0.001$). The final test showed an average of 49 ml/min•kg, which is 2 ml/min•kg more than the mean of healthy Norwegian men, 20–30 years old. Group 2 continued with the same training program in the second period, and the mean value in the final test was 40 ml/min•kg. Expressing averages of first and last tests as a percentage of normal values, the mean values increased from 76% to 104% for Group 1; for Group 2, a mean increase from 74.4% to 85.1% was observed when compared with the respective control groups (Figures 9 and 10).

DISCUSSION

Obesity was a common feature of these subjects. The sum of three skinfolds was almost 80% larger than the median for the control subjects (Skrobak-Kaczynski et al., 1973). Obesity is also common in other groups with mental retardation (Nordgren, 1970).

Reductions in body weight and thicknesses of subcutaneous fat seem to be related to periods of increased physical activity. However, it was not possible, using these subjects, to calculate a correlation between the number of training hours, training intensity, and reduction of fat tissue. This was due to the increased physical activity even in periods without active training for all subjects participating in the project. In addition, many of the parents tried to activate their children during weekends to a much higher extent during and after the program than before.

The recorded reductions in body weight and skinfold thicknesses in Group 1, and the decrease in body fat in Group 2, indicate that the obesity in this group of patients is caused by their habitual low level of physical activity. This can be corrected by adequate training.

The increase in height observed in our subjects when compared with older subjects (Brousseau, 1928—146 cm; Benda, 1956—149 cm; Dutton, 1958—150 cm) was most probably the secular trend noted in the general population caused by the improved standard of living. On the other hand, there was no explanation why these Oslo patients with Down syndrome were so much taller than the children with Down syndrome measured by Thelander and Pryor (1966), and Rarick and Seefeldt (1974). This difference is even more remarkable since a comparison of schoolchildren from both countries shows only minor differences.

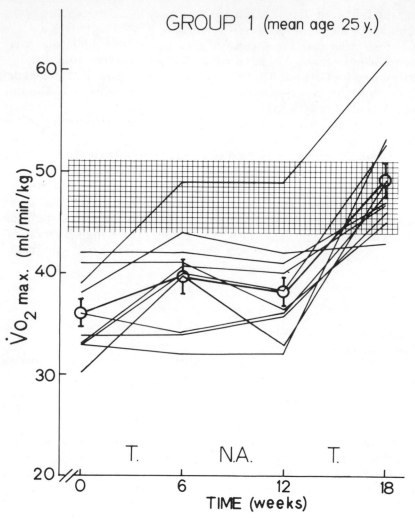

Figure 9.   Individual and mean values of maximal oxygen uptake of Group 1. Shaded area indicates the average of Norwegian children, ± 2 SD. Vertical bars indicate the range of 1 SE. T = training, NA = normal activity.

The relative increases in muscle strength were more pronounced in Group 2 than in Group 1. This can be explained by the fact that this group, at the beginning of the program, had a very low mean, much lower than Group 1. The average strength of the trunk flexor muscles in Group 2 was only 37% of the average for healthy schoolboys of the same age, whereas the average for Group 1 corresponded to 63% of the average for the general population. Strength of trunk extensors was 38% and 66% for Groups 2 and 1, respectively, when compared to the norm. Nordgren

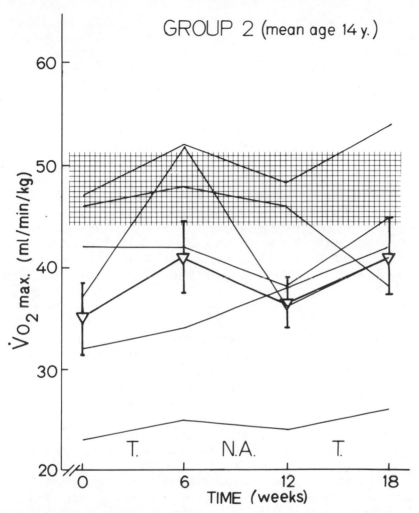

Figure 10.   Individual and mean values of maximal oxygen uptake of Group 2. Shaded area indicates the average of Norwegian children ± 2 SD. Vertical bars indicate range of 1 SE. T = training, NA = normal activity.

(1970) reported that, for 39 mentally retarded mature men (no specific ages were given), the forward flexion was found to be 70% and the backward extension to be 66% of the normal averages. These results are surprisingly close to the findings for Group 1 in this study. It is possible that the larger deviation from normal averages observed in Group 2 can be partly explained by their young age. Since patients with Down syndrome show considerably slower rates of growth and development than healthy persons, it is reasonable to assume that the group of boys, 11–16 years of age, was relatively more retarded than the group whose members were, on the average, 25 years old (Group 1). Group 1 matured later than the control group; but at the time of testing most of them had attained maturity. The better quality of the physical education program that Group 1 enjoyed during the last 4–5 years could be another explanation of the superiority of this group.

The final result obtained for Group 1 (extension, 90% and flexion, 81% of normal averages), and the considerable improvement in Group 2, prove that muscular strength in patients with Down syndrome approaching a level within or slightly below normal limits of the healthy population can be obtained with training. The possibility that muscular strength could be increased successfully indicates that the muscular weakness observed in this group is caused by lack of sufficient training.

The increase in aerobic working capacity was largest in Group 1. This group had a mean of 49 ml/min•kg in the final test. The mean value for Norwegian men 20–30 years of age is 47 ml/min•kg. These results can be compared with the results of Bjørke et al. (1978) after a 1-month training program at Beitostølen Health Sport Centre. They found that within this period the maximal oxygen uptake for the participating 18 mentally retarded boys increased from 75.9% to 86.1% of the average for the normal population.

For another group of mentally retarded children, additional training was carried out by a physiotherapist and a sport instructor for a period of one school year. The average maximal oxygen uptake, expressed as a percentage of the normal average, increased significantly from about 80% to about 104%. This is very much in accordance with our results. Since Bjørke et al. (1978) did not report the diagnoses of their subjects, a direct comparison between the two studies was not possible. In spite of this, their study confirms that mentally retarded children have a large potential for trainability in their aerobic capacities.

The differences in the increases between the two groups in this study can be explained by differences in the status of physical education programs in their respective institutions. Because of the poorly organized program for Group 2, the boys in this group had a lower attention span, lower threshold of anxiety, and greater difficulties in understanding verbal instructions. Because Group 1 was more familiar with physical training, less time was needed for motivation and instruction. This resulted in better utilization of the available time for physical training.

It is rather interesting to note that both of these groups, as well as the children studied by Bjørke et al. (1978) at Beitostølen, had nearly similar values of maximal oxygen uptake at the beginning of the training programs. Can this be interpreted as the typical value for retarded children who are not forced to stay in bed, but who, for a number of reasons (lack of stimulation, overprotection by parents and staff, lower level of spontaneous physical activity), have a low habitual physical activity level?

The observation that Group 1, in spite of being involved in systematic physical training for some length of time, had the same maximal oxygen uptake as the group not participating in such activities may indicate that, in order to improve this parameter, the training must be more specific and intense than what is commonly practiced in institutions.

The regression or stagnation in most of the parameters in the period of normal activity shows that continuity of training is necessary if one hopes to keep patients with Down syndrome on a higher level of physical fitness. The regression of physical status observed after cessation of the first training period seems to be the result of developmental training in children with Down syndrome, as reported by Aronson and Fällström (1977). Developmental training had a significant effect on the mental age of the trained children. However, in a follow-up study the beneficial effect was reduced in the trained group.

According to reports by staff and parents, participation in the training in this study also resulted in positive psychological effects. The same effect was reported by Bjørke et al. (1978).

CONCLUSIONS

The conclusions of this study are as follows:

1. Persons with Down syndrome have a large capacity for improving physical fitness. Physically mature males with Down syndrome can, within a relatively short time, reach a strength and endurance level that is within or close to normal values.
2. The obesity of patients with Down syndrome is caused by a low level of physical activity, but weight loss can be induced by physical training.
3. Positive and measurable physiological effects can be obtained only by a trained regimen that exceeds in intensity and duration that which is usually practiced in institutions.
4. Patients with Down syndrome tolerate and also enjoy physical training that is much more intense than what is normally practiced in institutions.
5. Disruption of training results in a regression in physical fitness. To achieve long-term benefits, the training must be a continuous process.

These results indicate the need for increased physical training, which must be given the same attention as the developmental training. It must be realized that this study was limited, but it is hoped that the study will stimulate the initiation of other controlled programs of physical training.

ACKNOWLEDGMENTS

We express our gratitude to the Department of Health for Mentally Retarded, Oslo Community, for financial support which made this study possible. We also thank Drs. Vislie and Dommerud for their interest and help in realizing the training programs, and Dr. Svein Oseid, of the College of Physical Education and Sport, for his assistance in writing this manuscript. Finally, we thank T. Nesse, H. Graff, and S. Hajdu for their highly skilled assistance in performing the training and testing programs.

REFERENCES

Aronson, M., and K. Fällström. 1977. Immediate and long-term effects of developmental training in children with Down's syndrome. Dev. Med. Child Neurol. 19:489–494.

Åstrand, J. 1960. Aerobic work capacity in men and women, with special reference to age. Acta Physiol. Scand. 49, Suppl. 169.

Benda, C. 1956. A comprehensive review of Mongolism. Arch. Pediatr. 73:391.

Bjørke, G., R. Hagen, H. Lie, and I. Kleive. 1978. Physical activation of mentally retarded children (in Norwegian). J. Norwegian Med. Assoc. 3:134–136.

Brousseau, K. 1928. Mongolism: A Study of the Physical and Mental Characteristics of Mongolian Imbeciles. Williams & Wilkins Co., Baltimore.

Brundtland, G. H., K. Liestøl, and L. Walløe. 1975. Height and weight of schoolchildren (in Norwegian). J. Norwegian Med. Assoc. 2:79–83.

Dutton, G. 1959. The physical development of Mongols. Arch. Dis. Child. 34: 46–50.

Lange-Andersen, K., and T. Nesse. 1979. Health and Work Environment. Part 3: Overload and Backache (in Norwegian). Postverkets Bedriftshelsetjeneste, Oslo.

Menolascino, F. J. 1965. Psychiatric aspects of Mongolism. Am. J. Ment. Defic. 69:653.

Nordgren, B. 1970. Physical capabilities in a group of mentally retarded adults. Scand. J. Rehabil. Med., Suppl. 125.

Rarick, G. L., and V. Seefeldt. 1974. Observations from longitudinal data on growth in stature and sitting height of children with Down's syndrome. J. Ment. Defic. Res. 18:63–78.

Skrobak-Kaczynski, J., T. Nesse, H. Olsen, and K. Lange-Andersen. 1973. Methods for Biological Evaluation of Growth and Development in Schoolchildren (in Norwegian). Landsrådet Fysisk Fostring i Skolen, Oslo.

Thelander, H. E., and H. B. Pryor. 1966. Abnormal patterns of growth and development in Mongolism. An anthropometric study. Clin. Pediatr. 5:493–501.

The Effects on Growth, Body Composition, and Circulatory Function of Anorexia Nervosa in Adolescent Patients

L. P. M. Fohlin

Anorexia nervosa (AN) is a serious disorder with a dubious prognosis. An increasing incidence has been reported in Sweden (Nylander, 1971) and other countries (Duddle, 1973; Crisp et al., 1976). Most of the common clinical symptoms of AN, such as bradycardia, low blood pressure, low body temperature, and amenorrhea, also occur during long-standing caloric restriction (Keys et al., 1950). However, there are also important differences: AN chiefly affects adolescent girls, many patients are hyperactive, and deficiency stages are often lacking.

In previous studies, body composition (Davies et al., 1978), cardiovascular function (Fohlin, 1978; Fohlin et al., 1978), and renal function (Aperia et al., 1978) were investigated. The effects of caloric restriction on the essential pubertal growth period are scarce because most published data on AN are concerned with adult patients.

The present study was undertaken to evaluate the influence of rehabilitation—resulting in the restitution of normal body weight—on body composition and circulatory function; and also to study the long-term effects of AN on growth.

SUBJECTS AND METHODS

Eight patients, three boys and five girls, with AN were studied before and after weight gain. All were included in a previously described investigation (Fohlin, 1977). They were studied after informed consent had been

Table 1. Physical characteristics of three boys and five girls with AN before (I) and after weight gain (II)

Patient	Age (years) I	II	Premorbid weight (kg)	Weight (kg) I	II	Lean body mass (kg) I	II	Height (kg) I	II
Male									
TT	16.0	18.9	72	56.7	76.0			188	188
AN	18.2	19.3	62	48.7	63.5	46	54.9	186	186
MS	17.1	17.8	62	51.0	62.5	48.2	53.8	184	184
Female									
HH	12.1	14.3	35	30.0	45.0	29.2	33.6	153	154
JJ	12.8	13.2	45	29.3	47.0	29.3	39.0	160	160
MSt	14.0	15.0	48	35.0	49.0	31.5	39.9	164	164
CP	14.2	16.0	41	34.5	43.3	31.4	35.9	157	157
AH	15.9	17.8	54	35.8	49.3	32.6	39.7	164	164
$\bar{x}$	15.0	16.5	52.4	40.1	54.5	35.5	42.4	170	170
±SD	2.1	2.2	12.4	10.4	11.6	8.1	8.5	14	14
p	<0.01			<0.001		<0.001		N.S.	

given by the Ethical Committee of the Karolinska Institutet. None of them had a history of overweight before the onset of AN. The average duration of AN at the first examination of weight loss was 1.0 year. The mean age at first examination was 17.1 years for the boys and 13.8 years for the girls. Their physical characteristics are shown in Table 1. The boys were postpubertal at the onset of the disease. Two girls had secondary amenorrhea, and the three others developed symptoms before the onset of menarche. The time interval to recovery varied between 0.4 and 2.9 years. All the patients were treated in a hospital for some time, and were regularly seen by a psychiatrist. None were on drug therapy.

When rehabilitated, the patients returned to their premorbid weight. They were reinvestigated immediately following rehabilitation except for one boy (TT), who had been rehabilitated for about 1.5 years and during that time had trained extremely hard with long-distance running. When rehabilitated, two girls were followed for 1–2 years with respect to their growth.

Blood volume (BV) was determined with ^{125}I-labeled albumin (Williams and Fine, 1961). Heart volume (HV) was measured in the prone position (Kjellberg et al., 1949). Skinfold thicknesses, at triceps and subscapular sites, were measured with a Harpenden caliper. From the sum of these measurements, lean body mass (LBM) was calculated (Parízková, 1977). Detailed information regarding the methods is given elsewhere (Fohlin, 1977). Exercise was performed with the patients sitting on an electrically braked bicycle ergometer (Siemens-Elema), with step-wise increases in work loads. The criteria for maximal exercise ($\dot{V}O_{2 \, max}$)

Table 2. Resting circulatory data and dimensions (individual values and $x \pm$ SD)—significance before (I) and after treatment (II) is given

Patient	Heart rate (b.p.m.)		Blood pressure (mm Hg)		Heart volume (ml)		Blood volume (l)		Blood lactate (mmol/l)	
	I	II	I	II	I	II	I	II	I	II
TT	38	78	110/80	140/60	769	1123	4.94	6.46	1.4	2.0
AN	63	80	110/65	115/70	545	682	2.80	4.10	3.9	1.7
MS	60	76	95/60	120/70	620	756	3.51	5.30	1.8	1.0
HH	47	84	90/60	105/60	362	479	2.37	3.27	2.0	1.0
JJ	57	105	80/60	115/70	391	541	3.00	3.80	1.2	1.4
MST	53	84	90/60	110/70	332	448	2.46	3.76	1.4	—
CP	53	57	105/80	105/70	406	499	2.90	3.46	1.7	1.8
AH	52	68	95/65	100/80	453	521	2.40	4.40	1.7	0.9
$\bar{x}$	53	79	97/65	114/71	485	631	3.05	4.32	1.9	1.4
$\pm$SD	8	14	97 ± 11^a 65 ± 7^b	114 ± 12^a 70 ± 8^b	150	225	0.86	1.07	0.9	0.4
p	<0.01		0.05^a N.S.^{b}		<0.01		<0.01		N.S.	

^{a}Systolic.
^{b}Diastolic.

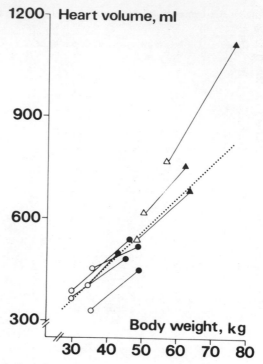

Figure 1.   Heart volume in relation to body weight in eight patients with AN. The dotted line represents 109 healthy children (Thorén, in preparation). ○ = girl, △ = boy; filled symbols signify postrehabilitation.

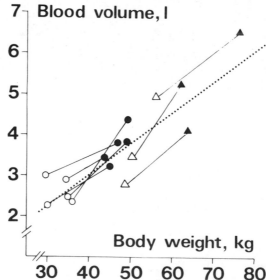

Figure 2.   Blood volume in relation to body weight in eight patients with AN. The dotted line corresponds to 75ml/kg of body weight (Karlberg and Lind, 1955). Symbols as in Figure 1.

Table 3.   Maximal exercise data ($\bar{x} \pm$ SD)—significance before (I) and after treatment (II) is given

Patient	Work load (W)		Heart rate (b.p.m.)		Oxygen uptake (l/min)		Oxygen uptake (ml/kg•min)	
	I	II	I	II	I	II	I	II
TT	130	330	175	200	1.75	4.12	31	54
AN	140	190	180	195	1.79	2.61	37	41
MS	130	230	175	195	1.65	3.10	32	50
HH	80	140	170	200	0.94	1.93	34	42
CP	110	140	180	185	1.38	1.77	40	41
AH	100	130	182	195	1.41	2.31	39	47
$\bar{x}$	115	193	177	195	1.49	2.64	36	46
$\pm$ SD	23	77	5	6	0.32	0.87	4	5
p	< 0.05		< 0.01		< 0.01		< 0.05	

were that blood lactate and respiratory quotient should exceed values of 9 mmol/liter and 1.0, respectively (Åstrand and Rodahl, 1970). Two girls failed to fulfill these criteria. The statistical significance of the observed values before and after rehabilitation was tested using the student's paired t test.

RESULTS

Basic data concerning the patients at rest before and after rehabilitation are given in Tables 1 and 2. Their mean weight loss was 25%. The boys had 6% of their total body weight as fat before treatment and 14% as fat after weight gain, when calculated from skinfold measurements (Table 2). Corresponding mean values for the girls were 6% and 19%. LBM increased significantly in all patients; the mean LBM was 35.5 kg at the first investigation, and 42.4 kg at the second investigation.

The height of the patients remained unchanged between the two observations. Heart and blood volumes increased significantly in all patients following weight gain (Figures 1 and 2), but the increase was, on the whole, proportional to the gain in weight. Mean values for blood volume per kg of body weight before and after treatment were 77 ml and 79 ml, respectively. At rest, the heart rate was significantly faster ($p < 0.01$) when the patients were rehabilitated, with a mean value of 79 b.p.m., compared to 53 b.p.m. before treatment. The mean oxygen uptake at rest increased from 0.015 liter/min to 0.020 liter/min after weight gain. Blood lactate at rest was not significantly changed after rehabilitation.

The responses to maximal exercise performance are shown in Table 3. The maximal exercise heart rate increased significantly ($p < 0.01$), from 177 to 195 b.p.m. The absolute $\dot{V}_{O_2 max}$ rose from 1.49 ± 0.32 liters/min to 2.64 ± 0.87 liters/min ($p < 0.05$) after weight gain. Expressed in terms of

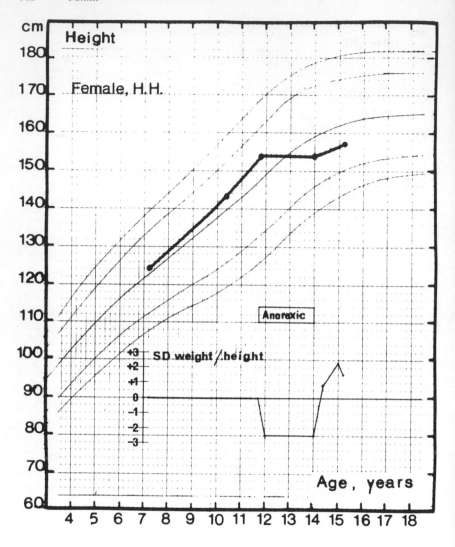

Figure 3a and b. Height in relation to age on Swedish standard height-weight curves (Broman et al., 1942) for two rehabilitated girls. The standard deviation of the relationship of weight to height is given.

body weight, the corresponding mean figures were 36 ml/kg•min and 46 ml/kg•min. Maximal blood lactate was 12.5 mmol/liter on both examinations. The height of the patients remained unchanged between the two examinations. Two of the prepubertal girls were followed for 1–2 years after they had been rehabilitated. Their height-to-age relationships are given in Figures 3a and b. Figure 4 is a photograph of one girl before and after treatment.

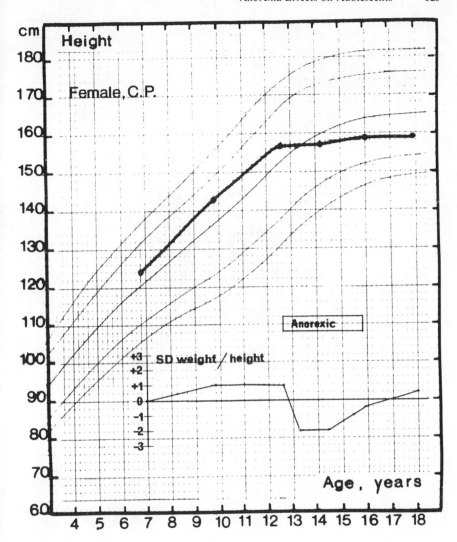

DISCUSSION

The semistarvation in AN has a marked effect on body composition. The decline in body weight was due not only to a reduction in fat, but also to a decrease in soft fat-free tissue. Similar findings have been reported from dietary treatment of obese subjects (Kjellberg and Reizenstein, 1970). LBM increased significantly in all patients after recovery. The effect of caloric restriction on body structure and function found in the present investigation is in good agreement with previous studies of experimental semistarvation (Keys et al., 1950). The bradycardia, hypotension, and

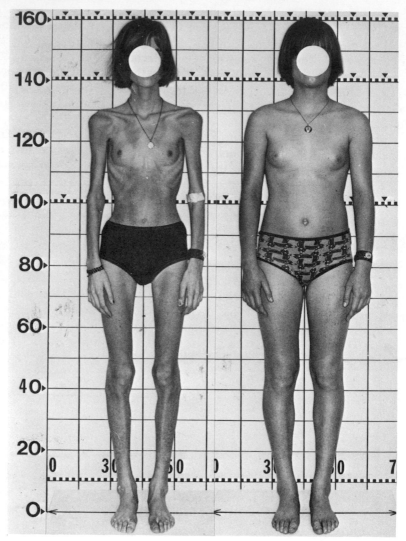

Figure 4.   A girl with AN, and four months later, after weight gain of 17.7 kg.

hypothermia found in AN patients were all normalized following rehabilitation with weight gain to normal and premorbid levels. This indicates that the pathophysiological findings may reflect the reduced energy supply per se. Heart and blood volume in AN patients showed a more marked adaptation to body weight than results obtained from a Minnesota study (Keys et al., 1950). Blood volume in that experiment hardly changed following 24 weeks of semistarvation, with a weight loss of about 24%. In AN the change of blood volume is influenced by the age of onset of the disease, the duration, and the degree of physical activity.

The responses to exercise showed that the maximal heart rate and $\dot{V}_{O_2\,max}$ were low. The decrease in $\dot{V}_{O_2\,max}$ was greater than expected with regard to weight loss, lean body mass, and circulatory dimensions (heart and blood volume). The reduction in $\dot{V}_{O_2\,max}$ in the present study is in good agreement with results of the Minnesota experiment (Keys et al., 1950), where $\dot{V}_{O_2\,max}$ per kg of body weight declined 26% in nine adult men following a 24% weight reduction.

The low maximal heart rate of the AN patients is hard to explain. The reduction of muscle mass found in AN, which contributes to loss of strength, undoubtedly affects the ability to perform maximal aerobic work, and may result in a low maximal heart rate. However, the respiratory quotient and blood lactate values indicate that the AN patients were at or very close to their "true" $\dot{V}_{O_2\,max}$. The low maximal heart rate may also be a reflection of the bradycardia seen at rest.

None of the prepubertal girls showed any growth in height, and no girl menstruated during this study. It is obvious from the data of the two girls who were followed after rehabilitation (Figures 3a and b) that long-standing caloric restriction during this essential growth period could have serious effects on growth. These two girls have closure of the epiphysial zones of the knees, resulting in a very small possibility for any further growth in height. Figures 3a and b show that there has been no catch-up growth, with reduced final height as a result.

These findings emphasize the importance of early recognition and proper treatment in young AN patients.

CONCLUSION

It is concluded from this study that the body of the adolescent patient with AN has considerable ability to adapt to varying degrees of caloric supply, and that caloric restriction in this age group could seriously affect growth.

REFERENCES

Aperia, A., O. Broberger, and L. Fohlin. 1978. Renal function in anorexia nervosa. Acta Paediatr. Scand. 67:219–224.

Åstrand, P.-O., and L. Rodahl. 1970. Textbook of Work Physiology. McGraw-Hill Book Co., New York.

Broman, B., G. Dahlberg, and A. Lichtenstein. 1942. Height and weight during growth. Acta Paediatr. Scand. 30:1–66.

Crisp, A. H., R. L. Palmer, and R. S. Kalucy. 1976. How common is anorexia nervosa? A prevalence study. Br. J. Psychiatry 128:549–554.

Davies, C. T. M., W. von Döbeln, L. Fohlin, U. Freyschyss, and C. Thorén. 1978. Total body potassium, fat free weight and maximal aerobic power in children with anorexia nervosa. Acta Paediatr. Scand. 67:229–234.

Duddle, M. 1973. An increase of anorexia nervosa in a university population. Br. J. Psychiatry 123:711–712.

Fohlin, L. 1977. Body composition, cardiovascular and renal function in adolescent patients with anorexia nervosa. Acta Paediatry. Scand. (Suppl. 268).

Fohlin, L. 1978. Exercise performance and body dimensions in anorexia nervosa before and after rehabilitation. Acta Med. Scand. 204:61–65.

Fohlin, L., U. Freyschuss, B. Bjarke, C. T. M. Davies, and C. Thorén. 1978. Function and dimensions of the circulatory system in anorexia nervosa. Acta Paediatr. Scand. 67:11–16.

Karlberg, P., and J. Lind. 1955. Studies on the total amount of hemoglobin and the blood volume in children. Acta Paediatr. Scand. 44:17–34.

Keys, A., J. Brozek, A. Henschel, O. Mickelsen, and H. L. Taylor. 1950. The Biology of Human Starvation. University of Minnesota Press, Minneapolis.

Kjellberg, S. R., U. Rudhe, and T. Sjöstrand. 1949. The amount of hemoglobin and the blood volume in relation to the pulse rate and cardiac volume during rest. Acta Radiol. 31:113–122.

Kjellberg, J., and P. Reizenstein. 1970. Effect of starvation on body composition in obesity. Acta Med. Scand. 188:171–178.

Nylander, I. 1971. The feeling of being fat and dieting in a school population. Acta Sociomed. Scand. 1:17–26.

Pařizková, J. 1977. Body Fat and Physical Fitness. Martinus Nijhoff B.V. Medical Division, The Hague.

Williams, I. A., and J. Fine. 1961. Measurements of blood volume with a new apparatus. N. Engl. J. Med. 264:842–848.

Perception of Exertion in Anorexia Nervosa Patients

C. T. M. Davies, L. Fohlin, and C. Thorén

Anorexia nervosa (AN) is recognized as a serious disorder that is primarily psychogenic in origin. It is characterized by an active refusal to eat and a severe loss of body weight. The disease therefore shares many of the common clinical and physiological symptoms seen in involuntary starvation, such as bradycardia, hypotension, hypothermia, acrocyanosis, decreased metabolic rate, and amenorrhea in girls (Fohlin, 1977). However, AN does differ in several important respects from severe inanition: it chiefly affects pubertal girls, there are seldom signs of protein or vitamin deficiency, and anemia is usually absent. In addition, the patients are known to have a disturbed perception of their own body image or disturbed mind-body relationship, which may be associated with a hyperactive state and a denial of exertion and fatigue following physical effort (Dally, 1969; Bruch, 1973).

In a series of previous studies from this laboratory (Aperia et al., 1978; Davies et al., 1978; Fohlin, 1978; Fohlin et al., 1978; Freyschuss et al., 1978), extensive reports on the clinical and physiological concomitants of the disease have been given. The purpose of the present investigation, therefore, was to examine these physiological aspects of anorexia by collecting data on the level of exercise perceived by patients with the disease under standardized conditions of exercise on a bicycle ergometer.

SUBJECTS AND METHODS

One male and eight female patients with AN were studied during prolonged exercise of one-hr duration performed on a bicycle ergometer. Their physical characteristics are given in Table 1. During the first and second

327

Table 1. Individual data on age, height; weight, weight loss from premorbid weight, lean body mass (LBM), heart rate, and maximal aerobic power ($\dot{V}o_{2\,max}$) for nine anorexia nervosa patients

Subject	Age (years)	Height (cm)	Weight (kg)	Weight loss (%)	LBM[a] (kg)	Heart rate (b.p.m.)		$\dot{V}o_{2\,max}$ (l/min)
						Rest	Max	
AN	18.2	186	48.7	31	45.7	63	180	1.79
CP	14.2	157	34.5	28	32.2	53	180	1.38
UN	16.9	180	41.8	20	37.2	42	175	1.45
ME	13.6	169	48.5	19	40.7	57	175	1.07
AL	15.5	132	26.9	20	23.7	49	—	0.85
HH	12.1	153	30.2	30	29.2	47	170	0.94
HH$_1$	13.2	168	40.5	31	35.0	55	180	1.07
MS	14.6	164	35.0	37	32.3	53	163	0.73
LP	17.6	162	42.5	22	36.2	54	177	1.22
$\bar{x}$	15.0	163	38.7	26.4	34.7	52.6	175.0	1.17
SD	2.1	16	7.7	6.4	6.4	6.0	5.9	0.33

[a]Calculated from skinfold thicknesses according to the method of Pařízková (1977).

30-min period of the experiment, oxygen intake was measured using the standard (Douglas bag) technique, oxygen and carbon dioxide concentrations of the inspired gas were determined by the micro-Scholander (chemical) method, and the rated perceived exertion (RPE) was assessed using the RPE scale of Borg and Linderholm (1967), as shown below:

6	11—fairly light	16
7—very, very light	12	17—very hard
8	13—somewhat hard	18
9—very light	14	19—very, very hard
10	15—hard	20

The patients were shown the chart at approximately 10-min intervals and were asked to indicate a number on the scale corresponding to the degree of exertion perceived. On a separate occasion, determination of their maximal aerobic power output ($\dot{V}O_{2\,max}$) was made using a progressive test outlined by Fohlin et al. (1978). The criteria for maximal performance were that the exchange ratio (R) should exceed unity and that blood lactate, which was determined enzymatically from a sample from a prewarmed fingertip on the immediate cessation of effort, should be >9 mmol/liter. For comparison, data previously collected on eight normal subjects using similar methods are presented. Eleven experiments were performed with the anorexic patients, and 21 with the normal subjects.

RESULTS AND DISCUSSION

The patients were all typical for AN, with a mean weight loss of 26.4% and a body weight less than 10% in excess of the lean body mass. The mean heart rates at rest, 52.6 b.p.m., and at maximal exercise, 175.0 b.p.m., were in accordance with earlier functional studies of AN (Fohlin et al., 1978). Their aerobic power in relation to body weight (30 ml/ kg•min) was also low, as expected.

After 10 min of prolonged exercise at a relative work load of approximately 62% $\dot{V}O_{2\,max}$, there was no significant difference in the mean rating of perceived exertion given by the patients compared with normal subjects (Table 2). The majority of the individual data points for both the patients and normal subjects lie within the lower limits of the linear relationship previously found for short-term progressive exercise (Figure 1). In only one anorexic patient is there any suggestion of "denial of exertion," but, since she was particularly difficult, this patient was suspected of being deliberately perverse in responding to the rating scale (which she subsequently admitted).

After 60 min of prolonged steady state exercise, mean RPE in the patients had risen by 2.1, which was slightly, but not significantly, greater than the rise of 1.1 seen in the normal control subjects (Table 2). Associated with this was a slight rise ($\sim 3\%$) in oxygen uptake ($\dot{V}O_2$) and rela-

Table 2. Rated perceived exertion (RPE), oxygen uptake ($\dot{V}O_2$), and relative work load (% $\dot{V}O_{2\,max}$) after 10 and 60 min of prolonged exercise[a]

Group	10-min exercise			60-min exercise		
	RPE	$\dot{V}O_2$ (l/min)	$\dot{V}O_{2\,max}$ (%)	RPE	$\dot{V}O_2$ (l/min)	$\dot{V}O_{2\,max}$ (%)
Anorexia nervosa ($N=9$)	13.0	0.81^{b}	64	15.1	0.84^{b}	66
	±2.4	±0.23	±9	±3.7	±0.23	±11
Normal subjects ($N=8$)	12.6	2.24	61	13.7	2.34	64
	±1.3	±0.53	±7	±1.7	±0.54	±8

[a] $\bar{x} \pm$ SD.
[b] $p < 0.001$.

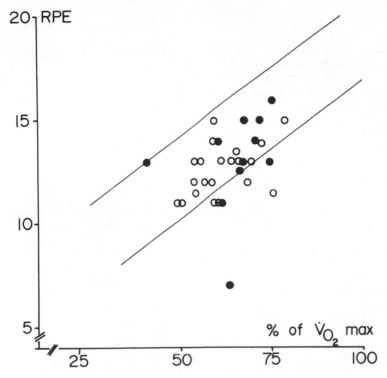

Figure 1.   Ratings of perceived exertion (RPE) in relation to work load. Solid circles represent AN patients; open circles represent normal subjects. Lines indicate the limits of linear regression found previously (Sargeant and Davies, 1973) for short-term progressive exercise.

tive work load (% $\dot{V}_{O_2 max}$). The mean heart rate for the AN group increased from 134.9 to 147.7 b.p.m.

Thus, these data extend previous observations made with normal men (Sargeant and Davies, 1973), and with patients with muscular atrophy of the lower limb(s) following fracture (Sargeant and Davies, 1977), where RPE was shown to increase linearly with relative work load. The data also support the usefulness and reliability of the Borg scale for the assessment of exertion in man. The data give no support to the view (Dally, 1969) that in anorexia nervosa there is a denial or loss of perception of exertion. The patient's verbal rating of exertion was qualitatively and quantitatively (if account was taken of the relative work load) similar to young healthy subjects without the disease. The self-restricted caloric intake and (involuntary) loss of working capacity that are associated with AN do not, at least in the teenagers in this study, impair the ability to discriminate accurately between work levels of similar duration, but different intensity.

REFERENCES

Aperia, A., O. Broberger, and L. Fohlin. 1978. Renal function in anorexia nervosa. Acta Paediatr. Scand. 67:219–224.

Borg, G., and H. Linderholm. 1967. Perceived exertion and pulse rate during graded exercise in various age groups. Acta Med. Scand. Suppl. 472:194–206.

Bruch, H. 1973. Eating Disorders: Obesity, Anorexia Nervosa and the Person Within. Basic Books, Inc., New York.

Dally, P. 1969. Anorexia Nervosa. William Heinemann Medical Books, London.

Davies, C. T. M., W. von Döbeln, L. Fohlin, U. Freyschuss, and C. Thorén. 1978. Total body potassium, fat free weight and maximal aerobic power in children with anorexia nervosa. Acta Paediatr. Scand. 67:229–234.

Fohlin, L. 1977. Body composition, cardiovascular and renal function in adolescent patients with anorexia nervosa. Acta Paediatr. Scand., Suppl. 268.

Fohlin, L. 1978. Exercise performance and body dimensions in anorexia nervosa before and after rehabilitation. Acta Med. Scand. 204:61.

Fohlin, L., U. Freyschuss, B. Bjarke, C. T. M. Davies, and C. Thorén. 1978. Function and dimensions of the circulatory system in anorexia nervosa. Acta Paediatr. Scand. 67:11–16.

Freyschuss, U., L. Fohlin, and C. Thorén. 1978. Limb circulation in anorexia nervosa. Acta Paediatr. Scand. 67:225–228.

Pařízková, J. 1977. Body Fat and Physical Fitness. Martinus Nijhoff B. V. Medical Division, The Hague.

Sargeant, A. J., and C. T. M. Davies. 1973. Perceived exertion during rhythmic exercise involving different muscle masses. Hum. Ergol. 2:3–11.

Sargeant, A. J., and C. T. M. Davies. 1977. Perceived exertion of dynamic exercise in normal subjects and patients following leg injury. In: G. Borg (ed.), Physical Work and Effort. Wenner-Gren International Symposium, Vol. 28, pp. 345–355. Pergamon Press, Oxford.

Physical Characteristics of Children with Congenital Heart Disease: Body Characteristics and Physical Working Capacity

S. de Knecht and R. A. Binkhorst

In pediatric cardiology three important questions are often asked:

1. What is the physical working capacity of a child with a congenital heart disease?
2. What is the child's daily physical activity?
3. Is it possible to improve the child's physical condition?

An impression of the working capacity and the daily activity is usually obtained by questioning the child and his parents. More objective data are often not available in the Netherlands, but do appear in foreign literature (Adams and Duffie, 1961; Hugenholtz and Nadas, 1963; Adams and Moss, 1969; Goldberg et al., 1969; Godfrey, 1970; Thorén et al., 1974; Mocellin and Bastanier, 1976).

In the Netherlands, a pilot study was conducted in which physical working capacity and daily physical activity of children with congenital heart disease were assessed. This report of the investigation includes the data on body characteristics and working capacity.

METHODS

Patients

Anthropometric data, diagnoses, Hb (HICN method), and some blood gas data at rest (capillary blood sample from arterialized earlobe, analyzed in a Corning apparatus) on the 39 subjects are presented in Table 1.

Table 1. Some characteristics and diagnoses of the subjects

Sex	Group	N	Age range (years)	Height range (cm)	Weight range (kg)	Hemoglobin range (mmol/l)	$Po_2{}^a$ range (mm Hg)	$Pco_2{}^a$ range (mm Hg)	Diagnosis	(N)
Boys	Cyanotic	10	9–14	130.5–163.5	21.0–43.6	9.2–14.4 (mean 11.1)	48–59 (94[b])	29–37	Tetr. of Fallot	(1)
									Tetr. of Fallot with shunt	(2)
									Pulm. atresia with VSD	(2)
									Single ventr., sing. atrium, TGA, Pulm. sten. with shunt	(1)
									Tricuspid atresia, pulm. atresia with shunt	(1)
									TGA, VSD, PAH	(1)
									VSD, PAH	(1)
									TGA, VSD, PDA, coarct. of the aorta, banding pulm. artery	(1)
Boys	Not cyanotic	9	9–14	135–182	25.0–59.3	7.8–9.5 (mean 8.7)	77–102	28–39	ASD I	(1)
									ASD II	(4)
									VSD	(3)
									Ebstein's anomaly	(1)

							Diagnosis	
Girls	Cyanotic	6	8–15	119.5–158.5	17.9–42.8	9.5–13 (mean 11.1)	43– 68	28–35	Ebstein's anomaly	(1)
									Tetr. of Fallot with shunt	(1)
									Tricuspid atresia with Glenn	(1)
									TGA, VSD, PAH	(1)
									VSD, banding pulm. artery	(1)
									Truncus arteriosus	(1)
Girls	Not cyanotic	14	8–15	129–168	23.9–63.7	7.6–9.8 (mean 8.7)	88–105	28–38	ASD I	(1)
									ASD II	(5)
									VSD	(8)

Abbreviations: VSD = ventricular septal defect; ASD I = atrial septal defect, primum type; ASD II = atrial septal defect, secundum type; TGA = transposition of the great arteries; PAH = pulmonary arterial hypertension; PDA = patent ductus arteriosus.

[a]Values at rest with normal pH (range 7.37–7.45).

[b]One subject evident cyanotic during exercise.

All the children were of normal intelligence, with the exception of one child; data for this child were excluded due to a lack of complete cooperation.

Physical Examinations

All physical examinations were performed by a pediatric cardiologist. Besides the data presented in Table 1, four skinfold thicknesses were taken (biceps, triceps, subscapula, and suprailiac) according to the method of Durnin and Ramahan (1967), using the Harpenden caliper. Furthermore, bone age was determined from x-ray of the left hand, using the Tanner-Whitehouse (TWI) method (1962).

Neurological Examination

Examinations of the nervous system revealed only minor distrubances in eight of the noncyanotic children, whereas 12 of the cyanotic children showed minor to modest disturbances, such as signs of spasticity or ataxia. All patients could perform the test without handicap due to these disturbances.

Lung Function

Lung functions were determined to exclude significant respiratory disorders; vital capacity, total and residual lung volumes, expiratory and inspiratory 1-sec values, and, mostly, the single breath CO transfer factor were measured. Vital capacity as a mean was 14% lower (range, +15% to −50%) for both cyanotic and noncyanotic patients as compared with normals. This is in accordance with values reported in the literature (Davies and Gazetopoulos, 1967; Howlett, 1972). The mean CO-transfer factor in both groups of patients was 6 ml•liter^{-1} of alveolar volume (range, 4.6 to 8.0), which was higher than for normals (4–5 ml•liter^{-1}); apparently, diffusion to the alveolar blood was not disturbed at rest (Bucci and Cook, 1961). The other data did not show significant differences from normal values. It can be seen in Table 1 that the patients showed a degree of hyperventilation (subnormal P_{CO_2}), with a normal pH, and, especially for the cyanotics, a high Hb concentration and a low P_{O_2}.

Motor Developmental Age

Motor development was assessed with the Oseretsky-Guilman method as modified by Verstappen (1970). It is applicable in the age range of 2–12 years, and contains tests for general static coordination, dynamic coordination, rapidity of movement, simultaneous movements, and dissociation of complex movements. This method can be used to obtain a general impression of the motor developmental age.

Exercise Test

Physical work was performed on an electronically-braked Lode bicycle ergometer, pedal frequency 60–70 rpm, with an increasing load of 10 W per minute.

Gas Exchange

Expired air was measured with the Douglas bag method; paramagnetic oxygen analysis (Servomex type OA 272), infrared carbon dioxide analysis (Uras), and volume with a Tissot spirometer.

Oxygen Uptake

$\dot{V}_{O_2 \, max}$ was determined in two-thirds of the subjects; in the others it had to be predicted from maximal load (using the relationship between maximal load and maximal oxygen uptake of the others) because they could not breathe through the mouthpiece while exercising at maximal load. Objective criteria for maximal exercise were age dependent: both maximal heart rate and blood lactic acid could be determined in only 28 subjects; lactic acid determination of the others failed.

Lactic Acid

Lactic acid was determined (Boehringer test kit) from blood obtained from the arterialized earlobe before exercise and 3–5 min after having reached maximal load.

Heart Function

The heart was monitored continuously before, during, and after exercise, using a unipolar V4-V5 ECG lead (reference electrode on the manubrium of the sternum). Every 30 sec a few beats were registered on a Hellige EK 75 recorder. Blood pressure was measured every third minute with a Doppler instrument (Arteriosonde, Roche, Switzerland). PWC_{170} power was calculated from heart rates between 130–170 b.p.m.

RESULTS AND DISCUSSION

Body Characteristics

Neurological disturbances were found more often in the cyanotic than in the noncyanotic group, which is in agreement with Tyler and Clark (1957). During obduction, Berthrong and Sabiston (1951) found arterial and venous occlusions in the brains of such patients. Reasons for these findings could be factors such as polycythemia, hyperviscosity of the blood, dimension of the right-to-left shunt, and condition after labor.

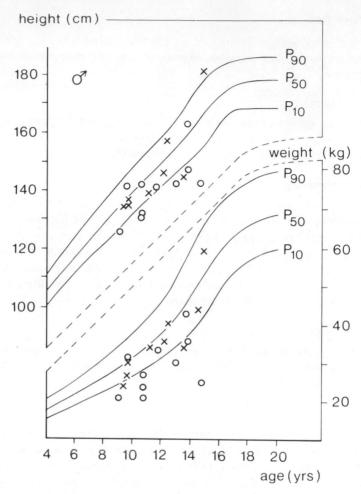

Figure 1.   Weight and height of boys in relation to calendar age. Data for normal boys (lines) from van Wieringen et al. (1968). O, cyanotic boys; X, noncyanotic boys.

Height and weight are plotted against age in Figures 1 and 2. These graphs show that, compared with normal Dutch children (van Wieringen et al., 1968), the patients, especially the cyanotic ones, were in general shorter and not as heavy. Weight seemed to be more affected than height, and this was more conspicuous in the boys than in the girls. This was in agreement with the findings of Linde et al. (1967), Pavilonis and Adomaitis (1977), and Levi et al. (1978).

The sum of four skinfold thicknesses as an indication of percentage of fat in 28 patients (no distinct difference between cyanotics and noncyanotics) were mostly below the 50th percentile for age- and sex-matched Dutch children (Luyken et al., 1977; van der Haar and Kromhout, 1978).

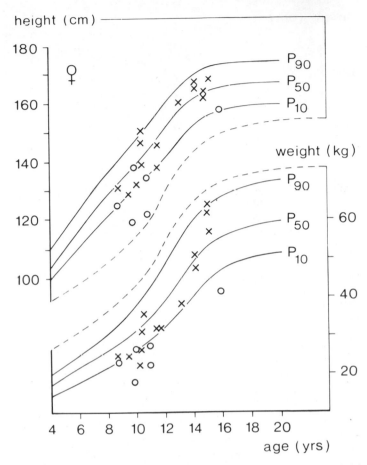

Figure 2.   Weight and height of girls in relation to calendar age. Data for normal girls (lines) from van Wieringen et al. (1968). O, cyanotic girls; X, noncyanotic girls.

This partly explains why body weight was relatively lower than normal at a certain age than height was (see Figures 1 and 2).

According to Linde et al. (1967) there is no correlation between the degree of cyanosis and the degree of growth retardation, but there is generally a delay in onset of puberty of 3 to 4 years, especially for the cyanotic patients.

Bone age of the patients in the experimental group showed a mean delay of about 1 year (range, $+1$ to -2 years) compared with normal Dutch children (Roede et al., 1976, unpublished data). When height and weight were plotted against bone age (Figures 3 and 4), the differences between these patients and normal Dutch children, as seen in Figures 1 and 2, were far less.

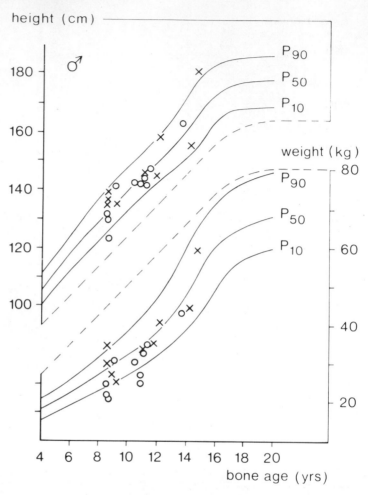

Figure 3.   Weight and height of boys in relation to bone age (Tanner-Whitehouse method, 1962). Data for normal boys (lines) from van Wieringen et al. (1968). O, cyanotic boys; X, noncyanotic boys.

       The results of the motor developmental test are presented in Figure 5. All patients showed a retardation in motor developmental age. The line of identity is drawn only up to 12 years; because the test is, in fact, only applicable for 2–12 year-old children. Also, if instead of calendar age, bone age (which was, as a mean, 1 year less in the patients) is plotted on the abscissa, the differences become smaller. In conclusion, it can be said that for certain purposes, bone age as well as calendar age should be used, since patients with congenital heart disease are often retarded in growth.

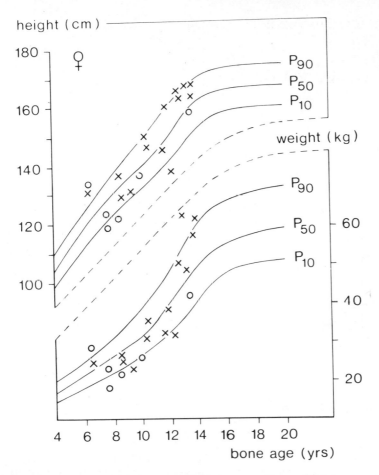

Figure 4. Weight and height of girls in relation to bone age (Tanner-Whitehouse method, 1962). Data for normal girls (lines) from van Wieringen et al. (1968). O, cyanotic girls; X, noncyanotic girls.

Physical Working Capacity

Above all, it should be mentioned that all patients performed a maximal test, although not all, especially of the cyanotics, reached the objective criteria for calling a test maximal; i.e., age dependent maximal heart rate and blood lactic acid. It will be seen from the figures that a considerable amount of normal data are lacking in the Netherlands (except data from Wafelbakker and Bink, 1971); normal data for other variables were obtained from the data reported in the literature in surrounding countries.

For lactic acid the criterion was set at 5 mmol·liter^{-1}, which is about the mean value minus 1 SD for the age of 9 years (Davies et al., 1972).

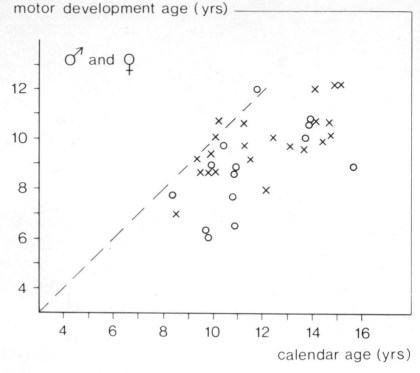

Figure 5.   Results of the Oseretsky-Guilman motor development test, related to calendar age for boys and girls. O, cyanotic; X, noncyanotic. The mean line of identity is dashed.

Although blood lactic acid concentration is age dependent in children, the differences in this value were so small (at 15 years about 7 mmol•liter^{-1}) that we chose one value.

For maximal heart rate, the criterion was set at 190 b.p.m., which is the mean minus 1 SD for the age group 9–16 years (Davies et al., 1972; Lindemann et al., 1973; Binkhorst and De Jong, unpublished data).

Maximal lactate concentration and maximal heart rate are plotted in Figure 6, in which the dotted lines correspond with the criteria. Of the cyanotic patients, only three met both criteria, whereas only five noncyanotics did not meet these criteria. One patient did not reach the criterion for maximal lactate, four did not achieve the maximal heart rate, and seven did not reach the values set for lactate and heart rate. One of the reasons could be that these limits (mean value minus 1 SD) are too high. On the other hand, it might be that these subjects deserve a somewhat deeper examination with regard to their physical activity, since it can be expected that they never push themselves to a reasonable intensity of exercise. A reason for not reaching a high lactate concentration might also be

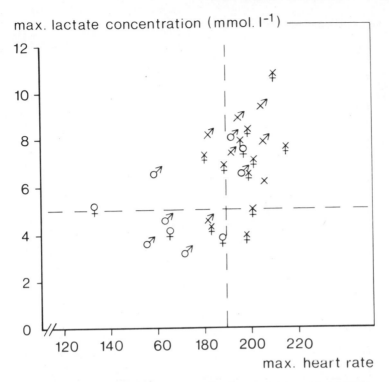

Figure 6.   Blood lactate concentration immediately after maximal work in relation to maximal heart rate for cyanotic girls (♀) and boys (♂), and for noncyanotic girls (⚥) and boys (⚦). Dotted lines represent the mean values minus 1 SD for normal subjects; heart rate for the age group (9–16 years) was calculated from data of Lindemann et al. (1973), Davies et al. (1972), and Binkhorst and De Jong (unpublished data); lactate concentration was calculated according to Davies et al. (1972). The value for lactate (mean − 1 SD; i.e., 5 mmol•liter^{-1}) is the lowest in the age group 9–16 years.

a low anaerobic energy–delivering capacity, as was shown for children by Eriksson (1972). It is also possible, at least in the cyanotic patients, that a very low arterial P_{O_2} (see Table 1 for resting values) develops in a short time during exercise, so that the work had to be stopped before anaerobic energy could be delivered substantially.

From Figures 7 and 8, it can be concluded that almost none of the cyanotic subjects had a normal maximal $\dot{V}_{O_2}$ uptake. This might be expected since they start with a very low P_{O_2} (see Table 1) and, therefore, they had to stop working at low work intensities. Only three noncyanotic boys and girls had low borderline values. Here again, these subjects might deserve special motivation with regard to their daily physical activity and training.

A high correlation ($r = 0.92$) was found between PWC_{170} and maximal $\dot{V}_{O_2}$ uptake per kg of body weight; this was higher than that found by

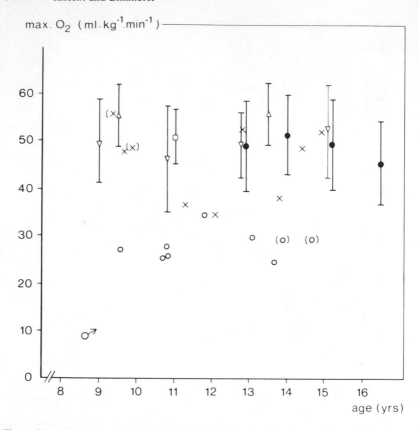

Figure 7.   Maximal oxygen consumption in relation to calendar age for cyanotic (O) and noncyanotic (X) boys. Symbols between bars predicted from maximal load. Mean and 1 SD of normal boys according to Lindemann et al. (1973), △; Davies et al. (1972), ▽; Binkhorst and de Jong (unpublished data), □; and Vos (unpublished data), ●.

Mocellin and Bastanier (1976) ($r = 0.74$). Nevertheless, it is the opinion of these authors that PWC_{170} should not be used instead of maximal load or maximal oxygen uptake unless these cannot be determined, or, as Mocellin and Bastanier (1976) suggested, to differentiate between groups of sick and healthy children.

It has been previously stated that children with low maximal values deserve special attention with regard to their physical activity and training. This means that in such cases a test battery, including maximal exercise, should be applied to assess whether the heart disease as such or a poor physical condition is the reason for low maximal values. If undertraining is the main factor, then a systematic training program should be followed. However, even when the heart disease itself is the main cause, it might be worthwhile to consider a training program to improve the residual capacities so that the child might live easier and probably have a happier daily life.

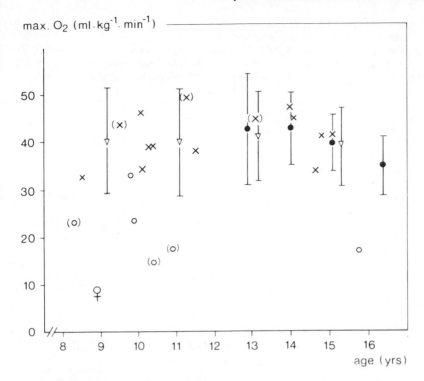

max. O_2 (ml·kg^{-1}·min^{-1})

age (yrs)

Figure 8.   Maximal oxygen consumption in relation to age for cyanotic (O) and noncyanotic (X) girls. Symbols between bars predicted from maximal load. Mean and 1 SD of normal girls according to Lindemann et al. (1973), △; Davies et al. (1972), ▽; Binkhorst and de Jong (unpublished data), □; and Vos (unpublished data), ●.

REFERENCES

Adams, F. H., and E. R. Duffie. 1961. Physical working capacity of children with heart disease. Lancet 81:493–496.

Adams, F. H., and A. J. Moss. 1969. Physical activity of children with congenital heart disease. Am. J. Cardiol. 24:605–606.

Berthrong, M., and D. Sabiston. 1951. Cerebral lesions in congenital heart disease. Bull. Johns Hopkins Hosp. 89:384–401.

Bucci, G., and C. D. Cook. 1961. Studies in respiratory physiology in children. VI. Lung diffusing capacity, diffusing capacity of pulmonary membrane and pulmonary capillary blood volume in congenital heart disease. J. Clin. Invest. 40: 1431–1441.

Davies, C. T. M., C. Barnes, and S. Godfrey. 1972. Body composition and maximal exercise performance in children. Hum. Biol. 44:195–214.

Davies, H., and N. Gazetopoulos. 1967. Lung function in patients with left-to-right shunts. Br. Heart J. 29:317–326.

Durnin, J. V. G. A., and M. M. Ramahan. 1967. The assessment of the amount of fat in the human body from measurements of skinfold thicknesses. Br. J. Nutr. 21:681–689.

Eriksson, B. O. 1972. Physical training, oxygen supply and muscle metabolism in 11–13 year old boys. Acta Physiol. Scand. Suppl. 384.

Godfrey, S. 1970. Physiological response to exercise in children with lung or heart disease. Arch. Dis. Child. 45:534–538.

Goldberg, S. J., F. Mendes, and R. Hurwitz. 1969. Maximal exercise capability of children as a function of specific cardial defects. Am. J. Cardiol. 23:349–353.

Howlett, G. 1972. Lung mechanisms in normal infants and infants with congenital heart disease. Arch. Dis. Child. 49:707–715.

Hugenholtz, P. G., and A. S. Nadas. 1963. Exercise studies in patients with congenital heart disease. Pediatrics 32(Suppl. 2):769–775.

Levi, R. J., A. Rosenthal, O. S. Miettinen, and A. S. Nadas. 1978. Determinants of growth in patients with ventricular septal defects. Circulation 57:793–797.

Linde, L. M., O. J. Dunn, R. Schireson, and B. Rasof. 1967. Growth in children with congenital heart disease. J. Pediatr. 70:413–419.

Lindemann, H., J. Rutenfranz, R. Mocellin, and W. Sbresny. 1973. Methodical research into indirect estimation of maximal oxygen consumption (in German). Eur. J. Appl. Physiol. 32:25–53.

Luyken, R., J. F. de Wijn, J. C. A. Zaat, and K. Schreinemakers. 1977. Somatometric data of Dutch adolescents and young adults (1960–1973) (in Dutch). Voeding 38:340–366.

Mocellin, R., and C. Bastanier. 1976. The W_{170} as a reliable measurement of the physical working performance of children with a heart disease (in German). Eur. J. Pediatr. 122:223–239.

Mocellin, R., J. Rutenfranz, and R. Singer. 1971. Normal values of the W_{170} for children (in German). Z. Kinderheilkd. 110:140–165.

Pavilonis, S., and A. Adomaitis. 1977. Sexual influence on physical development of the child with a congenital heart disease (in German). Anat. Anz. 141: 340–344.

Tanner, J. M., R. H. Whitehouse, and M. J. R. Healy. 1962. A New System for Estimating Skeletal Maturity from the Hand and Wrist, with Standards Derived from a Study of 2600 Healthy British Children. Centre International de l'Enfance, Paris.

Thorén, C., P. Herrin, and J. Vavrá. 1974. Studies of submaximal and maximal exercise in congenital complete heart block. Acta Paediatr. Belg. Suppl. 28: 132–141.

Tyler, H. R., and D. B. Clark. 1957. Incidence of neurological complications in congenital heart disease. Arch. Neurol. Psychiatry 77:17–22.

van der Haar, F., and D. Kromhout. 1978. Food uptake, nutritional anthropometry and blood chemical parameters in 3 selected Dutch school children populations. Thesis, Wageningen, Holland.

van Wieringen, J. A., F. Wafelbakker, H. P. Verbrugge, and J. H. de Haas. 1968. Diagram of growth in the Netherlands 1965; Second survey 0.24 years (in Dutch). Nederlands Instituut Praeventieve Geneeskunde, TNO. Wolters-Noordhoff, Groningen.

Verstappen. P. 1970. The Oseretsky Test. Instructions of the Department of Physical Therapy. University Hospital, Nijmegen, Holland.

Wafelbakker, F., and B. Bink. 1971. Physical working capacity at maximal levels of work of boys 8–23 years of age. Geneesk. Sport 4:9–13.

Exercise Performances of Children after Valvotomy of a Pulmonary Valvular Stenosis

R. Mocellin, C. Bastanier, and B. Kaltwasser

The natural history of patients with simple pulmonary stenosis depends on the severity of the obstruction between the right ventricle and the pulmonary artery. In cases of mild obstruction, cardiovascular performance capacity is usually normal, and the natural history is comparable to that of healthy people. The question is whether this is also valid for those patients with initially severe pulmonary stenosis in whom mild obstruction has persisted after surgical valvotomy of the pulmonary valve.

SUBJECTS AND METHODS

Twenty-one children, 10 boys and 11 girls between the ages of 8 and 14 years, were studied. Each had undergone surgery 6 months to 6 years before the study began. Mean values of weight and height did not differ significantly from those of healthy children. The patients were unselected, and were studied in the outpatient department after a routine clinical examination.

After right heart catheterization, the catheter was placed in the right pulmonary artery via a cubital vein, and a plastic cannula was inserted into the brachial artery. Central venous and arterial blood were collected simultaneously by a pump system. Determination of the oxygen content of the blood was performed by means of a coulometric method (Sinet, 1973). The Douglas bag method was employed for measurement of ventilation and oxygen uptake.

Measurements were carried out at rest in the recumbent position, and during work on a bicycle ergometer. The first work load was performed at

Table 1. Mean values and standard deviation of maximal oxygen uptake and stroke volume, as a percentage of height standard

	$\bar{x}$	SD
$\dot{V}_{O_2\,max}$ (%)	90	21
Stroke volume	94	23

about 1.5 W/kg of body weight, whereas the second load was selected such that maximal oxygen uptake was attained. This was considered to be achieved when marked increases in respiratory rate and excursion were observed, and when a marked increase in the ventilatory equivalent for oxygen, a gas exchange ratio greater than 1.0, and blood lactate values consistent with the expected values for the respective age groups were obtained. At the end of the first work load the catheter was withdrawn from the right pulmonary artery via the right ventricle into the right atrium and the superior vena cava, and pressure was measured during this procedure.

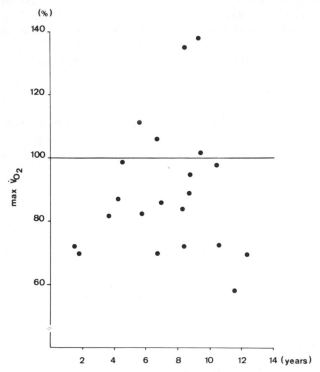

Figure 1. Maximal oxygen uptake ($\dot{V}_{O_2\,max}$), as a percentage of height standard, related to age at surgery.

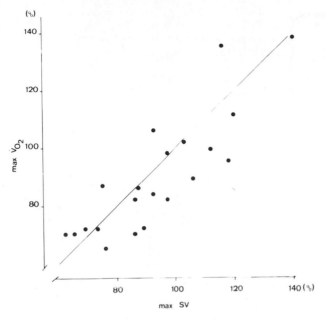

Figure 2.   Maximal oxygen uptake ($\dot{V}O_{2\,max}$), as a percentage of height standard, related to stroke volume (SV), as a percentage of height standard.

RESULTS

Heart rate was 83 ± 10 b.p.m. at rest, 152 ± 22 b.p.m. at submaximal, and 189 ± 13 b.p.m. at maximal load. The arteriovenous oxygen difference increased from 4.3 ml/100 ml at rest to 11.0 ml/100 ml at submaximal load. Stroke volume was approximately equal at rest in the recumbent position (57 ± 17 ml) and during submaximal load (58 ± 19 ml).

For better comparison, maximal oxygen uptake and stroke volume of all the children were expressed as a percentage of expected normal values for children of the same height. Table 1 shows that the mean values of both parameters were slightly depressed. In Figure 1, the individual values for maximal oxygen uptake, expressed as a percentage of height standard, are related to the age of the patients at the time of surgery. An above-average cardiovascular performance capacity was found only in five of the patients. The values varied independent of the age at surgery.

Figure 2 shows the relation between stroke volume and maximal oxygen uptake, in which all values were expressed as a percentage of expected normal values, according to body height. Most of the values were below the line of identity, but, nevertheless, as in healthy persons, stroke volume seems to be a determining factor of aerobic capacity.

Figure 3 depicts the mean values of right ventricular peak systolic pressure and peak systolic gradient between right ventricle and pulmonary

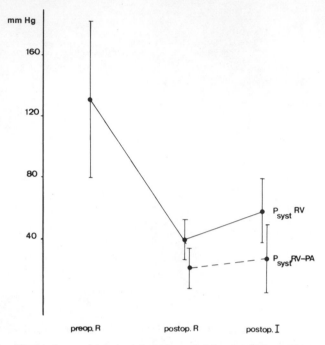

Figure 3. Mean values and standard deviations of right ventricular peak systolic pressure ($P_{syst}RV$) preoperatively at rest (preop. R), postoperatively at rest (postop. R), and at submaximal load (postop. I) and the respective postoperative values of peak systolic gradient between right ventricle and pulmonary artery.

artery. Mean right ventricular peak systolic pressure, which had been 131 mm Hg before operation, decreased to 40 mm Hg at rest and increased slightly to 59 mm Hg at submaximal load. The postoperative pressure gradient between right ventricle and pulmonary artery was 21 mm Hg at rest and 28 mm Hg at submaximal load, with large interindividual differences.

Figure 4 does not show any correlation between the individual values of right ventricular peak systolic pressure at submaximal load and aerobic capacity. A lack of correlation could also be demonstrated between pulmonary valve resistance and maximal oxygen uptake (Figure 5).

DISCUSSION

These results show that residual stenosis may persist after operation on an isolated pulmonary stenosis, and that an overproportional increase of right ventricular pressure during exercise can often be observed in these children.

In spite of this residual gradient, however, there was only slight cardiovascular dysfunction in most of these patients. A comparison of our results with those of other authors is difficult, because measurements (Campbell and Brock, 1955; Stone et al., 1974) were only performed at

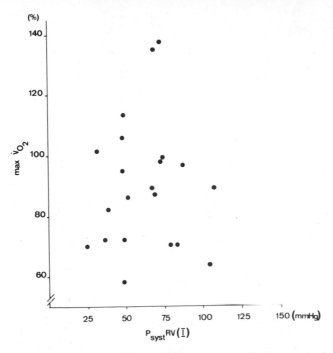

Figure 4.   Maximal oxygen uptake ($\dot{V}O_{2\ max}$), as a percentage of height standard, related to right ventricular systolic pressure at submaximal load.

relatively low loads, and consequently the functional capacity of the cardiovascular system could not be determined precisely. The conclusions of Hanson et al. (1958), however, agreed with the results of this study—that the differences in functional capacity are not simply correlated with the postoperative decrease in right ventricular pressure.

In this group of children, aerobic capacity was often less than could be expected from stroke volume. The reason may be that maximal heart rate was generally reduced to a mean value of 189 b.p.m.

Considering the lack of correlation between right ventricular pressure and aerobic capacity on the one hand and the good correlation between aerobic capacity and stroke volume on the other hand, stroke volume and right ventricular pressure can be assumed to vary independently of each other. This assumption is in agreement with the findings of other investigators (Lewis et al., 1964; Howitt, 1966; Ikkos et al., 1966; Moller et al., 1972; Finnegan et al., 1974; Stone et al., 1974) in patients with mild pulmonary stenosis. Only in the presence of severe, or at least moderate, stenosis could some kind of inverse relationship between right ventricular pressure and stroke volume be demonstrated (Johnson, 1962; Lewis et al., 1964; Jonsson and Lee, 1968; Möller et al., 1972). Nevertheless, marked increases in right ventricular pressure at exercise, together with decreases in stroke volume, may be found in individual patients with

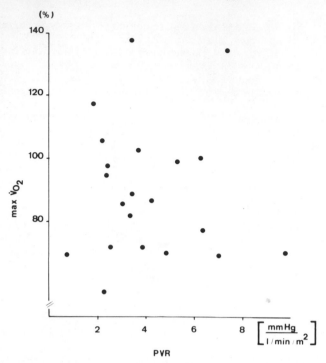

Figure 5.   Maximal oxygen uptake ($\dot{V}_{O_2 \text{ max}}$), as a percentage of height standard, related to pulmonary valve resistance (PVR).

even mild stenosis, as was illustrated in three of these children. Because right ventricular end diastolic pressure is often elevated at rest even after surgery, an additional increase at exercise, which was demonstrated by Stone et al. (1974) in some of their patients, may be the reason for a decrease in stroke volume. Reoperation must be considered in this small group of patients.

REFERENCES

Campbell, M., and R. Brock. 1955. The results of valvotomy for simple pulmonary stenosis. Br. Heart J. 17:229.

Finnegan, P., H. N. C. Ihenacho, S. P. Singh, and L. D. Abrams. 1974. Haemodynamic studies at rest and during exercise in pulmonary stenosis after surgery. Br. Heart J. 36:913.

Hanson, J. S., D. Ikkos, C. Crafoord, and C.-O. Ovenfors. 1958. Results of surgery of congenital pulmonary stenosis. Comparison of the transventricular and transarterial approaches. Circulation 18:558.

Howitt, G. 1966. Hemodynamic effects of exercise in pulmonic stenosis. Br. Heart J. 28:152.

Ikkos, D., B. Jonsson, and H. Linderholm. 1966. Effect of exercise in pulmonic stenosis with intact ventricular septum. Br. Heart J. 28:316.

Johnson, A. M. 1962. Impaired exercise response and other residua of pulmonary stenosis after valvotomy. Br. Heart J. 24:375.

Jonsson, B., S. J. K. Lee. 1968. Haemodynamic effects of exercise in isolated pulmonary stenosis before and after surgery. Br. Heart J. 30:60.

Lewis, J. M., A. C. Montero, S. A. Kinard, E. W. Dennis, and J. K. Alexander. 1964. Hemodynamic response to exercise in isolated pulmonic stenosis. Circulation 29:854.

Moller, J. H., S. Rao, and R. V. Lucas. 1972. Exercise hemodynamics of pulmonary valvular stenosis. Study of 64 children. Circulation 46:1018.

Sinet, S. 1973. A new method for measuring the oxygen content in blood. A comparative study with the manometric method of Van Slyke (in French). Dissertation, Paris.

Stone, F. M., B. F. Bessinger, R. V. Lucas, and J. H. Möller. 1974. Pre- and postoperative rest and exercise hemodynamics in children with pulmonary stenosis. Circulation 49:1102.

Unger, F., M. Deutsch, E. Domang, F. Helmer, H. Mösslacher, K. Steinbach, M. Wimmer, and E. Wolner. 1973. The hemodynamics after correction of isolated pulmonic stenosis (in German). Wien. Klin. Wochenschr. 85:732.

Maximal Treadmill Endurance Times of Children with Heart Defects Compared to those of Normal Children

G. R. Cumming

An ongoing clinical investigation has been seeking answers to the following questions about the exercise tolerance of children with heart defects: How frequently is exercise tolerance impaired in children with heart disease compared to normal children? Does exercise capacity reflect disease severity in children with heart defects? How much heart disease must exist before exercise capacity is reduced below normal? How does exercise capacity change with time and treatment in children with heart disease? The questions are simple, and information to partially answer them is now available.

A suitable protocol to assess what was labeled exercise capacity was chosen and evaluated (Bruce et al., 1973) and suitable normal values were obtained for a clinic population (Cumming et al., 1978). A sizable number of cardiac patients have now been tested.

METHODS

The Bruce treadmill protocol has been used almost exclusively in the clinical exercise area for the past 5 years, after a preceding 15-year experience using an electric bicycle ergometer (Cumming, 1977). After experimenting with a number of combinations of speeds and grades on the treadmill, it was found that the most suitable combinations were very similar to those used in the Bruce test, which is used in many adult exercise laboratories in North America. It would have been foolish to develop a slightly

Work supported by the Children's Hospital of Winnipeg Research Foundation

different program for the sake of being original, and it has been of value to have a single standardized protocol.

Children are tested without any prior practice, unless they happen to have been tested in a preceding medical visit. Children 4 to 6 years of age are a little fearful at the start, but the slow speed during the first stage, only 2.7 km/hr, soon allays these fears. Because Stage I of the test requires 18 ml of oxygen/kg/min, it may be too difficult a work load for severely disabled patients. The exercise test is done to observe the children during exercise and really has no value in measuring whether they are disabled or not. In order to allow the children with severe disability to exercise for at least 6 min, two auxiliary stages have been added to the Bruce protocol, Stage A-I, which is zero grade and 2.7 km/hr, and Stage A-II, which is 5% grade and 2.7 km/hr. These auxiliary stages are not added to the endurance time that starts with Stage I of the test. The 3-min duration of the stages of the Bruce protocol is not so long that boredom sets in. Also, it does not allow a steady state to satisfy some of the purists, but 3 min is a compromise between that and what is practical for clinical purposes, and it does provide reasonable indices of the response to submaximal loads.

The stages and oxygen cost for performing the Bruce test are shown in Table 1. As shown by Åstrand (1952), young children require more oxygen for the same exercise on the treadmill. The use of the treadmill for following the child longitudinally can be criticized because the oxygen requirements may decrease with age, but this is the only disadvantage of using the treadmill. This disadvantage is outweighed by many advantages, including: 1) ease of calibration; 2) same protocol with the same mechanical work loads for all subjects ages 4 years and up and for subjects of body weight varying from 12 to 100 kg; and 3) the built-in motivation of working close to exhaustion on the treadmill, since the subject who fails to keep running is obviously propelled backwards. This is quite different than trying to encourage the young child to maintain a pedaling frequency on the bicycle ergometer, and the technicians with considerable experience in both bicycle and treadmill exercise in children in a medical setting clearly prefer the treadmill for this reason.

Maximal exercise in a cardiac patient should be the same as maximal exercise for the normal subject as long as the exercise is not endangering life. It is difficult not to feel some compassion for the cyanotic child in whom exercise frequently leads to a severe headache. It is difficult not to worry a little about maximal exercise in the child with significant aortic stenosis, and it is difficult not to prematurely stop an exercise test in a small child slated for a septal defect repair in a day or two when that child complains of fatigue or produces a few tears. However, if the maximal exercise capacity of the patients is to be compared to the maximal exercise capacity of normal subjects, those supervising the exercise test must over-

Table 1. Bruce treadmill test for cardiac patients

Stage	Speed (km/hr)	Grade (%)	Oxygen requirement of third min (ml/kg/min)					
			Children				Adults	
			7 years	9 years	11 years	14 years	Male	Female
A-I	2.7	0	—	—	—	12.0	—	—
A-II	2.7	5	—	—	—	14.6	—	—
I	2.7	10	20.2	18.6	18.1	18.2	17.4	17.1
II	4.0	12	26.4	25.5	24.3	25.9	24.8	24.0
III	5.5	14	40.2	36.5	35.2	37.7	34.3	33.3
IV	6.8	16	—	—	47.3	46.9	—	—
V	8.0	18	—	—	57.7	56.5	—	—
VI	8.8	29	—	—	65.2	64.0	—	—

Table 2.   Severity classification[a]

	Mild	Moderate	Severe
ASD	FR ≤ 1.5 and PA < 30	FR 1.6–2.5 and PA ≤ 50	FR > 2.5 and/or PA > 50
VSD	FR ≤ 1.3 and PA < 30	FR 1.4–2.0 and PA ≤ 50	FR > 2.0 and/or PA > 50 or PA Band
AS	PSG ≤ 30	PSG 31–45	PSG > 45
PS	PSG ≤ 30	PSG 31–55	PSG > 55

[a]Symbols: FR = pulmonary blood flow/systemic blood flow; PA = pulmonary artery systolic pressure; and PSG = peak systolic gradient.

come their misgivings and compassion and conduct the tests with confidence and firmness, yet kindness. Failure to sufficiently encourage children with cardiac disease to exercise maximally will exaggerate the frequency of impaired exercise performances and give a false indication of maximal heart rates in children with cardiac problems. Exercise tests in most cardiac children can be continued until the child stops for the same reason as the normal child stops, and only infrequently is it necessary to terminate an exercise test because of symptoms or ECG changes. We have not terminated an exercise test in children because of exercise-induced S-T segment changes. Ventricular tachycardia has been rare in most children, including those with serious cardiac malformations, so that exercise tests are seldom discontinued because of arrhythmia. There have been a few instances of exercise-induced ventricular tachycardia in which the test was terminated, a few instances of chest pain in patients with aortic stenosis leading to termination of the test, and a few instances of exercise-induced complete AV block, but there have been no alarming complications or morbidity during 20 years of experience of maximal exercise testing in children with heart disease.

Classification of Cardiac Patients

Cardiac patients have been classified as mild, moderate, or severe (Table 2). Patients with small ventricular septal defects, mild aortic stenosis, and pulmonary stenosis on clinical grounds who did not have catheterization studies were all placed in the mild category. Patients with rheumatic heart disease were classified as mild when cardiac enlargement was minimal or absent, and moderate if enlargement was present and there were auscultatory signs of severe regurgitation at the aortic and/or mitral valve.

Unsatisfactory Test

In this series of tests on children with cardiac problems, nine tests had to be discarded because the technologist supervising the test felt that the

Table 3.   Endurance time results in children with heart defects

	Number of tests	Mean age (years)	Percentage of subects with endurance times falling		
			Under 10th percentile	11th–50th percentile	Over 50th percentile
VSD					
Mild	123	10	6	43	52
Moderate	39	8	18	23	59
Severe	21	8	29	53	19
Postop	44	12	9	34	47
ASD					
Mild	27	10	11	34	56
Moderate	37	10	3	35	62
Severe	9	5	33	55	11
Postop	43	13	9	49	43
PDA					
Postop	10	12	0	50	50
AS					
Mild	51	10	0	48	54
Moderate	20	9	0	45	55
Severe	14	7	14	50	35
Postop	27	12	22	60	19

PS					
Mild	61	11	11	52	35
Moderate	16	8	19	31	41
Severe	5	9	0	80	20
Postop	15	12	20	60	20
COA					
Preop	24	7	13	37	67
Postop	23	12	22	60	17
Tetralogy					
No operation	12	6	67	33	0
Post shunt	10	6	90	10	0
Post open heart	37	12	19	60	22
Other Cyanotic	71	10	92	7	0
Post Rheumatic Fever					
Normal heart	25	11	8	40	52
Mild RHD	51	13	12	34	56
Severe RHD	15	12	47	53	0
Totals or Mean	830	10	21	40	38

child did not make a maximal effort. These were tests that were performed either by very young children 4 to 5 years of age, or teenage girls— the two groups where there are sometimes problems in motivation in the clinical setting.

Establishment of Normal Standards

Cumming and Hnatiuk (these proceedings) detail the problems of establishing normal values against which to compare children attending a hospital clinic. The normal data used in this report were obtained using patients seen in the cardiac clinic in whom no evidence of organic heart disease could be detected.

RESULTS

A total of 830 tests in cardiac patients were reviewed. The patients were divided into the various diagnostic categories, and the percentile distribution of their endurance times was found by plotting the results on charts. The number of tests and the percentile distribution of endurance times are summarized in Table 3. Low fitness was arbitrarily defined as an endurance time below the 10th percentile for the normal children. The lesions and categories where more than 18% of the subjects (twice the expected) had low fitness were ventricular septal defect (VSD), moderate and severe; atrial septal defect (ASD), severe; aortic stenosis (AS), postoperative; pulmonary stenosis (PS), moderate and postoperative; coarctation of the aorta (COA), postoperative; all cyanotic heart disease; and severe rheumatic heart disease (RHD). The overall frequency of low fitness in the 830 tests was 21%. Only the cyanotic lesions resulted in over 50% of the subjects being in the low fitness category.

Many patients with significant cardiac disease had fitness levels above the 50th percentile level established for the normal children. Lesions where over 40% of the subjects had endurance times above this 50th percentile level were VSD and ASD mild, moderate, and postoperative; AS mild and moderate; PDA postoperative; PS moderate; COA preoperative (but not postoperative); and patients with a past history of acute rheumatic fever who had either no cardiac lesion or mild valvular disease.

Unfortunately, the normal standards do not as yet include a body build factor, and this important determinant of endurance time should be factored out. Some of the cardiac patients were very lean and petite and had the ideal build to do well in a treadmill test. Other cardiac patients were obese, and their obesity rather than their cardiac lesions may have been the cause of the low endurance time.

Another shortcoming of the data was that the physical activity habits of the normal and patient groups were not recorded or taken into account. Nearly all of the cardiac patients were encouraged to take part in

Table 4.   Mean maximal heart rates: noncyanotic lesions

Severity	VSD	ASD	PS	AS	PDA	COA	RHD
Mild	204	201	200	203	—	—	204
Moderate	202	200	206	207	—	197	199
Severe	196	200	198	198	—	—	181
Postop	197	198	197	198	200	204	—

normal physical pursuits, or at least to try their best, but low exercise capacities in some of the subjects might be the result of low habitual activity rather than of their cardiac lesions.

The choice of the 10th—rather than the customary 3rd—percentile as being the lower limit of normal was an arbitrary one; it was based on the relatively small number of subjects (20–40) in the normal groups, and the conviction that fitness levels below the 10th percentile standards are less than desirable. Optimally, the normal series will eventually be expanded to include over 1000 subjects with the minimum of 100 subjects in each group.

MAXIMAL HEART RATES

In Table 4 the maximal heart rate data in noncyanotic patients are summarized. Mean maximal rates were over 190 b.p.m. in all patient groups except those with severe rheumatic heart disease. The mean maximal rates were the same as for the normal subjects. Prior reports suggesting that the maximal heart rates for children with heart disease are lower than normal may have included only subjects with very severe disease, or, as is more likely, many of the subjects studied in these reports did not perform near-maximal exercise.

Overall, only 22 of the noncyanotic patients (3%) had maximal heart rates below 180 b.p.m. (Table 5), and several of these subjects had nodal rhythm. None of the normal group had maximal heart rates less than 180 b.p.m.

Maximal heart rates were definitely reduced in the subjects with cyanotic congenital heart disease (Table 6). Some of these patients may

Table 5.   Number of tests with maximal heart rates less than 180 b.p.m.: noncyanotic lesions

Severity	VSD	ASD	PS	AS	PDA	COA	RHD
Mild	2	0	2	1	—	—	0
Moderate	2	0	0	0	—	0	3
Severe	3	0	0	0	—	—	4
Postop	2	1	1	0	1	0	—

Total, 22 (3%)

Table 6.   Mean maximal heart rates for cyanotic lesions

	Maximal heart rates $(\bar{x} \pm SD)$ b.p.m.	% below 180
Tetraloy		
no operation	178 ± 8	83
post shunt	192 ± 7	10
Other cyanotic lesions	175 ± 14	75
Total below 180 (64/93), 70%		

not have exercised maximally, but all exercised until severe symptoms appeared. Many of the subjects, even though cyanosed and considerably distressed, had maximal heart rates in excess of 170 b.p.m. The mean maximal heart rate of the cyanotic patients was still 175 b.p.m.

DISCUSSION

Most cardiac patients seemed to stop exercising for the same reason as did the normal subjects—severe leg fatigue developed, and they did not wish to punish themselves any further. Dyspnea and dizziness were less common complaints and were seldom volunteered. Patients with cyanotic heart disease stopped because of severe leg fatigue, severe generalized fatigue, dyspnea, headache, and an "all-in" feeling that was very uncomfortable. Knowledge of the unpleasantness of their symptoms when they had exercised close to maximally on previous occasions frequently led the subject to terminate subsequent exercise tests prior to the development of such severe symptoms.

Potential limiting factors in the cardiac patient include: 1) limited cardiac output with decreased perfusion of the working muscles; 2) dyspnea from lungs made stiff from arterial or venous congestion; 3) pulmonary transudation, or pulmonary hypertensive changes; 4) chest pain from myocardial hypoxia, as in coronary anomalies or aortic stenosis; 5) dizziness from altered cerebral blood flow or hyperventilation; and 6) cardiac arrhythmias and changes in blood gases causing symptoms or limiting oxygen delivery. Indirect causes of diminished endurance times include: 1) a decrease in exercise habits and fitness; 2) increased body fatness; and 3) fear of maximal work by the patient or on the part of those conducting the test.

Patients with resting pulmonary artery systolic pressures over 50 mm Hg uniformly had low fitness. Only a few patients with aortic stenosis developed angina—a dramatic example is shown in the ECG in Figure 1.

Because of the many factors responsible for the endurance time (including motivation, aerobic and anaerobic systems, body build, past and current exercise habits, muscular factors, technician factors, equipment

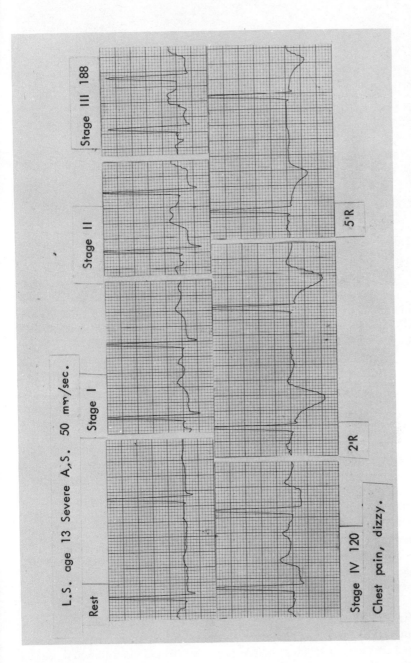

Figure 1.   Exercise ECG recorded at 50mm/sec for a 13-year-old girl with valvular aortic stenosis, peak resting systolic gradient 94 mm Hg. Heart rate was 188 b.p.m. for Stage III; after 30 sec at Stage IV there were chest pains, near syncope, and a slowing of the heart rate to 120 b.p.m.

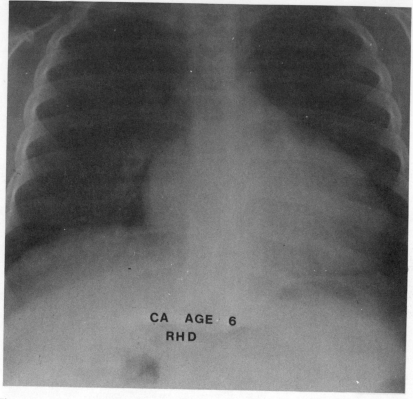

Figure 2.   Chest roentgenogram of a 6-year-old boy with severe mitral regurgitation, on digoxin for past heart failure. Endurance time was 13 min (95th percentile), with a maximal heart rate of 203 b.p.m.

calibration, and treadmill know-how), it would be very surprising if the simple measurement of exercise capacity would separate out children with mild or even moderate heart disease from normal children, as has been claimed by Goldberg et al. (1969).

The results presented indicate that even children with severe heart disease frequently may have exercise capacities well within the normal range. The chest roentgenograms of three children with severe rheumatic heart disease shown in Figures 2 to 4 emphasize this point. In addition, the exercise test failed to differentiate between patients with mild, moderate, and severe hemodynamic derangements (ASD, VSD, AS, PS, or RHD) with sufficient precision to be of any clinical value.

In the absence of $\dot{V}O_2$ measurements in these patients, it must be assumed that the cardiac patients have the same oxygen requirements as normal children in performing the exercise; this has been shown to be true by others (Bruce et al., 1973). Energy requirements can be met by anaerobic sources for less than 60 sec, and there is no indication that cardiac

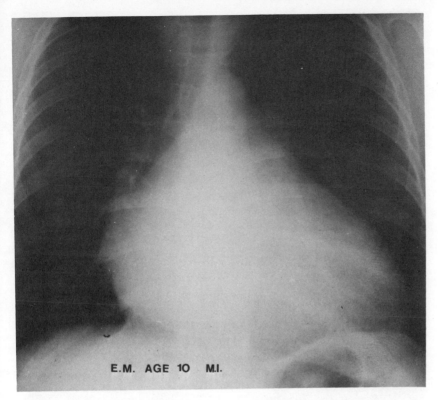

Figure 3.   Roentgenogram of a 10-year-old boy with severe rheumatic mitral regurgitation and previous atrial fibrillation who was receiving digoxin. Endurance time was 10 min (about the 10th percentile), with a maximal heart rate of 176 b.p.m.

patients have a greater capacity for anaerobic work than normal children. When cardiac output is limited, cardiac patients can compensate by extracting more oxygen and widening their arteriovenous oxygen difference to maintain a normal Vo_2 for each work load. It would seem that moderate and severe congenital defects may not limit performance because the healthy myocardium is able to provide the additional work necessary. In patients with aortic regurgitation, the decrease in diastolic time and the reduction in systemic vascular resistance that occur with exercise reduce the regurgitant volume and the hemodynamic burden so that exercise may be well tolerated until myocardial weakness occurs (Marshall and Shepherd, 1968). A similar compensation may occur in some patients with atrial and ventricular septal defects (Bruce and John, 1957). In patients with obstructive lesions (AS, PS, COA) the healthy myocardium seems to be capable of generating the added work necessary for intense physical exercise of short duration.

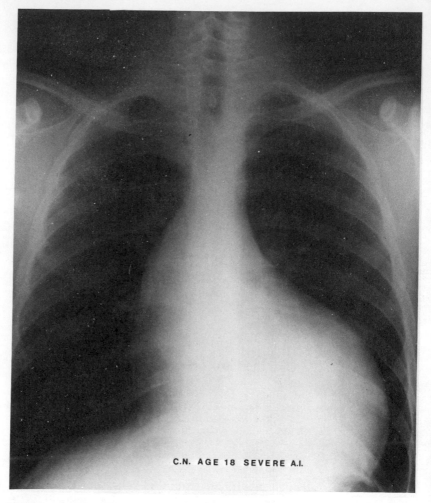

C.N. AGE 18 SEVERE A.I.

Figure 4.   Roentgenogram of an 18-year-old boy with severe rheumatic aortic regurgitation and gallop rhythm on no medication. Endurance time was 12 min (30th percentile) with a maximal heart rate of 196 b.p.m.

    The normal range of endurance times established for our clinic population for ages 8–16 years requires maximal oxygen uptake in the range of 42–60 ml/kg/min for boys and 35–55 ml/kg/min for girls, similar to those reported in most population studies (Cumming, 1967). If the normal values had been higher, more of the cardiac patients would have fallen in the low fitness group.

    A child with a significant defect but with favorable body build and genetic factors may have a high exercise capacity in the absence of participation in intense sport activities. Children with mild myocardial dis-

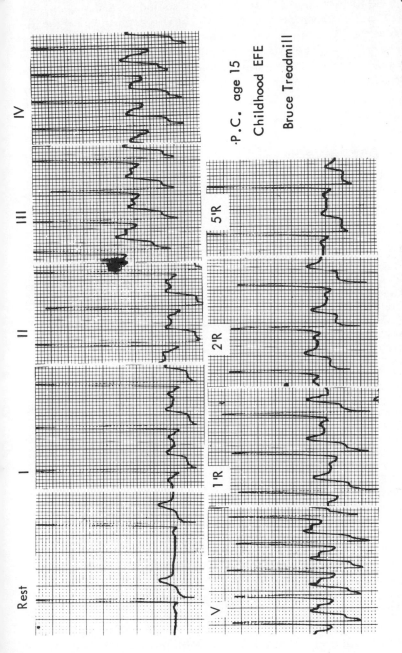

Figure 5.   Exercise ECG of a 15-year-old boy who had severe cardiomegaly and heart failure in infancy. Current x-ray and resting ECG were normal. Endurance time was 16 min (90th percentile) despite the fact that he had never taken part in competitive sports or intense physical training. Severe exercise S-T segment changes are not necessarily an indication to stop an exercise test in children.

ease and children with moderately severe aortic stenosis have been advised to avoid competitive sports. It is not unusual to find normal or even high-normal exercise capacities in children who have complied with these recommendations. The boy whose exercise ECG is shown in Figure 5 had never engaged in competitive sports or intense physical training, and yet he was able to finish Stage V of the Bruce protocol ($\dot{V}O_{2\,max}$ in excess of 56 ml/kg/min). This major degree of S-T segment depression is most unusual; S-T changes are not necessarily an indication to terminate an exercise test in children.

ACKNOWLEDGMENTS

All the exercise tests were carried out by a dedicated staff: L. Hastman (RT), J. McCort (RT), S. McCullough (RN), and D. Everatt (RN).

REFERENCES

Åstrand, P.-O. 1952. Experimental Studies of Physical Working Capacity in Relation to Sex and Age. Ejnar Munksgaard, Copenhagen.

Bruce, R. A., and G. G. John. 1957. Effects of upright posture and exercise on pulmonary hemodynamics in patients with central cardiovascular shunts. Circulation 16:776–783.

Bruce, R. A., F. Kusumi, and D. Hosmer. 1973. Maximal oxygen intake and nomographic assessment of functional aerobic impairment in cardiovascular disease. Am. Heart J. 85:546–562.

Cumming, G. R. 1967. Current levels of fitness. Can. Med. Assoc. J. 96:868–876.

Cumming, G. R. 1977. Exercise studies in clinical pediatric cardiology. In: H. Lavallée and R. Shephard (eds.), Frontiers of Activity and Child Health, pp. 17–45. Proceedings of the VIIth International Symposium of Pediatric Work Physiology. Editions du Pélican, Ottawa.

Cumming, G. R., D. Everatt, and L. Hastman. 1978. Bruce treadmill test in children: Normal values in a clinic population. Am. J. Cardiol. 41:69–75.

Cumming, G. R., D. Goulding, and G. Baggley. 1969. Failure of school physical education to improve cardiorespiratory fitness. Can. Med. Assoc. J. 101:69–73.

Epstein, S. E., G. D. Beiser, R. E. Goldstein, D. R. Rosing, D. R. Redwood, and A. G. Morrow. 1973. Hemodynamic abnormalities in response to mild and intense upright exercise following operative correction of an atrial septal defect or tetralogy of Fallot. Circulation 47:1065–1075.

Goldberg, S. J., F. Mendes, and R. Hurwitz. 1969. Maximal exercise capability of children as a function of specific cardiac defects. Am. J. Cardiol. 23:349–353.

Marshall, R. J., and J. T. Shepherd. 1968. Cardiac Function in Health and Disease, p. 286. W. B. Saunders, Philadelphia.

Direct $\dot{V}_{O_2\,max}$ in Children with Congenital Heart Disease

F. W. Kasch

The increase in the incidence of some forms of congenital heart disease (CHD) has created a need for continued careful evaluation and management of such patients (Anderson et al., 1978). The control of such factors as environmental conditions, sports, and recreational participation, as well as education and occupation, are all challenging factors to the attending physician in his care of the patient. Evaluation of the immediate and long-term effects of surgical and other therapeutic interventions is also extremely important in the successful management and treatment of patients with CHD (Kitterman et al., 1972; Friedman et al., 1977; Stevenson, 1977). Periodic patient re-evaluation is also an important consideration for the attending physician. This study was undertaken as a means of aiding the physician in his appraisal and management of the patient with CHD.

It was the aim of this study to measure the $\dot{V}_{O_2\,max}$ of children with CHD for comparison with a normal population. Fourteen children, five girls and nine boys, with a mean age of 10.9 years (± 4.3), were studied. Four patients had ventricular septal defects (VSD), four had pulmonary stenosis, three had aortic stenosis, two had patent ductus arteriosus, and one had transposition of the great vessels. Body weight averaged 40.0 kg (± 12.8) and height, 148 cm (± 19.7) (Table 1). Resting arterial blood oxygen saturation was near normal, 95.8%. Since $\dot{V}_{O_2\,max}$ indicates the functional capacity of the circulation and has a linear relationship to cardiac output, it was used as the criterion measurement for comparison of CHD patients with normal subjects (Åstrand and Rodahl, 1970; Folkow and Neil, 1971).

Table 1.   Physical characteristics of patients with congenital heart disease ($N = 14$)[a]

Age (years)	10.9	(6–20)
Height (cm)	148	(112–179)
Weight (kg)	40	(19.6–63.0)
HR rest (b.p.m.)	88	(60–135)
Systolic BP (mm Hg)	111	(82–148)
Diastolic BP (mm Hg)	71	(44–92)

[a]Values in parentheses denote range.

METHOD

Each patient entered the laboratory in the early morning after a 12-hr fast. An informed consent was signed by the parent, after which height, weight, resting heart rate (HR) and blood pressure (BP) were measured. An Ensco oximeter with a Varian recorder was employed for determining the blood oxygen saturation. The instrument was calibrated with span gases and filters, and the patient breathed the various gases during calibration. The oxygen-sensing cell was fastened to the patient's ear and held firmly in place by an elastic band and lacings to minimize movement during exercise. Headgear held a one-way-flow mouthpiece assembly, with a high velocity valve, for collection of expired air into 150 liter collection bags. A shunt system permitted the collection of serial bags, which were timed by a stopwatch. Exercise was performed on a step bench varying from 20–40 cm in height depending on the patient's stature (Kasch et al., 1965). The stepping rate ranged from 24–47 per min at maximal rate depending on the patient's ability to perform work. Exercise duration ranged from 2.5 to 9.0 min, with a mean of 4.8 min. Exercise HR was monitored by a special stethoscope device securely strapped to the patient's chest over the pericardium. An examiner recorded the HR each 10 sec throughout exercise and recovery. Reliability of the examiner's HR measurements was determined at another time using an ECG ($\pm 2\%$).

RESULTS

$\dot{V}_{O_2 max}$ averaged 32.1 ml/kg·min (± 10.1). The mean for the five girls was 31.4 (± 3.5), and the nine boys' mean was 32.4 (± 11.9), or approximately 80% and 65% of the $\dot{V}_{O_2 max}$, respectively, when compared to data on normal American children (Cassels and Morse, 1962; Knuttgen, 1967; Skinner et al., 1971). Mean HR_{max} was 176 b.p.m. (± 15.3), and $\dot{V}_E$ was 30.4 (± 17.7) liters/min at STPD.

Resting oxygen saturation was 95.8% (97.0%–93.7%) and at maximal work it averaged 90.8% (95.0%–70.0%). $\dot{V}_E$ was 29.0 liters/min (± 8.4). $\dot{V}_{E_{max}}$ was 37.3 liters/min at BTPS (± 21.7).

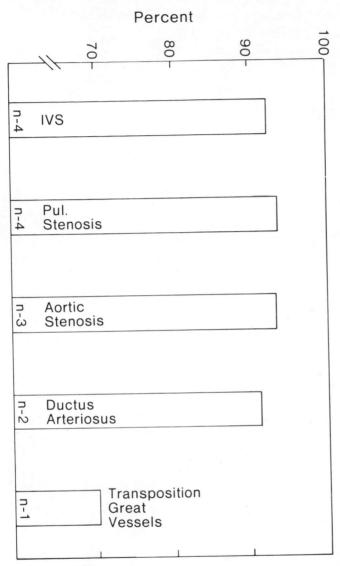

Figure 1.   Defects and oxygen saturation at maximal work in patients with CHD.

DISCUSSION

It can readily be seen from the $\dot{V}_{O_2\,max}$ measurements that the girls were about 20% below their counterparts, whereas the boys were 35% below. Perhaps this can be explained by the low standard for American girls in relation to that for boys; i.e., 39.0 compared to 50.0 ml/kg•min.

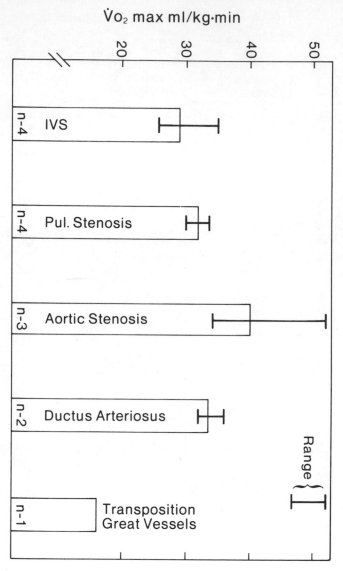

Figure 2. $\dot{V}_{O_2\,max}$ in CHD patients, by defect group.

During exercise there were three cases with oxygen saturation below 90%: they were 89.7%, 87.1%, and 70.0%. The latter, case no. 14, had transposition of the great vessels and the lowest $\dot{V}_{O_2}$, 17.7 ml/kg•min (Figure 1). It appears that his low PWC was a result of oxygen desaturation. Undoubtedly this patient would need special attention in physical education in school and would be restricted in competitive sports.

Table 2. METS required for participation in selected competitive sports

Archery	3–4	Golf	2–4
Bowling	2–4	Swimming	4–8
Cycling	3–8	Tennis	3–6
Dancing	3–7	Volleyball	3–6
Ventricular Septal Defect	8.4		
Pulmonary Stenosis	9.0		
Ductus Arteriosus	9.6		

The cases of VSD, pulmonary stenosis, and patent ductus arteriosus had similar aerobic capacities, 29.4%, 31.5%, and 33.7%, respectively (8.4–9.6 METS) (Figure 2). From these data there appeared to be very little difference in the aerobic power of these types of defects in these subjects. Probably all of these cases could participate in instructional physical education in school and, to a limited degree, in some of the less aerobic competitive sports, i.e., archery, bowling, golf, swimming, tennis, and volleyball (see Table 2, METS).

The relatively low HR_{max} of 176 b.p.m. (± 15.3) can be expected in subjects with congenital heart defects, as was reported by Goldberg (1970), who gave a maximal figure of 171 b.p.m. He also stated that there was no explanation for this lower HR in CHD. One-half of these patients had an HR_{max} over 180 b.p.m. and all but two were above 161 b.p.m., which means that 12 of 14 patients were above 1 SD below the mean. Several investigators (Cassels and Morse, 1962; Knuttgen, 1967; Skinner et al., 1971) have reported an HR_{max} of about 197 b.p.m. for this age group in normal subjects. Cassels and Morse (1962) reported an HR_{max} of 123 b.p.m. for boys and 116 b.p.m. for girls with acyanotic type CHD, and 135 b.p.m. for boys and 120 b.p.m. for girls with cyanotic type CHD. The work levels of these subjects undoubtedly were not maximal.

When the measured $\dot{V}_{O_2 \, max}$ was compared with an estimated $\dot{V}_{O_2}$ from the kpm of stepping, a very close relationship was found, 32.1 and 33.0 ml/kg•min, respectively. Thus, the kpm of work and the oxygen uptake are nearly alike. This in turn helps to substantiate the validity of the $\dot{V}_{O_2}$ measurements, as does the HR_{max} of 176 b.p.m.

CONCLUSIONS

CHD patients, acyanotic at rest, are partially limited in PWC as seen by the results of 14 cases with five types of lesions. An arterial blood oxygen saturation of 91% appears to be a limiting factor during exercise. Such patients probably can participate in moderate physical activities, but not in competitive sports. $\dot{V}_{O_2 \, max}$ is a noninvasive evaluation procedure that objectively differentiates between the PWC of patients with CHD and normal subjects and is seen as a safe and excellent clinical measurement in the immediate and subsequent appraisal of the functional capacity of the circulatory system. By this method, the physician can periodically evaluate surgical and other therapeutic media and, thereby, more easily manage each patient with CHD.

REFERENCES

Anderson, C. E., L. D. Edmonds, and J. D. Erickson. 1978. Patent ductus arteriosus and ventricular septal defect. Am. J. Epidemiol. 107(4):281–289.

Åstrand, P.-O., and K. Rodahl. 1970. Textbook of Work Physiology. McGraw-Hill Book Co., New York.

Cassels, D. E., and M. Morse. 1962. Cardiopulmonary Data for Children and Young Adults. Charles C Thomas, Springfield, Ill.

Folkow, B., and E. Neil. 1971. Circulation. Oxford University Press, New York.

Friedman, W., M. Heymann, and A. Rudolph. 1977. New thought on an old problem—Patent ductus arteriosus in premature. J. Pediatr. 90:338. Editorial.

Goldberg, S. J. 1970. Functional evaluation of children with congenital heart disease by response to maximal exercise. In: F. H. Adams, H. J. C. Swan, and V. E. Hall (eds.), Pathophysiology of Congenital Heart Disease. University of California Press, Los Angeles.

Kasch, F. W., W. H. Phillips, J. E. L. Carter, W. D. Ross, and J. L. Boyer. 1965. Maximum work capacity in middle-aged males by a step test method. J. Sports Med. Phys. Fitness 5(4):198–202.

Kitterman, J. A., L. H. Edmunds, G. A. Gregory, et al. 1972. Patent ductus arteriosus in premature infants. Incidence, relation to pulmonary disease, and management. N. Engl. J. Med. 287:473–477.

Knuttgen, H. E. 1967. Aerobic capacity of adolescents. J. Appl. Physiol. 22:655.

Skinner, J. S., O. Bar-Or, V. Bergsteinova, C. W. Bell, R. Royer, and E. R. Buskirk. 1971. Comparison of continuous and intermittent tests for determining maximal oxygen intake in children. Acta Pediatr. Scand. 217:24–28.

Stevenson, J. G. 1977. Fluid administration in the association of patent ductus arteriosus complicating respiratory distress syndrome. J. Pediatr. 90:257–261.

Adrenergic Activity at Rest and During Exercise in Normotensive Boys and Young Adults, and in Hypertensive Patients

G. Koch

The sympathetic-adrenergic innervation constitutes the most important regulatory principle for the cardiovascular system. This is true not only under physiological conditions but also for several cardiovascular conditions in which the adrenergic response elicited by the disease process may play a decisive role in its course and final outcome. Typical examples of this are myocardial infarction and heart failure.

Epinephrine is mainly released from the adrenal medulla and norepinephrine from the sympathetic nerve endings. Although this is a very complex process, particularly because of the re-uptake of norepinephrine by the nerve endings, the levels of circulating catecholamines appear to reflect adrenergic activity in a reliable way (Cryer, 1976). However, plasma concentrations of catecholamines are extremely low, and only the very recent development of enzymatic isotope–derivative methods has provided a sensitive tool for the measurement of epinephrine and norepinephrine in plasma and tissues, and hence for the study of adrenergic physiology and pathophysiology.

During the last few years, a method based on this principle has been developed in our laboratory, allowing simultaneous determination of epinephrine, norepinephrine, and dopamine in 0.1-ml samples. This paper describes the application of the method for the study of the adrenergic response in association with submaximal and maximal exercise in normotensive adolescents and young adults, and in young hypertensive patients.

This study was supported by a grant from the Deutsche Bundesinstitut für Sportwissenschaft (German Federal Republic Institute of Sport Science).

SUBJECTS AND PROCEDURES

There were 16 healthy volunteers, 10 men and 6 women, ages 22–34 years; a group of 9 physically well-trained ($\dot{V}o_2$ max 59 ml/kg of body weight) boys, ages 15–16 years; and a group of hypertensive patients, ages 24–46 years, who were studied. WHO Grade 1 essential hypertension was diagnosed in all the patients; in most of them it was the borderline type.

Plasma renin activity, plasma epinephrine, and norepinephrine were measured in blood samples obtained via in-dwelling venous catheters at rest after lying supine for 10 min and after standing upright for 2 min, as well as during and after steady state exercise sitting on a bicycle ergometer. Exercise was performed on at least four but usually five increasing work loads, the highest one corresponding to about 85%–90% of the individual's maximal working capacity in the adults, and to 95%–100% in the group of adolescents. Exercise lasted for 6 min during each load; thus, the total period of exercise exceeded 24 min in every case. Loads were 35, 70, 100, 135, and 170 W for the females and 50, 100, 150, 200, and 250 W for both the men and boys. Heart rates were obtained by continuous ECG recording, and blood pressures by the Riva-Rocci cuff method.

ANALYTICAL METHODS

Catecholamines

Basically the assay consisted of:

1. Conversion of epinephrine (E), norepinephrine (NE), and dopamine (DA) into their respective methyl derivatives in the presence of catechol-O-methyltransferase (COMT) and S-adrenosyl-methionin-[³H]methyl
2. Extraction of the methylated tritium-labeled amines with diethyl ether
3. Separation by thin-layer chromatography
4. Measurement in a β-radiation scintillation counter

The method has been shown to have a high degree of sensitivity, specificity, and precision, allowing measurement of catecholamine concentrations in the range of 0.1 pmol/ml with a coefficient of variation of approximately 5%–8%. Details of the method are reported elsewhere (Koch et al., in preparation).

Plasma Renin Activity (PRA)

Another hormone related to adrenergic activity is renin. It is produced in the juxtaglomerular apparatus of the kidneys and can easily be evaluated by measuring plasma renin activity by radioimmunoassay methods. The method used was that described by Fyhrqvist et al. (1976).

RESULTS

In the normotensive subjects there were no significant changes in PRA, E, and NE after standing upright for 2 min compared with resting values in the supine position, although there was a trend toward higher levels in the upright position. PRA, E, and NE increased during exercise in parallel with the work load, peak values being attained at the highest load or immediately after cessation of exercise. Ten min after work, NE and PRA were still significantly higher than the initial resting values, while E had approached the initial level. Peak values of PRA, E, and NE showed approximately three-, six-, and tenfold increases, respectively, in the normotensive adults (Figure 1) and rose as high as four-, ten-, and twentyfold in the group of boys (Figure 2).

Resting PRA and NA levels were higher in the hypertensive than in the normotensive adults, and the hypertensives showed a significant increase of NE after 2 min of standing upright. Submaximal, but not peak, NE values were higher in the hypertensive adults compared with the normotensive adults at corresponding work loads and heart rates. Thus, hypertensives show a significantly steeper rise in NE in relation to both heart rate and systolic pressure increases (Figures 3 and 4). Even E has a tendency to increase more rapidly in relation to heart rate in the hypertensives (Figure 4). It should be noted that the boys showed a trend similar to that of the hypertensive adults with respect to NE and a much steeper E increase in relation to heart rate and systolic pressures than both groups of adults (Figures 3, 4, and 5).

DISCUSSION

Catecholamines and PRA in normotensive adults have consistently been shown to increase on changing from supine to erect posture. However, substantial increments in levels of circulating hormones are not observed until the subjects have remained in the erect position for about 4–5 min (Cryer, 1976; Koch, 1977; Koch et al., in preparation). The hypertensive patients not only showed higher adrenergic activity in terms of NE levels, in both the supine and erect positions, but the onset of NE increase during standing was significantly more rapid. Increased levels of total plasma catecholamines (Christensen and Brandsburg, 1973) and of NE (Häggendahl et al., 1970) have previously been observed in connection with exercise. The absence of detectable levels of E in the series of Häggendahl et al. (1970) was probably due to the obvious lack of sensitivity and speci-

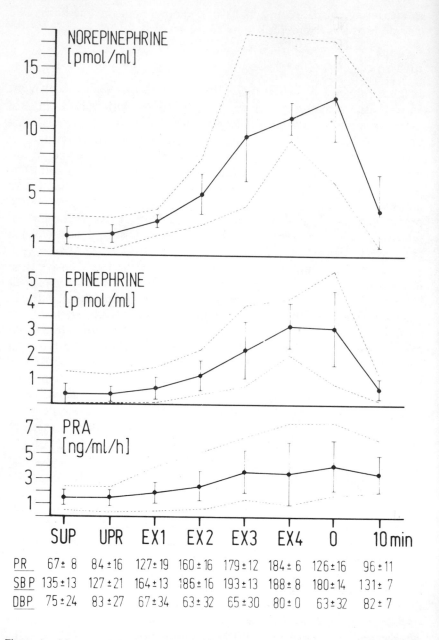

Figure 1.   Means, standard deviations, and ranges of norepinephrine, epinephrine, and plasma renin activity (PRA) at rest in the supine and upright positions as well as during and after steady state exercise in 16 healthy young adults. PR = pulse rate (means and standard deviations), SBP = systolic blood pressure, DBP = diastolic blood pressure.

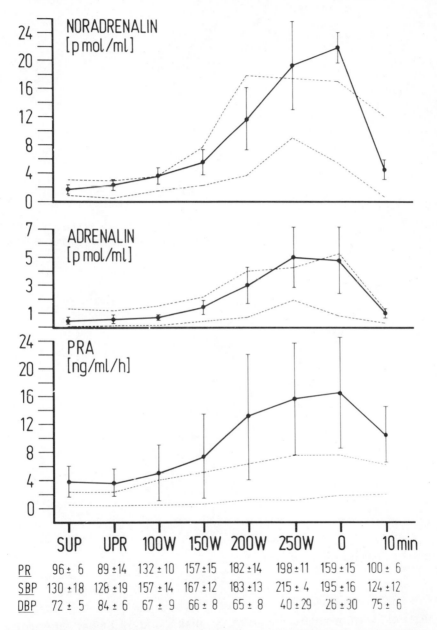

	SUP	UPR	100W	150W	200W	250W	0	10 min
PR	96± 6	89 ±14	132 ±10	157±15	182±14	198±11	159 ±15	100± 6
SBP	130 ±18	128 ±19	157 ±14	167±12	183 ±13	215± 4	195±16	124 ±12
DBP	72 ± 5	84 ± 6	67 ± 9	66 ± 8	65 ± 8	40 ±29	26 ±30	75 ± 6

Figure 2. Means, standard deviations, and ranges of norepinephrine (noradrenalin), epinephrine (adrenalin), and plasma renin activity (PRA) at rest in the supine and upright positions as well as during and after steady state exercise in 9 well-trained boys ages 15–16 years. PR = pulse rate (means and standard deviations), SBP = systolic blood pressure, DBP = diastolic blood pressure.

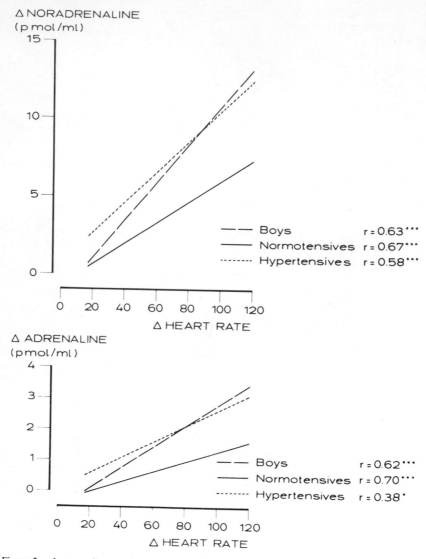

Figure 3. Increase in norepinephrine (noradrenaline) and epinephrine (adrenaline) during submaximal work in relation to increase in heart rate (r = coefficient of correlation).

ficity of the fluorometric method used. In this study, a similar pattern of increases in E, NE, and PRA was observed in all three groups of subjects, although the rate of NE increase was much higher than that of E, particularly at work levels exceeding 70% of the maximal work capacity.

It should be noted that the boys had significantly higher peak levels of E and, in particular, of NE, and higher PRA levels under all conditions. This probably reflects on age-correlated higher basal and peak sym-

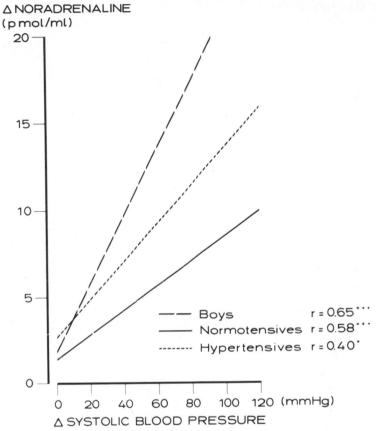

Figure 4.   Increase in norepinephrine (noradrenaline) during submaximal work in relation to increase in systolic blood pressure (r = coefficient of correlation).

pathetic activity in the younger age group. However, a higher relative work intensity in the boys (maximal heart rate 198 ± 11 b.p.m. as opposed to 184 ± 6 b.p.m. in the normotensive adults) is presumably a contributory mechanism. The significantly higher PRA values at rest and during exercise in the younger age group are especially noteworthy. They may partly reflect the higher adrenergic activity. The correlation between adrenergic stimulation and renin secretion is well established (Wiener et al., 1971) and was also found in this study (the coefficient of correlation between peak NE and peak PRA values ranging between 0.63 and 0.71 [$p < 0.001$] in the three groups).

There is a large body of indirect evidence that adrenergic overactivity is an important triggering mechanism in early essential hypertension and that the dysregulation of central and renal hemodynamics and of renal salt and water handling, and the blood volume changes that are typical of essential hypertension are secondary manifestations. In particular, the hyperkinetic high-output normal-resistance circulation regularly seen

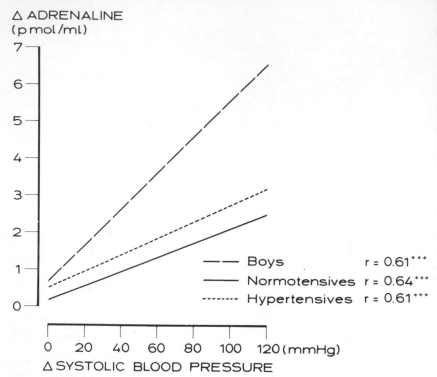

Figure 5.   Increase in epinephrine (adrenaline) during submaximal work in relation to increase in systolic blood pressure (r = coefficient of correlation).

during the initial stage of essential hypertension can be satisfactorily explained as being due to sympathetic overdrive.

However, attempts aimed at actually proving adrenergic overactivity by measuring plasma catecholamines in hypertension have been rather disappointing; only about 30% to 50% of the hypertensives studied showed significantly increased levels of NE or E, or both (De Champlain et al., 1976; Franco-Morselli et al., 1977; Sever et al., 1977). The present results, showing significantly increased adrenergic activity in terms of NE during rest conditions but, particularly, during light and moderate exercise, give substantial support to the hypothesis that increased adreno-sympathetic activity is associated with at least the early stages of hypertension.

CONCLUSIONS

The following conclusions can be drawn from the data presented:

1. The increase in adrenergic activity during exercise and the peak adrenergic activity are age dependent and are higher in adolescents 16–17 years old than in adults ages 22 to 34 years.

2. Young adult hypertensives have higher levels of circulating NE during resting conditions, both in the supine and upright posture, and a steeper increase of adrenergic activity in terms of NE in relation to the rise in heart rate and systolic pressure during light and moderate work. No significant differences appear to exist with respect to peak adrenergic activity as evaluated during maximal exercise.

3. These findings further suggest that increased sympathetic activity is an important—and under certain circumstances possibly causative—factor in essential hypertension.

REFERENCES

Christensen, N. J., and O. Brandsburg. 1973. The relationship between plasma catecholamine concentration and pulse rate during exercise and standing. Eur. J. Clin. Invest. 3:299–306.

Cryer, P. E. 1976. Isotope-derivate measurements of plasma norepinephrine and epinephrine in man. Diabetes 25:1071–1082.

De Champlain, J., L. Farley, D. Cousineau, and M.-R. von Amerigen. 1976. Circulatory catecholamine levels in human and experimental hypertension. Circ. Res. 38:109–114.

Franco-Morselli, R., J. L. Elghazi, E. Joly, S. Di Giulio, and P. Meyer. 1977. Increased plasma adrenaline concentrations in benign essential hypertension. Br. Med. J. 2:1251–1254.

Fyhrqvist, F., P. Soveri, L. Puutula, and U.-H. Stenman. 1976. Radioimmunoassay of plasma renin activity. Clin. Chem. 22(2):250–256.

Häggendahl, J., L. H. Hartley, and B. Saltin. 1970. Arterial noradrenaline concentration during exercise in relation to the relative work levels. Scand. J. Clin. Lab. Invest. 26:337–342.

Koch, G. 1977. Plasma renin activity, epinephrine and norepinephrine at rest and during exercise in young adults and boys. Scand. J. Clin. Lab. Invest. 37 (Suppl 147):107.

Sever, P. S., B. Osikowska, M. Birch, and R. D. G. Tunbridge. 1977. Plasma-noradrenaline in essential hypertension. Lancet 1:1078–1081.

Wiener, N., D. S. Chokshi, and W. G. Walkenhorst. 1971. Effects of cyclic AMP, sympathomimetic amines, and adrenoreceptor antagonists on renin secretion. Circ. Res. 29:239–243.

Physiological Changes in a Child with Ductus Arteriosus, Pre- and Postsurgery (Three-Year Follow-up)

F. W. Kasch

The repair of patent ductus arteriosus has been considered a relatively simple surgical procedure for many years. It is generally considered successful in 100% of the cases. The patient usually is capable of performing normal physical activities, including vigorous sports, postsurgically. The degree of success of the intervention can be measured by the physical working capacity (PWC) of the patient. PWC is readily determined by the criterion measurement known as $\dot{V}O_{2\,max}$ (Simonson and Enzer, 1942; Mitchell et al., 1958). Thus, $\dot{V}O_{2\,max}$ can show the degree of success pre- and postoperatively. It was the aim of this study to measure the $\dot{V}O_{2\,max}$ in a 14-year-old female with patent ductus arteriosus in order to evaluate the surgical procedure.

SUBJECT

A 14.4-year-old Caucasian female with patent ductus arteriosus diagnosed by heart catheterization was followed for 3 years beginning just before and continuing after surgical intervention. Her initial weight was 29.0 kg and her height was 142 cm. Resting heart rate (HR) was elevated slightly; blood pressure (BP) remained normal (see Table 1).

METHOD

The patient entered the laboratory in the morning at 8 A.M. after a 12-hr fast. An informed consent was signed by one parent. After height and weight measurements, resting HR and BP were taken. The subject had previously been given a preliminary test to accustom her to all of the pro-

Table 1.   Anthropometric data in ductus arteriosus, female subject

Age (years)	Height (cm)	Weight (kg)	Months	Rest HR (b.p.m.)	BP (mm Hg)
14.4	142	29.0	0[a]	99	97/64
15.1	147	31.4	8	91	102/72
15.4	147	32.2	12	83	108/70
15.7	149	35.0	15	92	98/72
17.5	154	42.3	36	90	100/70

[a]Presurgery.

cedures. The oximeter earpiece (Water's) was then attached to the patient's ear and held securely in place by a cap, laces, and an elastic band. The Ensco oximeter with Varian recorder was calibrated with span gases of 100% oxygen, 8% oxygen, and room air, and with filters. A chest strap fitted with a special stethoscope was securely fastened to the patient's chest for HR determination. HR measurements were validated by ECG on another day.

Expired gases were collected serially for 1 min in meteorological balloons. Air samples were drawn into 50-ml oiled glass syringes with special fittings for double Scholander analysis. Ventilation ($\dot{V}E$) volumes were measured in a calibrated wet-test gas meter and corrected for STPD.

Exercise was performed to maximal rate on a 30-cm padded step bench at increasing rates from 24 to 40 steps per min (Kasch et al., 1965). The duration of each test was 6 min. BP was measured by auscultation over the left brachial artery at rest and during 5 min recovery. The criterion for maximal work was a leveling off or an actual decline in $\dot{V}O_2$ with a further increase in physical work.

RESULTS AND DISCUSSION

$\dot{V}O_{2\,max}$ initially was 36.0 ml/kg•min or 1.05 liters/min and rose to 37.2 ml/kg•min after 8 months postoperatively (Figure 1). It remained slightly above that level throughout the 3-year postsurgical period (see Table 2).

HR_{max} was 191 b.p.m. at the initial evaluation and rose to 200 b.p.m. by the 36th month. $\dot{V}E$ increased from 34.4 to 68.9 liters/min BTPS, primarily as a result of growth (Figure 2).

Table 2. $\dot{V}O_{2\,max}$, ductus arteriosus, female subject

$\dot{V}O_{2\,max}$	Months				
	0	8	12	15	36
ml/kg•min	36.0	37.2	39.3	40.0	38.2
l/min	1.045	1.169	1.257	1.399	1.619

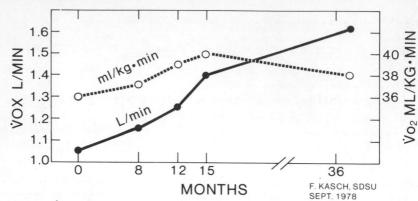

Figure 1. $\dot{V}O_{2\ max}$ in a female subject with ductus arteriosus.

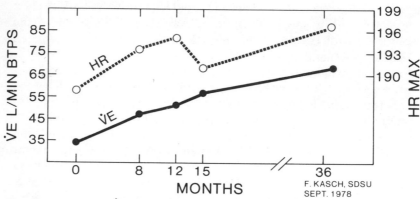

Figure 2. HR_{max} and $\dot{V}E$ in a female subject with ductus arteriosus.

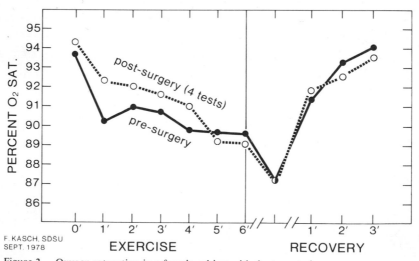

Figure 3.   Oxygen saturation in a female subject with ductus arteriosus.

Table 3. $\dot{V}E$, ductus arteriosus, female subject

	Months				
	0	8	12	15	36
$\dot{V}E/\dot{V}O_2$	32.9	40.2	47.9	49.2	42.6

Resting arterial oxygen saturation prior to surgery was 93.7% and ranged from 93.4% to 95.2% over the ensuing 36 months. During exercise, the oxygen saturation dropped to 87.1% during the first evaluation and remained near that level for the 3-year interim (Figure 3). From the small changes seen in $\dot{V}O_2$ and oxygen saturation, it appears that less improvement occurred than might be expected in these two parameters.

HR_{max} was within the range of normal for age (Cassels and Morse, 1962; Knuttgen, 1967; Skinner et al., 1971). It was not depressed, as is usually the case (Goldberg, 1970) in congenital heart disease. Resting HR and BP showed little change, the former ranging from 90–99 b.p.m. and the latter from 97/64 to 100/70 mm Hg.

$\dot{V}E$ was 33 at the initial test, 49 at 15 months and 43 at 36 months (Table 3).

The growth pattern remained below average, with greater improvement occurring in stature than in body weight (Figure 4). The height decrement improved from a negative 11% to negative 5%, whereas the weight decrement gained from a negative 42% to a negative 22% during the 36-month period. Figure 5 relates normal growth with the decrement of growth in the patient with ductus arteriosus. Did the need for growth and energy prevent a change in PWC and arterial oxygen saturation? Or was there a further small lesion that caused the oxygen saturation and $\dot{V}O_{2\ max}$ to remain relatively constant? Or could it be a lack of physical fitness due to lack of physical exercise?

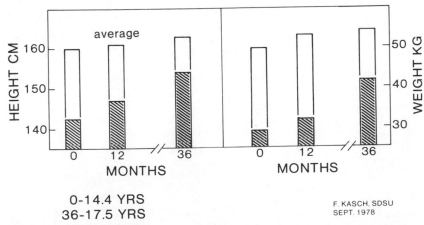

0-14.4 YRS
36-17.5 YRS

F. KASCH, SDSU
SEPT. 1978

Figure 4.   Growth pattern of a female subject with ductus arteriosus.

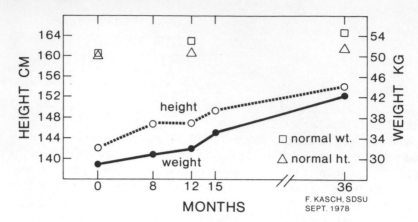

Figure 5.   Height and weight of a female subject with ductus arteriosus compared to normal values.

CONCLUSION

In conclusion, it appears that surgery for patent ductus arteriosus helped the child's growth, but the relative inability to improve the oxygen saturation and $\dot{V}_{O_{2}\,max}$ was somewhat disappointing.

REFERENCES

Cassels, D., and M. Morse. 1962. Cardiopulmonary Data for Children and Young Adults. Charles C Thomas Publisher, Springfield, Ill.

Goldberg, S. J. 1970. Functional evaluation of children with congenital heart disease by response to maximal exercise. In: F. H. Adams, H. J. C. Swan, and V. E. Hall (eds.), Pathophysiology of Congenital Heart Disease. University of California Press, Los Angeles.

Kasch, F. W., W. H. Phillips, J. E. L. Carter, W. D. Ross, and J. L. Boyer. 1965. Maximum work capacity in middle-aged males by a step test method. J. Sports Med. Phys. Fitness 5:198–202.

Knuttgen, H. G. 1967. Aerobic capacity of adolescents. J. Appl. Physiol. 22:265.

Mitchell, J., B. Sproule, and C. Chapman. 1958. The physiological meaning of the maximal oxygen intake test. J. Clin. Invest. 37:538–547.

Simonson, E., and N. Enzer. 1942. Physiology of muscular exercise and fatigue in disease. Medicine 21:345–419.

Skinner, J. S., O. Bar-Or, V. Versteinova, C. W. Bell, R. Royer, and R. Buskirk. 1971. Comparison of continuous and intermittent tests for determining maximal oxygen intake in children. Acta Pediatr. Scand. Suppl. 217:24–28.